IMMUNOLOGY OF THE LIVER

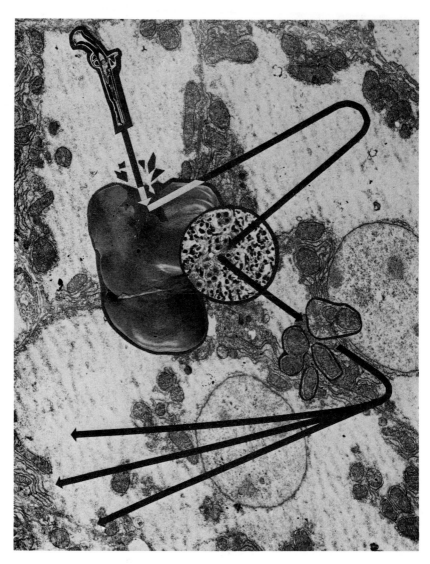

Frontispiece
*(Flintlock pistol by permission of the trustees
of the Wallace Collection.)*

IMMUNOLOGY

OF

THE LIVER

Martin Smith
and
Roger Williams

Proceedings of an International Meeting held
at King's College Hospital Medical School London,
on 6th and 7th July, 1970

Published by
WILLIAM HEINEMANN MEDICAL BOOKS LTD
LONDON

First published 1971

ISBN 0 433 30725 0

Printed by photo-lithography and made in
Great Britain at the Pitman Press, Bath

EDITORS' FOREWORD

Once involved in liver transplantation, it was perhaps not surprising that
The Liver Unit at King's should also become interested in auto-immune liver disease.
After an investigation of cell mediated responses during rejection, it became
clear to us that such processes might also be involved in active chronic hepatitis
and in primary biliary cirrhosis. There is also a high incidence of serum auto-
antibodies in these conditions, but their exact role in pathogenesis has not so far
been determined. The idea then began to grow of holding a meeting in which
laboratory workers and clinicians with interests in this field would come together
and discuss the basis of immune reactions in liver disease. To hold such a meeting
seemed doubly important in view of the increasing use of immunosuppressive
agents in the treatment of patients with apparently different clinical types of
liver disease but which, according to current thinking, are attributable to auto-
immunity.

The success of such a meeting depends so much on the ability of the chairmen
and speakers and to them we express our sincere thanks. Dr. G. Dobias from
Hungary, Dr. V. Pipitone from Italy and Dr. N. D. C. Finlayson from New York
were unavoidably detained at the last moment but have allowed their papers to
be published. Indeed, we are grateful to all those who came from overseas and we
hope that this book represents a truly international account of auto-immune
liver disease at the present time.

We are very much aware in publishing this symposium of the dangers of delay
and we are most grateful to Heinemann's who have achieved such rapid
publication. The meeting was generously sponsored by Beecham Research
Laboratories and Mr. D. Goodchild, Liaison Officer, gave invaluable assistance.
Many members of the Liver Unit helped in the organisation in different ways. It
is not possible to mention them individually, except Dr. Adrian Eddleston who
was responsible for a major share of the ideas and organization of the meeting.

Finally, without the untiring efforts of my personal secretary, Miss Margaret
Skellern, and the Unit secretaries — Mrs. Jean Rowles and Miss Gillian McNay — the
meeting and the publication of the proceedings would never have come to
fruition.

Martin Smith
Roger Williams

Liver Unit,
King's College Hospital,
London, S.E.5.

CONTENTS

PARTICIPANTS

CHAIRMEN AND SPEAKERS

Dr. J. R. Batchelor (Queen Victoria Hospital, East Grinstead, U.K.)
Professor R. Y. Calne (Addenbrooke's Hospital, Cambridge, U.K.)
Professor G. C. Cook (The University of Zambia, Lusaka, Zambia)
Professor J. De Groote (Akademisch Ziekenhuis, St. Rafael, Leuven)
Dr. Hans Diederichsen (Klovervaenget, Odense, Denmark)
Professor Gyorgy Dobias (Postgraduate Medical School, Budapest, Hungary)
Dr. Deborah Doniach (The Middlesex Hospital, London, U.K.)
Dr. D. C. Dumonde (Kennedy Institute of Rheumatology, London, U.K.)
Dr. A. L. W. F. Eddleston (King's College Hospital, London, U.K.)
Dr. N. D. C. Finlayson (The New York Hospital — Cornell Medical Centre, New York, U.S.A.)
Dr. R. A. Fox (The Royal Free Hospital, London, U.K.)
Dr. M. G. Geall (King's College Hospital, London, U.K.)
Dr. L. E. Glynn (Canadian Red Cross Memorial Hospital, Taplow, U.K.)
Dr. P. L. Golding (The London Hospital, London, U.K.)
Dr. J. Knolle (University of Mainz, Germany)
Dr. M. H. Lessof (Guy's Hospital, London, U.K.)
Dr. B. P. MacLaurin (University of Otago and the Medical School, Birmingham, U.K.)
Dr. K. H. Meyer zum Büschenfelde (University of Mainz, Germany)
Dr. Christine Mitchell (King's College Hospital, London, U.K.)
Dr. A. P. Pagaltsos (University of Thessaloniki and King's College Hospital)
Dr. Vincenzo Pipitone (Institute of Medical Pathology, Bari, Italy)
Professor Hans Popper (Mount Sinai School of Medicine, New York, U.S.A.)
Professor A. E. Read (Bristol Royal Infirmary, Bristol, U.K.)
Professor I. M. Roitt (The Middlesex Hospital, London, U.K.)
Dr. Alison Ross (The Royal Free Hospital, London, U.K.)
Professor S. J. Saunders (University of Cape Town, South Africa)
Professor Fenton Schaffner (Mount Sinai School of Medicine, New York, U.S.A.)
Dr. P. J. Scheuer (The Royal Free Hospital, London, U.K.)
Dr. M. G. M. Smith (King's College Hospital, London, U.K.)
Dr. M. Søborg (Rigshospitalet, Copenhagen, Denmark)
Professor N. Tygstrup (Rigshospitalet, Copenhagen, Denmark)
Dr. Marta Velasco (Hospital Salvador, Santiago, Chile)
Dr. J. G. Walker (The Middlesex Hospital, London, U.K.)
Dr. D. I. Williams (King's College Hospital, London, U.K.)
Dr. Roger Williams (King's College Hospital, London, U.K.)
Dr. Ralph Wright (Radcliffe Infirmary, Oxford, U.K.)

MEMBERS OF SYMPOSIUM

Miss Stephanie Barnes (King's College Hospital, London, U.K.)
Dr. G. Bendixen (Rigshospitalet, Copenhagen, Denmark)

Dr. J. P. Benhamou (Hospital Beaujon, Clichy, France)
Dr. M. C. Berenbaum, (St. Mary's Hospital, London, U.K.)
Dr. Barbara H. Billing (Royal Free Hospital, London, U.K.)
Professor C. R. B. Blackburn (University of Sydney, Australia)
Dr. R. Bown (St. Bartholomew's Hospital, London, U.K.)
Dr. B. E. Boyes (Southern General Hospital, Glasgow, U.K.)
Dr. H. Bunjé (Medical Research Council, London, U.K.)
Dr. M. Carrella (University of Naples, Italy, and King's College Hospital, London)
Dr. M. Clark (St. Bartholomew's Hospital, London, U.K.)
Professor M. Coltorti (University of Naples, Institute of Medical Pathology, Italy)
Dr. A. M. Dawson (St. Bartholomew's Hospital, London, U.K.)
Dr. W. Doe (Hammersmith Hospital, London, U.K.)
Dr. F. Dowling (Nottingham University Medical School, U.K.)
Mr. F. P. Doyle (Beecham Research Laboratories)
Dr. J. D. Dudley (Royal Free Hospital, London, U.K.)
Dr. P. W. Dykes (The General Hospital, Birmingham, U.K.)
Dr. I. W. Dymock (King's College Hospital, London, U.K.)
Dr. S. G. Elkington (King's College Hospital, London, U.K.)
Dr. S. Erlinger (Hospital Beaujon, Clichy, France)
Dr. L. J. Farrow (West Middlesex Hospital, London, U.K.)
Professor René Fauvert (Hospital Beaujon, Clichy, France)
Dr. Denise Fauvert (Hospital Beaujon, Clichy, France)
Dr. K. Federlin (Kennedy Institute, London, U.K.)
Dr. René Fiasse (Cliniques Universitaires St. Pierre, Leuven, Belgium)
Dr. R. Fleisher (King's College Hospital, London, U.K.)
Dr. G. Goertz (Pomeranian Medical Academy, Poland, and King's College
    Hospital, London)
Dr. J. M. Grainger (The Royal Free Hospital, London, U.K.)
Dr. A. H. Griffith (Burroughs Wellcome Ltd., London, U.K.)
Mr. R. Hague (King's College Hospital, London, U.K.)
Dr. K. Havemann (Medizinische Universitätsklinik, Marburg, Germany)
Dr. M. Hellier (St. Bartholomew's Hospital, London, U.K.)
Dr. Rosemary Hickman (University of Cape Town, South Africa)
Dr. J. O. Hunter (King's College Hospital, London, U.K.)
Dr. S. Jain (Dudley Road Hospital, Birmingham, U.K.)
Professor R. A. Joské (University of Western Australia, Perth, Australia)
Miss Angela Kemp (King's College Hospital, London, U.K.)
Dr. R. P. Knill-Jones (King's College Hospital, London, U.K.)
Dr. E. T. Knudsen (Beecham Research Laboratories)
Mr. J. Kolthammer (King's College Hospital, London, U.K.)
Dr. P. Kumar (St. Bartholomew's Hospital, London, U.K.)
Dr. R. Lendrum (Central Middlesex Hospital, London, U.K.)
Dr. D. Marleau (Hospital Beaujon, Clichy, France)
Dr. R. N. M. MacSween (Western Infirmary, Glasgow, U.K.)
Dr. H. Malchow (Medizinische Universitätsklinik, Marburg, Germany)
Dr. J. D. Maxwell (King's College Hospital, London, U.K.)
Dr. N. McIntyre (The Royal Free Hospital, London, U.K.)
Dr. D. B. L. McLelland (Royal Infirmary, Edinburgh, U.K.)
Dr. V. Melikian (Dudley Road Hospital, Birmingham, U.K.)

Dr. Joanna Miller (King's College Hospital, London, U.K.)
Dr. A. P. Mowat (King's College Hospital, London, U.K.)
Dr. I. M. Murray-Lyon (King's College Hospital, London, U.K.)
Dr. G. Neale (Royal Postgraduate Medical School, London, U.K.)
Dr. N. Nicoloupoulos (University of Thessaloniki, Greece, and Central Middlesex Hospital)
Dr. Z. M. Nooman (The London School of Hygiene and Tropical Medicine, London, U.K.)
Dr. P. Papanagyioutou (University of Athens and West Middlesex Hospital, London, U.K.)
Dr. I. W. Percy-Robb (Royal Infirmary, Edinburgh, U.K.)
Dr. K. Pettingale (King's College Hospital, London, U.K.)
Dr. M. Podda (Royal Postgraduate Medical School, London, U.K.)
Dr. J. D. Price (Beecham Research Laboratories)
Dr. M. O. Rake (King's College Hospital, London, U.K.)
Dr. K. Ramsøe (Rigshospitalet, Copenhagen, Denmark)
Dr. L. Ranek (Rigshospitalet, Copenhagen, Denmark)
Dr. Reimara Roessler (University of Tubingen, West Germany)
Dr. Otto Roessler (University of Tubingen, West Germany)
Dr. P. J. Roylance (Beecham Research Laboratories)
Dr. P. Sharpstone (King's College Hospital, London, U.K.)
Dr. K. B. Shilkin (King's College Hospital, London, U.K.)
Dr. G. Sladen (St. Bartholomew's Hospital, London, U.K.)
Dr. C. P. Sodomann (Medizinische Universitätsklinik, Marburg, Germany)
Mr. D. Stewart (King's College Hospital, London, U.K.)
Dr. J. S. Stewart (The West Middlesex Hospital, London, U.K.)
Dr. A. S. Tavill (Royal Free Hospital, London, U.K.)
Dr. Dudley Tee (King's College Hospital, London, U.K.)
Dr. J. Terblanche (University of Cape Town, South Africa)
Dr. D. Trigger (Radcliffe Infirmary, Oxford, U.K.)
Dr. Joan Trowell (Royal Postgraduate Medical School, London, U.K.)
Dr. M. D. Turner (Strong Memorial Hospital, Rochester, New York, U.S.A.)
Dr. J. Ungar (Swiss Serum and Vaccine Institute, Berne, Switzerland)
Dr. R. J. Walker (Western General Hospital, Edinburgh, U.K.)
Professor H. K. Weinbren (Nottingham University Medical School, U.K.)
Dr. M. Willoughby (St. Bartholomew's Hospital, London, U.K.)
Mr. J. Winch (King's College Hospital, London, U.K.)
Dr. R. Zeegen (Westminster Hospital, London, U.K.)

OPENING ADDRESS BY THE DEAN OF KING'S COLLEGE HOSPITAL MEDICAL SCHOOL — DR. D. I. WILLIAMS

At the end of January, 1860, an eminent physician was called to see a patient in South Wales. This was Sunday, January 29. On his way back he spent the night in Gloucester and while there he was seized with haematemesis and vomited three pints of blood. He did not rest but took the early train back to London and although feeling very ill he managed to see several patients. At 1 p.m. haematemesis violently came on again and prostrated him completely. Despite the attendances of five of his colleagues he died at 8 p.m. in his consulting room at the age of 50. He had been aware for at least a year of his inevitable doom; indeed, you can read all about it in Thackeray's "Roundabout Papers", where he is thinly disguised as "Mr. London". At the postmortem it was found that he had hypertrophic cirrhosis of the liver, the disease in fact sometimes called after him. Shortly before his death, he had collected a number of lectures which were later published. The last chapter in the book treats of "the therapeutical action of alcohol". "Some of you", he said, "would doubtless be surprised at seeing that a good deal of wine and brandy is administered to many of my patients". Some of you may think to salve your consciences when you hasten to agree with his statement that "alcohol possesses its stimulating property because it is a form of aliment, appropriate to the direct nourishment of the nervous system and its preservation, and its especial adaptation to this system gives it an immediate, exciting power superior to any other kind of food".

I may say, he stresses its value in very much divided doses. "Taken too much at one time, the patient will become more or less intoxicated or, in common language (he says), drunk." His potion is a most palatable mixture of Tinct. Canella,* brandy, syrup and water, and, judging by the accounts of the hospital, he prescribed it very often.

Now, this was a great teacher, a great physiologist and a great clinician. But his greatest contribution was to found this Hospital in 1839, and his statue, by Noble, was erected by colleagues, pupils and friends and now stands on Denmark Hill. His name was Professor Robert Bentley Todd, and our present Liver Unit, by chance rather than design, is in Todd Ward.

Before 1839, King's College — that is, King's College, London, not the Hospital — had medical students but no hospital: Todd was the power behind the foundation of the new Hospital, close to Lincoln's Inn Fields, alongside the graveyard of St. Clement Dane's Church and adjacent to the slaughterhouse of Butchers, Row. "Its locality is fine", the *Medical Times* said, "shambles on one side and a churchyard on the other — butchers within and without, prayers for the living and for the dead". In 1864 a second hospital was built on the old site, where W. H. Smith's are now, and in 1913 we came out to Denmark Hill. In 1909 the Medical School became a School of Medicine of the University of London.

In 1845 there was published a book on "Diseases of the Liver" by George Budd, like Todd, a Fellow of the Royal Society, and herein he describes the case of a man who died in King's in February, 1844, with "inflammation of the hepatic vein". Curiously, he too says, "The patient had for many years been in the habit of drinking enormous quantities of gin", and it was to this that Budd

* Wild cinnamon.

attributed the inflammation. In 1912, another great man, Samuel Kinnier Wilson, wrote on progressive lenticular degeneration — 'Wilson's Disease', and he came on the staff of this hospital in 1919. On a personal note, may I say that I had the honour of being his house physician, but this was later, in 1937.

This exciting meeting arises, therefore, almost as a natural progression in the study of liver disease at this hepatophilic Hospital. But not quite so. It has arisen, really, on the initiative of my colleague and namesake, Dr. Roger Williams, who gets all my cheques while I get his bills, who conceived the idea and who has worked so hard to bring it into the world, and it is up to the rest of you to give life to this conception. On behalf of the Medical School, I am therefore very happy to welcome you to this meeting, and I hope you will enjoy it.

The Dean then repeated the welcome in German, Italian, Spanish, French, Australian and American.

PART I
Clinical, Morphological and Virological Aspects

CLINICAL SPECTRUM OF AUTO-IMMUNE LIVER DISEASE
A. E. Read

Over the past twenty years, those interested in liver disease have gradually accepted the idea that certain chronic liver disorders may represent either partially or completely the effects of auto-immune damage. In opening this symposium, it is my task to review with you the clinical features of the diseases which have come under auto-immune "suspicion", admitting that, on the one hand, there is really no clear proof that any one of these diseases is of auto-immune aetiology and on the other, it is equally possible that I shall leave out some disorders which will later turn out to be clearly of this aetiology. However, I propose to start by reviewing the features of so-called "Primary auto-immune" disease, that is, auto-immune disease where specific organ antibodies are found and where these antibodies are thought to cause damage to the target organ. These have been reviewed very ably by Dr. Doniach (1970) recently and some of the features that she has set out are shown in Table 1. Primary auto-immune

Table 1

Features of Primary Auto-immune Diease

(Doniach 1970)

(1) No known cause
(2) Female preponderance
(3) Protracted course
(4) Appropriate serum antibodies
(5) Histology shows immune hyperactivity
(6) Familial aggregation
(7) Association with other auto-immune conditions
(8) Variable clinical picture.

disease has no known cause, often a female preponderance and a protracted course; there are appropriate specific serum antibodies, the histology shows immune hyperactivity, there is often familial aggregation of cases, there is an association with other auto-immune conditions, and lastly, the clinical picture is sometimes variable.

HEPATIC DISEASES FULFILLING CRITERIA OF PRIMARY AUTO-IMMUNE DISORDERS

Now let us see what diseases might fit into this pattern, or a similar sort of pattern, when we are dealing with the liver. Table 2 shows those conditions where auto-immunity may, in the light of present knowledge, have a part to play in hepatic damage. Firstly, active chronic hepatitis — known by a wide variety of names, most of them stressing some clinical or pathological feature of the disease. Secondly, primary biliary cirrhosis and thirdly, a rare syndrome for which I have found no name, first adequately described by Craig, Schiff and Boone in 1955, in which chronic liver disease exists in an environment of auto-immune disease affecting the adrenal gland, the parathyroid, etc. Some of these cases are

1

Table 2

Clinical spectrum of auto-immune liver disease

(1)   Active Chronic Hepatitis.

              Lupoid hepatitis
              Waldenström's active chronic hepatitis
              Plasma cell hepatitis
              Juvenile cirrhosis.

(2)   Primary biliary cirrhosis.

              Chronic non-suppurative destructive cholangitis.

(3)   Craig-Schiff-Boone Syndrome (1955).

              Chronic hepatitis, hypoparathyroidism.
              Addison's disease. Moniliasis.

(4)   ? Cryptogenic cirrhosis.

(5)   Liver disease in collagen diseases

              (a) Systemic sclerosis
              (b) Rheumatoid arthritis – Felty's Syndrome
              (c) Sjögren's syndrome, etc.

complicated by systemic Candida infections. Fourthly, it is possible that some cases of cryptogenic cirrhosis, of the sort commonly seen in this country, belong to this group. Lastly, one must look for evidence of liver disease in the collagen disorders as the latter are already suspected of an auto-immune aetiology, and it is therefore reasonable to examine these cases for evidence of liver involvement. The ones that have been particularly investigated are systemic sclerosis, rheumatoid arthritis with Felty's syndrome, and Sjögren's syndrome.

ACTIVE CHRONIC HEPATITIS

This is a disease of great interest, one which has an international flavour (Table 3), for various features have been described from various parts of the

Table 3

Landmarks in the history of A.C.H.

(1)   1948 (Australia) Wood *et al.* "*Chronic Infectious Hepatitis*".
(2)   1950 (Sweden) Waldenström. *Age Sex.*
(3)   1950 (U.S.A.) Kunkel. *Serum proteins.*
(4)   1955 (Australia) Joske and King, *LE cell.*
(5)   1956 (U.S.A.) Bearn *et al. Generalised Disease.*
      1957 (Australia) Gajdusek. *Immunology.*
(6)   1960 (U.S.A.) Page & Good. *Histology.*
(7)   1963 (England) Read *et al. Multiorgan involvement.*
(8)   1965 (England) Johnson *et al. S. M. Antibody.*

world. In Australia, this was thought to be chronic infectious hepatitis by Wood
et al. (1948). Waldenström(1950) pointed out the particular age and sex
incidence, the serum protein changes were described by Kunkel and Labby
(1950). Joske and King (1955) in Australia first showed that some patients have
an LE cell phenomenon, hence one of its alternative names, lupoid hepatitis.
In the United States (Bearn *et al.* 1956) and England (Read *et al.* 1963), it was
realised that this was a multisystem disease and not just one confined to the
liver. Gajdusek (1958) in Australia found nonspecific antibodies in the serum and
Page and Good (1960) were particularly interested in the plasma cell infiltrate in
the liver. Lastly, the smooth muscle antibody was described by Johnson *et al.*
(1965) in a fair percentage of patients with this disease, whereas it was not
found in patients with disseminated lupus.

There are two particularly interesting facets to this disease:

Multisystem involvement

Firstly, many organs apart from the liver may be involved. I do not propose to
give you a comprehensive list of the conditions that can occur, but joint and skin
involvement, disorders of the lungs, gut disease, particularly ulcerative colitis,
valvular heart disease, various types of glomerular and tubular renal lesions,
endocrine disorders and blood disease, are well recognised. The important thing
is that evidence of organ involvement may precede that in the liver. I should also
remind you of the systemic manifestations more recently described. In the
kidney, one should mention renal tubular acidosis; in the lungs one might mention
fibrosing alveolitis (Turner Warwick, 1968), and perhaps also pulmonary
nypertension (Cohen and Mendelow, 1965), as being the most recent additions to
the crime sheet.

Prognosis

The second interesting factor about this disease concerns the prognosis. When
we looked some years ago, at a series of 82 cases with respect to the prognosis,
dividing patients into males and females, and also into those who had received
corticosteroids — because this was the only form of therapy known at the time —
and those who had not, we found very little evidence of a beneficial effect of
corticosteroids on the mortality. The average expectation of life in both groups
seemed to be of the order of three and a half years. There were, however, a
number of cases, mostly female, and often those who had not been treated with
corticosteroid drugs, in which there was an extremely long survival, where
apparently the liver cell lesion gradually burnt itself out. Recently Page *et al.*
(1969) have reported their results of immunosuppressive therapy with
6-mercaptopurine and corticosteroids and point out that they have a twelve-year
survival of almost 30 per cent. So perhaps there is a variability, either natural or
due to therapy, of the survival of patients with this disease. I would like to
mention two examples of this, to show how variable the disease may be.

The first is a patient who initially presented at the age of 12, with liver cell
jaundice. Because this lasted a number of weeks she was investigated surgically
and the diagnosis of active chronic hepatitis was made at laparotomy and biopsy.
She was treated at that stage with corticosteroid drugs. At the age of 19 she had
a Coombs positive haemolytic anaemia; at 22 she developed alopecia and also at
22 she had Stevens-Johnson syndrome of considerable severity due to drug-
sensitivity. At the same age she had a splenectomy because the corticosteroid
drugs failed to control completely her haemolytic anaemia — she also had severe
arthralgia; at 24 she had at least two attacks of staphylococcal septicaemia, but
by the age of 26, that is fourteen years later, she is well working perhaps rather

inappropriately as a barmaid, and with a barium swallow showing no varices! So after 14 years, perhaps because of treatment, perhaps despite it, the patient, with all these multiple vicissitudes, is well.

Contrast this with the second patient: a female aged 61 who in 1964 developed two-weeks jaundice and was found to have LE cells in her serum and was given corticosteroids. In 1966 she had splenomegaly and, two and a half years from the beginning, she had a haematemesis which led to her death, despite ligation of varices. At autopsy there was a fully developed macronodular cirrhosis of the liver and portal vein thrombosis.

These then are the extremes of the disease and this is one of the problems that worries me: how one tells what is going to happen to an individual patient. Various investigators have suggested that patients with an acute onset, with LE cells in the blood, and with multiple organ involvement are likely to do well with treatment. But then others have put forward exactly the same findings as indices of a poor prognosis. Personally, I find the age of great importance and I think, on the whole, that the younger patient with this syndrome does much better than the older one.

PRIMARY BILIARY CIRRHOSIS

This again is a disease which may be of auto-immune aetiology and I wonder if we could consider Dr. Doniach's requirements for a primary auto-immune disease and see how they fit this condition.

Indeed, this is a disease of unknown cause with a female preponderance and a protracted course. One observer at least has found specific antibodies (Paronetto *et al.* 1964) but many people have only found nonspecific serum antibodies. The histological picture is of immune hyperactivity, both in the liver and in the draining lymph node; there is a familial aggregation of cases and of antibody changes. There is a variable clinical picture in some of these patients but until recently I had not thought that this was a disease which was associated with other auto-immune conditions. I refer to the recent paper by Reynolds *et al* (1970), where they said "Is this a new syndrome?" They were describing five female patients, all with a positive mitochondrial antibody test, with the combination of systemic sclerosis, primary biliary cirrhosis and hereditary telangiectasia. I would remind you that systemic sclerosis is a disease in which clinicians have felt that auto-immunity might be important, and here it is allied with a genetically determined disease of the blood vessels (hereditary telangiectasia). Quite how these fit together is difficult to say but at least here was a disease occurring with primary biliary cirrhosis, so perhaps primary biliary cirrhosis is a multi-organ disease.

CRAIG-SCHIFF-BOONE SYNDROME

Now perhaps I could discuss an extreme rarity: I refer to the cases of multiple immunological endocrine disease, some of which have been accompanied by liver disorder. The history of this is quite interesting. In 1955, Reissner and Ellsworth described a number of patients with idiopathic hypoparathyroidism and pernicious anaemia. Some of these patients also had idiopathic Addison's disease and Candida infection. In 1931, Rowntree and Snell had already described 20 cases of non-tuberculous Addison's disease occurring with pernicious anaemia and they pointed out that some of these patients had Monilial infection and idiopathic hypoparathyroidism. Then Leonard (1946) gave the first suggestion that liver involvement occurred in patients with Addison's disease and hypoparathyroidism. We have two patients, a brother and sister, with this syndrome, under the care of Professor Bruce Perry and more recently, of my colleague Dr. Martin Hartog. I would like to show you their clinical histories because I think these are of interest.

The picture shows the children when they were aged five and seven (Fig. 1). Sarah and Peter, now aged 15 and 13, have clinical histories of great interest which are almost identical. They started life with keratitis; they were found to have hypoparathyroidism, both were found to have liver disease based on abnormal liver function tests, with mild jaundice in one of them — and now one

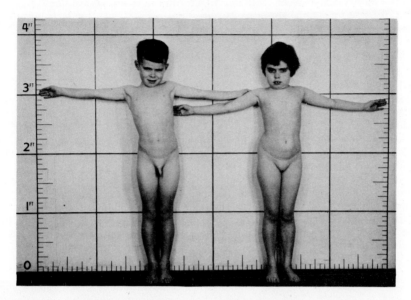

Fig. 1. Sarah and Peter at the ages of 5 and 7 respectively

has gone on to develop adrenal cortical failure. They both have a wide variety of antibodies against many tissues, but the parents apparently have no serum auto-antibodies. Other clinical features are recurrent monilial infections of the mouth, perhaps again of immunological significance (Valdimarsson *et al.* 1970) and the dental abnormality due to hypoparathyroidism. The liver biopsy findings were those of active chronic hepatitis.

One of the interesting things about this syndrome is the extreme variability of the liver disease, and in the literature there are patients who have fully developed cirrhosis of the liver, others who have just lymphoid infiltration in portal tracts, and others who have expansion of the portal zone with fibrosis. In these two patients, at the moment the liver disease does not seem to be very important, but then of course one is already on corticosteroid drugs for adrenal replacement therapy.

OCCURRENCE OF LIVER DISEASE IN THE "COLLAGEN DISORDERS"

Now we can look at the collagen disorders to see if there is evidence of liver disease.

FELTY'S SYNDROME

This condition of lymphoid hyperplasia complicating rheumatoid arthritis, has been known for a number of years occasionally to be complicated by hepatic involvement. From this Hospital in 1970 (Blendis *et al.*) came a paper describing the hepatic findings in twelve patients with this disease, eight of them female incidentally, and three of them in one family. The findings were of interest; 8 had

abnormal liver function tests, 5 on hepatic biopsy showed lymphocytic
infiltration in the liver, 3 had gone on to periportal fibrosis, and 1 had a fully
developed macronodular cirrhosis. The group of investigators were at pains to
point out that they were not sure of the significance of some of these findings,
and wondered whether increased blood-flow through the liver, perhaps related
to the very enlarged spleen, could be a factor in the abnormal histology. Nevertheless, there was a hepatic abnormality and abnormal liver function tests in this
disease.

Sjögren's Syndrome

This syndrome was recently reinvestigated from the hepatic point of view, by
Whaley *et al.* (1970). They approached the problem by taking patients with a
positive mitochondrial antibody test and looking for the incidence of positive
tests in patients with Sjögren's syndrome, in those with rheumatoid arthritis and
Sjögren's syndrome combined, and in those with rheumatoid arthritis alone.
They found a high incidence of mitochondrial antibodies in Sjögren's syndrome
(6 per cent) and an increased incidence in patients with rheumatoid arthritis and
Sjögren's syndrome. A slightly increased incidence was found in rheumatoid
arthritis patients who had that disease alone. They then examined 10 patients
with a positive test for clinical and biochemical evidence of liver disease. They
found 3 patients with hepatomegaly and 5 patients with biochemical liver
disease – they did no liver biopsies. One of these patients was of interest because
he had the biochemical features of cirrhosis with cholestasis and might have had
primary biliary cirrhosis.

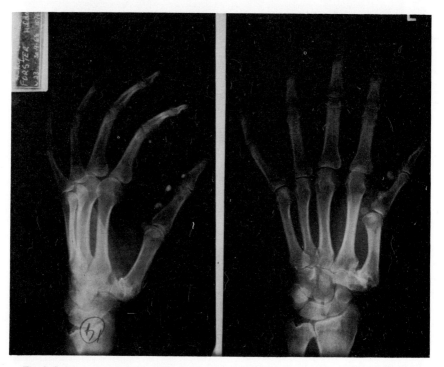

Fig. 2. Subcutaneous calcific deposits in a patient with systemic sclerosis and portal
        hypertension

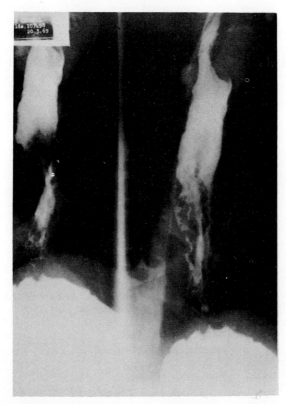

Fig. 3. The barium swallow from the patient referred to in Fig. 2.

Systemic Sclerosis

Here we are in difficulties because at least two major reviews of cases have suggested that there is no increased incidence of liver disease in this condition. The review of D'Angelo *et al.* (1969) of 58 cases revealed only 5 with an abnormal liver, i.e. rather less than in the control population – these were autopsy studies. The review of the Mayo Clinic (Bartholomew *et al.* 1964) of a large number of cases – 727 cases of systemic sclerosis – showed only 8 with an abnormal liver. These observers thought, quite reasonably, that there was no evidence to suggest that the liver was involved in this condition.

One cannot help, however, questioning these reports because there are other reports which do suggest a relationship between liver disease and this disorder. The liver can in fact show lymphoid infiltration or fibrosis, and even cirrhosis, and I have already pointed out that occasionally there is a link-up with primary biliary cirrhosis. Clinically, this disorder nearly always manifests itself as portal hypertension. There is one case in the literature of rupture of the liver (McCoy, 1967) and this the observers thought, was due to involvement of the blood vessels in the sclerotic process which led to haematoma formation and eventual rupture. The gall-bladder can also be involved in this syndrome; fibrosis is not unusual and this may give rise to abnormal contraction of the organ on X-ray visualisation, and also a condition of ischaemic ulceration of the bile duct has been reported (Wildenthal *et al.* 1968), progressing to obstructive jaundice.

We have seen 4 or 5 patients with systemic sclerosis, all of them with portal hypertension. Figures 2 and 3 illustrate the calcific subcutaneous deposits and tapering of the fingers, and the abnormal barium swallow found in one of these cases. This particular patient had a fully developed cirrhosis with regeneration nodules and cellular fibrous tissue between the tracts. The other interesting thing about the liver histology was that under high power fairly obvious piecemeal necrosis could be seen at the edge of the regeneration nodules, perhaps a further hallmark of auto-immune liver disease.

PROBLEMS FOR THE FUTURE

I have said nothing of the possibility that cryptogenic cirrhosis of the type commonly seen in this country, could be a manifestation of auto-immune liver disease. The close correlation pointed out by Walker *et al.* (1970) between a positive mitochondrial antibody test and the presence of biochemical or histological evidence of liver disease, makes this very possible, and of course, cryptogenic cirrhosis is silent in its progression. The patient usually presents with one of the complications of the disease, and I suppose it is possible that an auto-immune process could be responsible for this long and silent period.

I have tried to review the liver diseases in which there is evidence of auto-immunity but I would say two things in closing. Perhaps I have stressed much too much the compartmentalisation of these diseases. It is almost certain that one flows into another, and that types of disease intermediate between those that I have described, exist. The other aspect that needs explanation is the extreme variability of the clinical features of these diseases, ranging from gross evidence of liver cell failure at one end (perhaps the active chronic hepatitis end) – through portal hypertension (perhaps due to a disease like systemic sclerosis) – through to patients who apparently have only a few lymphocytes or a little extra fibrosis in their livers. The reason for these differences defies explanation by me, but perhaps some light might be shed in the discussion.

REFERENCES

Bartholomew, L. G., Cain, J. D., Winkelmann, R. K. and Bagenstoss, A. H. (1964) Amer. J. of Dig. Dis. 9, 43.
Bearn, A. G., Kunkel, H. G. and Slater, R. J. (1956) Amer. J. Med. 21, 3.
Blendis, L. M., Ansell, I. D., Lloyd Jones, K., Hamilton, E. and Williams, R. (1970) B.M.J. 1, 131.
Cohen, N. and Mendelow, H. (1965) Amer. J. Med. 39, 127.
Craig, J. M., Schiff, L. H. and Boone, J. E. (1955) Amer. J. Dis. Child. 89, 669.
D'Angelo, W. A., Fries, J. F., Masi, A. T. and Shulman, L. E. (1969) Amer. J. Med. 46, 428.
Doniach, D. (1970) Proc. Roy. Soc. Med. 63, 527.
Gajdusek, D. C. (1958) Arch. Int. Med. 101, 9.
Johnson, G. D., Holborow, E. J. and Glynn, L. E. (1965) Lancet 2, 878.
Joske, R. A. and King, W. E. (1955) Lancet 2, 477.
Kunkel, H. G. and Labby D. H. (1950) Ann. Int. Med. 32, 433.
Leonard, M. F. (1946) J. Clin. Endocrinol. 6, 496.
McCoy, D. G. (1967) J. Inst. Med. Ass. 60, 474.
Page, A. R. and Good, R. A. (1960) Amer. J. Dis. Child. 99, 288.
Page, A. G., Good, R. A. and Pollard, B. (1969) Amer. J. Med. 47, 765.
Paronetto, F., Schaffner, F., Mutter, R. D., Kniffen, J. C. and Popper, H. (1964) J. Amer. Med. Assoc. 187, 503.
Read, A. E., Harrison, C. V. and Sherlock S. (1963) Gut 4, 378.
Reissner, D. J. and Ellsworth, R. M. (1955) Ann. Int. Med. 43, 1116.
Reynolds, T. B., Denison, E. K., Frankl, H. D., Lieberman, F. L. and Peters, R. L. (1970) Proc. of the meeting of the Amer. Assoc. for the Study of Liver Diseases Oct. 1969; (1970) Gastroenterology 58, 290.

Rowntree, L. G. and Snell, A. M. (1931) A clinical study of Addison's Disease p. 81.
     Saunders. Philadelphia.
Turner Warwick, M. (1968), Quart. J. Med. 37, 133.
Valdimarsson, H., Holt, L., Riches, H. R. C. and Hobbs, J. R. (1970) Lancet, I, 1259.
Waldenström, J. (1950) Leber Blutproteine und Nahrungseweiss. Stoffwechs-Krh
     Sonderband : XV Tagung Bad Kissingen p. 8.
Walker, J. G., Doniach, D. and Doniach, I. (1970) Quart. J. Med. 39, 31.
Whaley, K., Goudie, R. B., Williamson, J., Huki, G., Dick, W. C., and Buchanan, W. W.
     (1970) Lancet 1, 861.
Wildenthal, K., Schenker, S., Smiley, J. D. and Ford, K. L. (1968) Arch. In. Med. 121, 365.
Wood, I. J., King, W. E., Parsons, P. J., Perry, J. W., Freeman, M. and Limerick, L. (1948)
     Med. J. Aust. 1, 249.

DISCUSSION
Chairman: Dr. Roger Williams

ROITT

On what grounds can you reject the findings on 727 patients with systemic sclerosis at the Mayo Clinic who showed no association with primary biliary cirrhosis? Why are they less likely to represent the truth than your very few patients, in whom you have found a concordance?

READ

Of course, one cannot dismiss the findings in so large a series of cases. However, the harder one looks the more likely one is to find liver involvement in patients with systemic sclerosis. There is indeed a difference of opinion across the Atlantic, but I have no figures comparable with theirs to make a statistical comparison.

CHAIRMAN

In support of this association, we have had 2 patients with primary biliary cirrhosis, both with mitochondrial antibodies in the serum, associated with systemic sclerosis and calcinosis. However they did not have portal hypertension.

READ

To confuse the situation still further, our patient with portal hypertension and scleroderma did not have the mitochondrial antibody.

GEALL

You are looking prospectively at patients in whom the suspicion of liver disease had already been raised by the finding, for example, of an increased alkaline phosphatase. On the other hand the Mayo Clinic study was a retrospective analysis of a large number of cases of systemic sclerosis who had not been examined specifically for liver involvement.

DONIACH

Much the same occurred with thyroid disease. In the classical papers on primary biliary cirrhosis, there was no mention of Hashimoto's thyroiditis or thyrotoxicosis. Now that we have started to look for these associations we find them quite frequently.

SAUNDERS

A few weeks ago, at the National Institute of Health Bethesda, Dr. Chalmers showed me a patient with Sjögren's syndrome and primary biliary cirrhosis. The following week Dr. Trey showed me the same syndrome in Boston.

MACSWEEN

In Glasgow we have biopsied the liver in 8 cases of Sjögren's syndrome. The histology in one resembled that of primary biliary cirrhosis and in two others there was marked lymphocytic inflammation. So there is a morphological counterpart for the recent finding of a high incidence of mitochondrial antibody in Sjögren's syndrome

MacLAURIN

The syndrome described by Reynolds of systemic sclerosis, primary biliary cirrhosis and hereditary telangiectasia represents an interesting combination. In another disease with telangiectasia — ataxia telangiectasia — there is gross impairment of cellular immunity. Studies on this aspect might be worthwhile in Reynold's patients.

MURRAY–LYON

The telangiectasia in scleroderma are identical, histologically and macroscopically, with those that occur in Osler's disease. Unless there was a clear family history of Osler's disease in these patients, one cannot say that they had three separate conditions. The telangiectasia were probably part of the scleroderma.

NEALE

Can the prognosis of 'auto-immune' liver disease be related to the degree of immunological reactivity, measured by serum gamma globulin concentrations or by the finding of various serum antibodies?

READ

Not at the moment, although it has always been said that people with a high gamma globulin respond well to treatment.

THE PATHOLOGY OF CHRONIC HEPATITIS
By P. J. Scheuer

In recent years it has become common practice to separate chronic hepatitis pathologically into two distinct varieties, chronic persistent hepatitis and chronic aggressive hepatitis, (De Groote *et al.,* 1968). The justification for this sharp separation is that the clinical course and prognosis of these two conditions are quite different. Before describing their pathological features, however, I must emphasize that there may be considerable diagnostic overlap, both histological and clinical, between chronic aggressive hepatitis and a third condition, primary biliary cirrhosis. This is one reason why it is necessary to discuss primary biliary cirrhosis together with these two varieties of chronic hepatitis. There is also some evidence, which you will no doubt hear over the next two days, that primary biliary cirrhosis shares pathogenetic features with other forms of chronic hepatitis.

CHRONIC PERSISTENT HEPATITIS

The characteristic feature of chronic persistent hepatitis is that pathological changes are more or less confined to the portal tracts. There is an inflammatory lesion involving the portal tracts which does not extend to any appreciable extent into the adjacent parenchyma. Piecemeal necrosis, the process in which liver cells at the junction between mesenchyme and parenchyma are gradually destroyed, is either slight or absent. As a result, the architecture of the liver lobules is preserved and there is little or no scarring except in the portal tracts. The prognosis is therefore good, and it is very unusual for this condition to progress to cirrhosis, (Becker *et al.,* 1970).

Chronic persistent hepatitis may be difficult to distinguish pathologically from a late stage of resolution of acute viral hepatitis. Nonspecific reactive hepatitis, which accompanies a number of systemic disorders, is also histologically similar. Not all cases of chronic persistent hepatitis have a recognizable acute episode, some presenting with quite vague symptoms. A firm diagnosis must therefore be based on both pathological and clinical data.

CHRONIC AGGRESSIVE HEPATITIS

The characteristic feature of this condition is piecemeal necrosis. Chronic inflammation is again found in the portal tracts but now it extends into the adjacent parenchyma in association with piecemeal necrosis of variable degree. Probably as a result of this process, fibrous tissue is formed within the liver lobules, there is distortion of lobular architecture and this condition tends to progress to cirrhosis with regeneration nodules.

There are variable degrees of activity and the prognosis is not always bad. In mild cases the pathological process may resolve and the patient recover. However, in severe cases with dense cellular infiltration and gross distortion of the hepatic parenchyma resolution is no longer possible. The liver cells became swollen and may be arranged in cylinders sometimes with a central lumen; in cross section these are seen as gland-like formations or rosettes. This is the classical pathological picture which has been associated with the clinical syndrome variously called active chronic hepatitis, lupoid hepatitis or juvenile cirrhosis.

Professor Read has already mentioned that the pathological features seen in cases of active chronic hepatitis are variable. Some patients show severe chronic

11

aggressive hepatitis on liver biopsy and others have fully developed cirrhosis, whereas in a minority liver biopsy shows only portal inflammation. Whether this represents a true variation in the pathology of the syndrome, or sampling error, or whether it represents the evolution of the disease process, the fact is that there may not be close correspondence between the pathological picture and the clinical findings. This is one reason why it is preferable to reserve the term "active chronic hepatitis" for the clinical syndrome and separate it from "chronic aggressive hepatitis", a pathological process.

PRIMARY BILIARY CIRRHOSIS

This is the third condition that should be mentioned in any discussion on chronic hepatitis. It is important to recognise that primary biliary cirrhosis has a distinct evolution from a florid duct lesion right through to cirrhosis. It is because only the late stages are cirrhotic that Rubin and co-workers proposed the the more accurate descriptive term "chronic non-suppurative destructive cholangitis", (Rubin *et al.*, 1965). Failure to recognize this evolution can easily lead to failure to recognize the disease on liver biopsy.

In the early stages, primary biliary cirrhosis is essentially a portal tract disease. Typically, the hyperplastic or ruptured epithelium of a damaged bile duct is surrounded by a cellular reaction of two kinds, the first consisting of a cuff of lymphocytes and plasma cells with some eosinophils, and the second of histiocytes or epithelioid cell granulomas with or without giant cells. In our experience, the overall incidence of these granulomas in primary biliary cirrhosis is around 30 per cent. However, when one considers the earliest stages of the disease in which only the florid duct lesion is present, the incidence of granulomas rises to nearly 80 per cent. This is an important diagnostic point since granulomas are extremely rare in other forms of chronic hepatitis.

In the later stages of primary biliary cirrhosis there may be considerable parenchymal involvement by piecemeal necrosis, and it is then easy to confuse the pathological appearances with those of chronic aggressive hepatitis. Mixed cases occur, having the histological features of both diseases.

INTERRELATIONS OF ACUTE AND CHRONIC HEPATITIS

Table 1 shows the possible pathological sequelae of acute hepatitis. There are two dotted lines; one is with respect to liver cell carcinoma, because although liver-cell carcinoma has been shown in patients carrying the hepatitis-associated (Australia) antigen in their serum, (Sherlock *et al.*, 1970), this could simply mean that these are cases of cirrhosis who have secondarily developed liver-cell carcinoma. There is no evidence as yet that this can occur directly as a result of acute hepatitis. Secondly, the development of primary biliary cirrhosis is represented by a dotted line for although this may be the end of acute hepatitis, the majority of cases of primary biliary cirrhosis have no clinically obvious antecedent cause.

All the remaining conditions have not only been shown to occur after acute hepatitis but have also been shown to occur after acute hepatitis in the presence of the hepatitis-associated antigen. There may be resolution or sometimes recurrence with the pathological features of simple acute hepatitis. Post-hepatitic scarring is another complication, which tends to be forgotten; strictly speaking this is not chronic hepatitis, but it no doubt exists as a potential cause of portal hypertension. Patients may die or they may develop chronic aggressive hepatitis and cirrhosis. The sequence of acute hepatitis, chronic aggressive hepatitis and cirrhosis has been seen in a patient whose serum contains hepatitis-associated antigen (Sherlock *et al.*, 1970).

Table 1

Possible Sequelae of Acute Hepatitis

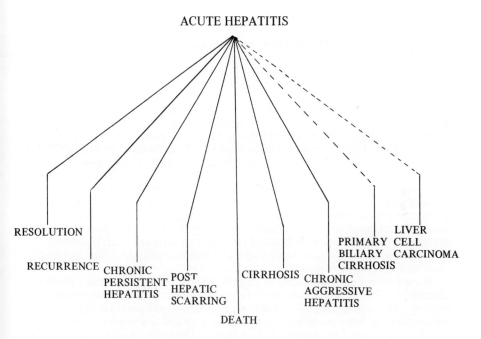

ACUTE HEPATITIS

RESOLUTION

RECURRENCE

CHRONIC PERSISTENT HEPATITIS

POST HEPATIC SCARRING

DEATH

CIRRHOSIS

CHRONIC AGGRESSIVE HEPATITIS

PRIMARY BILIARY CIRRHOSIS

LIVER CELL CARCINOMA

Primary Biliary Cirrhosis and Acute Hepatitis

This is at present a tenuous relationship and most cases of primary biliary cirrhosis are not preceded by a recognizable episode of acute hepatitis. However, Poulsen and Christoffersen from Copenhagen have recently published a series of 83 liver biopsies from cases of acute and chronic hepatitis, of which 14 showed biliary lesions on biopsy (Poulsen and Christoffersen, 1969). The striking point about these cases is that whereas the whole series included patients of both sexes and all ages the cases with biliary lesions were all middle aged or older females — the classical age and sex distribution of primary biliary cirrhosis.

Primary Biliary Cirrhosis: Definition

The old view of primary biliary cirrhosis as a rare icteric disease of middle-aged women may need revision. In a series of 41 cases of primary biliary cirrhosis studied by Fox and Sherlock (to be published), at the Royal Free Hospital, 22 per cent were anicteric at the onset, although many complained of pruritus. One of these patients remained anicteric for twelve years. Zeegen *et al.,* (1969), have shown that among 250 patients undergoing portacaval shunt for portal hypertension, as many as 23 had primary biliary cirrhosis and of these 15 presented with bleeding from oesophageal varices without jaundice or pruritus.

Furthermore some cases with the pathological features of the disease are asymptomatic and their liver disease is discovered incidentally, (Sherlock *et al.,* 1969). One such patient, a 23 year old girl, was attending a gynaecological clinic for menorrhagia. She was found to have a palpable liver, and subsequently to have a high serum alkaline phosphatase and mitochondrial antibodies. A liver biopsy showed classical changes of early primary biliary cirrhosis with granuloma formation.

How then, if the symptons are so variable, is "primary biliary cirrhosis" to be defined, and where do the limits of this disease lie? It would be unwise to rely entirely on the pathological features because it is not always easy to find a diagnostic lesion in a small needle biopsy. Nor can one rely on the mitochondrial antibody test, since it has been shown repeatedly that although this test is positive in a high proportion of cases of primary biliary cirrhosis, it is also positive in some 30 per cent of cases of active chronic hepatitis and of cryptogenic cirrhosis, (Doniach *et al.*, 1966). This phenomenon has been studied by Ross *et al*, who analysed data on 41 cases of cryptogenic cirrhosis. These were separated arbitrarily into those in which there were no pathological features in any way reminiscent of primary biliary cirrhosis, and those in which there were some features also found in primary biliary cirrhosis, such as granulomas, lymphoid aggregates or peripheral cholestasis. Among these 41 cases, there were more men than women, more without mitochondrial antibodies than with, and a similar number with and without extensive piecemeal necrosis. In the group with no histological features of primary biliary cirrhosis, there were many more men than women, more without mitochondrial antibodies, and now more cases without much piecemeal necrosis. However, in the group with some features of primary biliary cirrhosis all these factors were reversed; there were now more women than men, more with mitochondrial antibodies, and strikingly more with piecemeal necrosis.

These findings could be taken to mean that there are many different kinds of chronic liver disease which have some factor in common, perhaps piecemeal necrosis, (Doniach and Walker, 1969). An alternative explanation is that primary biliary cirrhosis has a much wider symptomatology and is a much less rare disease than has previously been supposed. Although I believe that there is some truth in both hypotheses I am inclined to favour the latter view.

REFERENCES

Becker, M. D., Scheuer, P. J., Baptista, A. and Sherlock, S. (1970) Lancet *i*: 53.
De Groote, J., Desmet, V. J., Gedigk, P., Kort, G., Popper, H., Poulsen, H., Scheuer, P. J.,
    Schmid, M., Thaler, H., Uehlinger, E. and Wepler, W., (1968), Lancet *ii*: 626.
Doniach, D., Roitt, I. M., Walker, J. G. and Sherlock, S. (1966), Clin. Exp. Immunol. *1*: 237.
Doniach, D. Walker, J. G. (1969). Lancet, *i*: 813.
Fox, R. A. and Sherlock, S. To be published.
Poulsen, H. and Christoffersen, P. (1969) Acta Path. Microbiol. Scand. *76*: 383.
Ross, A., Doniach, D., Scheuer, P. J. and Sherlock, S. To be published.
Rubin, E., Schaffner, F. and Popper, H. (1965) Amer. J. Path. *46*, 387.
Sherlock, S., Fox, R. A., Scheuer, P. J. and Doniach, D. (1969) Gastroenterology *56*: 1222.
Sherlock, S., Fox, R. A. Niazi, S. P. and Scheuer, P. J. (1970) Lancet, *i*: 1243.
Zeegen, R., Stansfeld, A. G., Dawson, A. M. and Hunt, A. H. (1969) Lancet *ii*: 9.

DISCUSSION
Chairman: Dr. Roger Williams

CHAIRMAN

How many of your patients with primary biliary cirrhosis had a history of infective hepatitis at the beginning of their illness? Secondly, in what percentage are granulomas found in cryptogenic cirrhosis, or in active chronic hepatitis? I had thought that granulomas were confined to primary biliary cirrhosis.

SCHEUER

A minority of cases of primary biliary cirrhosis, about 15 per cent, have a clearly defined history of acute hepatitis. How significant this is, occurring twenty years beforehand, is difficult to know, just as it is in any form of cirrhosis.

The finding of a granuloma in cryptogenic cirrhosis is exceedingly rare; I can recall perhaps two or three cases among several hundred. This is certainly also true of active chronic hepatitis; in fact, I do not remember any case with all the clinical and histological criteria of active chronic hepatitis which showed granulomas. They may, of course, be so very characteristic of primary biliary cirrhosis because we are using them as one of the defining features.

FOX

The incidence of acute hepatitis at the onset of primary biliary cirrhosis is very low, in our series of over 40 patients it occurred perhaps in only one case. However in the same series 15% had had hepatitis at sometime in the past.

DAWSON

Looking back to that series of patients with cryptogenic cirrhosis and a high alkaline phosphatase that you described some years ago with Professor Sherlock, how many of them were cases of true primary biliary cirrhosis?

SCHEUER

All of them might have been, and I suspect that some of them were! However I must emphasize that we have no sure way of diagnosing or delineating this condition at the moment. There is a great deal of overlap between different forms of chronic hepatitis.

CHAIRMAN

Five years ago an operative liver biopsy on a patient of ours showed classical primary biliary cirrhosis. But although the mitochondrial antibody is still present a recent liver biopsy shows only cirrhosis with no diagnostic features of primary biliary cirrhosis.

What do you now feel about that international study at Kansas in which a group of us examined sections from different types of cirrhosis? There was so much observer variation that we could not even write it up! (Laughter).

SCHEUER

The main object of that study was to delineate anatomical types of cirrhosis, and it did lead to a simplification of the classification. Dr. Popper and his group now refer to "regular" and "irregular" cirrhosis; we refer to "micronodular" and "macronodular" cirrhosis. However, the significance of this classification is strictly limited, for when you have said that the cirrhosis is micronodular you are not much further forward.

BLACKBURN

Dr. Scheuer said that patients with chronic aggressive hepatitis do not recover; however we have a patient in which this diagnosis was proven by biopsy who has certainly recovered both clinically and histologically.

SCHEUER

I did not mean to imply that all of them progress to cirrhosis. The prognosis is generally bad compared with chronic persistent hepatitis, which is why the two were separated. But one is surprised to hear of Professor Read's case who after some twelve years, is clinically well and without portal hypertension. In such cases I cannot believe that the liver is normal but presumably the patient has compensated from the mechanical and immunological point of view.

LESSOF

In Dr. Scheuer's last slide, he classified the histological characteristics of primary biliary cirrhosis and then showed a view of piecemeal necrosis.

SCHEUER

Those cases were patients with cryptogenic cirrhosis who had some of the features that one associates with primary biliary cirrhosis. I did not say that they *had* primary biliary cirrhosis. Otherwise, they would never have been put in the cryptogenic group. When we reviewed these cases we were surprised at the frequency with which features such as lymphoid aggregates or granulomas were observed.

MacLAURIN

It is possible to produce granulomata and giant cells experimentally using inbred strains of rats. A liver homogenate from one strain is used to immunize rats of a second strain. Sensitised spleen cells from a parent rat are then injected directly into the liver of an F_1 hybrid. The resulting granulomatous lesion may be produced as a result of a double immunological challenge: the cells injected are not only sensitive to the liver but also to some of the histocompatibility antigens present in the F_1 hybrid.

MORPHOLOGICAL AND IMMUNOLOGICAL STUDIES ON CHRONIC AGGRESSIVE HEPATITIS AND PRIMARY BILIARY CIRRHOSIS

Hans Popper

INTRODUCTION

The speakers before me have clearly illustrated the major problems and Dr. Scheuer has really covered the main points which I expected to discuss. I am very grateful for this because it gives me the opportunity to improvise a talk rather different from the standard discussion on chronic aggressive hepatitis and primary biliary cirrhosis that I have given only too often in my own country, all over the world and at least three times already in London! I now intend to conduct a reappraisal of two terms, both originating from Mount Sinai, that have been repeatedly used in our previous reports, namely piecemeal necrosis (Popper *et al.,* 1962a) and "chronic destructive non-suppurative cholangitis" (Popper *et al.,* 1962b).

I must first apologize for the term "piecemeal necrosis". This was intended to indicate a destruction of the parenchyma at the junction with the portal tracts, with loss of individual hepatocytes, associated with inflammation reflected in accumulation of lymphocytes, plasma cells or macrophages and with proliferation of bile ductules. It is now clear that the histological changes, and particularly piecemeal necrosis, do not provide a reliable prognostic index. Neither are the results of various immunological reactions, in particular the serological tests, any more reliable in predicting the prognosis, or the likely results of therapy.

CLASSIFICATION OF CHRONIC HEPATITIS

The tremendous polymorphism that exists within this group of diseases makes it clear that a dogmatic presentation of sharply defined entities is a description of prototypes. However, bearing in mind the frequent overlap of these prototypes in the individual patients. I would like to present a classification of chronic hepatitis (Popper and Orr, 1970), rather similar to Dr. Scheuer's (Fig. 1). In addition to the groups of persisting (portal) hepatitis, and aggressive (periportal)

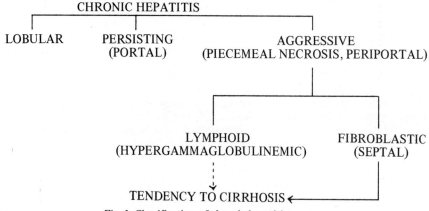

Fig. 1. Classification of chronic hepatitis.

17

hepatitis we have included a third, characterized by inflammatory changes in the lobular parenchyma. These intralobular changes by themselves do not differ in their conventional and fine structural characteristics from those found in acute hepatitis (Schaffner, 1969). In chronic hepatitis, if this lobular form occurs with the persisting (portal) or aggressive (periportal) form, no prognostic assumptions can be made. As long as intralobular changes are present, there is no way of knowing whether the portal or periportal alterations are merely a reaction to the intralobular cellular necrosis. Only when portal or more particularly periportal changes persist, after the lobular changes have subsided, can a "self perpetuation" be assumed. In the periportal form this then suggests that a transition to cirrhosis is likely.

ANALYSIS OF CHRONIC AGGRESSIVE HEPATITIS WITH SPECIAL REFERENCE TO PIECEMEAL NECROSIS

In this form of hepatitis, we have previously described two main components which frequently are present together. The first is the lymphoid component, evidenced by the lymphocyte and plasma cell infiltration. Clinically, this element is usually associated with hypergammaglobulinaemia. The second is the fibro-blastic component, reflected in excess connective tissue and, more especially, in septa formation. We have repeatedly emphasized (Popper and Orr, 1970) that this fibroblastic component is of greater importance to the prognosis than the lymphoid component. However the latter, in all probability an immunological reaction, is of greater diagnostic importance than the insidious fibroblastic response. It is likely that the impressive serological reactions are related in kind to this lymphoid element and possible that the manifestations in other organs are due to the deposition of antigen/antibody complexes.

Plasma Cells

There are several cellular components of piecemeal necrosis. The first is the plasma cell, which is found between hepatocytes and recognized by the large amount of rough endoplasmic reticulum that it contains, indicating protein secretion. Later in the meeting we shall doubtless hear about the various circulating antibodies — antinuclear, antismooth muscle, antimitochondrial and so on — produced by these cells both in the liver and elsewhere. I need not refer to the diagnostic importance of these and other immunoglobulins, however I must emphasize that the pathogenetic significance of any circulating antibody remains to be established in chronic aggressive hepatitis. It is possible to use immune (but not to my knowledge auto-immune) methods to produce experimental chronic liver injury. For instance, injections of pig serum elicit a diffuse fibrosis in rats (Paronetto and Popper, 1966). Under these circumstances, both antigen and antibody as immune complexes have been demonstrated in the liver by immunofluorescence. Nevertheless, Dr. Paronetto has not been able to demonstrate immune complexes in the human liver in chronic aggressive hepatitis.

Lymphocytes and the Anabolic Reaction in the Liver

The second cell component of piecemeal necrosis is the lymphocyte. It is quite possible that these cells may cause immunological liver injury as part of a delayed hypersensitivity reaction. Both in chronic aggressive hepatitis and in primary biliary cirrhosis, circulating lymphocytes can be transformed in tissue culture to lymphoblasts by exposure to autologous liver (Tobias et al., 1967). During this transformation several interesting morphological changes in the lymphocytes occur, the nucleus becomes larger and contains more DNA, the nucleoli enlarge, and the cytoplasm shows increased basophilia.

You are all familiar with this "anabolic" reaction, as I would like to call it, which is presumably initiated by an alteration of the plasma membrane of the lymphocyte. I submit that in piecemeal necrosis, some hepatocytes, especially those in the peripheral portion of the parenchyma in contact with lymphoid cells, show a similar "anabolic" reaction. Some of these changes can also be seen in the hepatocytes of cirrhotic nodules undergoing destruction. All these cells show large nuclei, large nucleoli, dense basophilic cytoplasm and PAS-positive non-glycogenic cytoplasmic granules, presumably lysosomes (Fig. 2). Binucleated

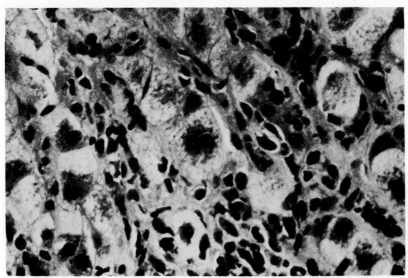

Fig. 2. "Anabolic" reaction of hepatocytes in chronic aggressive hepatitis. Note large nucleus and nucleolus, dark cytoplasm with granular material, presumably lysosomes. The hepatocytes are in close contact with lymphoid cells (H+E, 400 x.)

cells are often seen, and even mitoses. Taking the analogy to its logical conclusion, I suggest that this hepatocytic "anabolic" reaction is the result of a cell membrane change possibly related to an immunological interaction.

Similarities to Biliary Obstruction

On further analysis there are a series of other characteristic changes to be seen which I believe may be more relevant to the development of cirrhosis than the "anabolic" reaction. These changes mainly involve hepatocytes in the limiting plate, and those separated from the bulk of the parenchyma and located in the connective tissue of the portal tracts and septa. This type of cell also is frequently found in cirrhotic nodules undergoing destruction. The cells may be large, but their nuclei are small and they do not exhibit lysosomal granules. Their cytoplasm shows a peculiar vacuolization (Fig. 3), identical to the appearance of the cytoplasm of hepatocytes in cholestasis referred to as feathery degeneration (Gall and Dabrogorski, 1964); however, bile pigment need not be present in these cells in piecemeal necrosis.

Sometimes hyaline deposits can be seen in these cells which cannot be morphologically differentiated from the classical alcoholic hyaline of Mallory (Fig. 4). Like alcoholic hyaline, it stains blue with aniline blue and is PAS-negative. I should emphasize that, when there is bilirubin retention in hepatocytes, PAS-positive material may be recognized adjacent to the hyaline which had prompted some of us, including myself, to wrongly assume that the hyaline itself is PAS-positive. The occurrence of hyaline similar to alcoholic

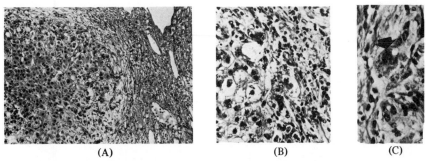

(A)   (B)   (C)

Fig. 3. Chronic aggressive hepatitis. (A) "Anabolic" manifestations in the peripheral portion
of the parenchyma and "cholate-static" changes on the junction between parenchyma
and the enlarged portal tract which shows considerable fibrosis. (H+E, 50 x.)
(B) Feathery degeneration of hepatocytes on the junction. They have small nuclei and
a vacuolated, almost empty cytoplasm. (H+E, 120 x.) (C) Hyaline resembling alcoholic
hyaline (arrow) in hepatocytes in the portal tract. Note segmented leukocytes around
them. (H+E, 200 x.)

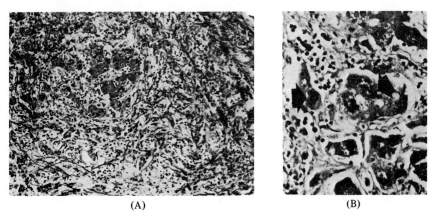

(A)   (B)

Fig. 4. (A) Cirrhosis in a young girl (non-alcoholic). Nodule undergoing degeneration.
(Mallory's aniline blue. 60 x.) (B) Hyaline, stained blue, (arrows) in hepatocytes.
(Mallory's aniline blue, 260 x.)

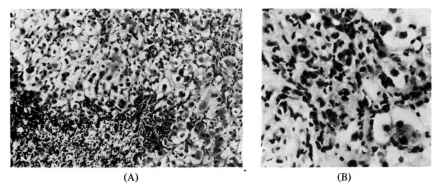

(A)   (B)

Fig. 5. Chronic aggressive hepatitis, Australia antigen positive. (A) Typical piecemeal necrosis
and erosion of the limiting plate. (H+E, 60 x.) (B) Close-up, showing many neutrophilic
segmented leukocytes. (H+E, 200 x.)

hyaline in mechanical biliary obstruction and even in bile infarcts is now fully recognized. Another very interesting observation is that around these cells in piecemeal necrosis, segmented leucocytes are found just as frequently as around alcoholic hyaline (Fig. 5). I must apologize that in our original and subsequent descriptions of piecemeal necrosis we entirely overlooked the presence of these polymorphonuclear leucocytes. The probable reason was that they are not found in the parenchyma, but on the junction with septa and portal tracts and, particularly, within the connective tissue.

The fact that these altered hepatocytes share similar morphological features (except for the frequent absence of retained bilirubin) with cells seen in mechanical biliary obstruction may give a clue to their pathogenesis. It is likely that these cells, which are isolated and trapped in the connective tissue, though presumably able to secrete bile pigment, are not able to secrete other biliary compounds. Currently our group in New York is finding that the characteristic alteration of the cytochrome P 450 dependent biotransformation system in the endoplasmic reticulum that occurs in experimental cholestasis (Hutterer *et al.,* 1970), can be produced *in vitro* by bile acids, in particular by chenodeoxycholic acid, as well as by some anionic detergents (Hutterer *et al.,* 1970). It could be that retained bile acids, through a detergent effect, are in this way responsible for the described morphological changes in the cells in piecemeal necrosis — cells that we now speculatively refer to as cholate-static.

We thus believe that in addition to the "anabolic" reaction in the parenchyma, a "cholate-static" phenomenon exists which stimulates leucocytic inflammation and fibrosis rather like alcoholic hyaline does, although in the.latter case the changes are mainly centrilobular (Edmondson *et al.,* 1963).

Other Cell Types in Piecemeal Necrosis

A third type of hepatocyte is found in active chronic hepatitis. These hepatocytes, sometimes called biliary hepatocytes, are arranged in acinar or rosette forms, with five or six cells surrounding a bile canaliculus as opposed to the norm of two or three (Fig. 6). Around such hepatocytes a basement

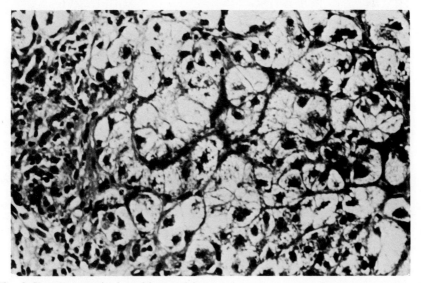

Fig. 6. Chronic aggressive hepatitis, septal form. Acinar arrangement, or rosette formation of the hepatocytes. (Mallory's aniline blue, 240 x.)

membrane can be demonstrated under the electron microscope, and even under the conventional microscope many collagenous fibres are seen to surround them. The fourth type of cell seen in piecemeal necrosis form the well known proliferated bile ductules. These are also surrounded by fibrosis.

To summarize thus far — I believe that an intralobular inflammatory response to hepatocellular degeneration and necrosis may lead to two types of portal reaction (Fig. 7). In the first type some macrophages, presumably derived from the intralobular inflammatory reaction, reach the portal tract and lymphoid cells accumulate. This represents what we call the persisting or portal form of chronic hepatitis. By contrast, in the aggressive form four types of cellular reaction develop, all of which combine to produce piecemeal necrosis. The first is a conspicuous periportal accumulation of lymphocytes and/or plasma cells with neighbouring hepatocytes showing the "anabolic" reaction. We think that this hepatocytic "anabolic" reaction is related to the lymphoid reaction. The second cell type is "cholate-static" showing small nuclei and feathery cytoplasm and sometimes even hyaline. Bile pigment may be present but is not essential. Segmented leucocytes gather round these cells. The third is the hepatocytes in acinar arrangement and the fourth is the proliferated bile ductules.

I submit that the last three components are more important for fibroplasia and that they stimulate the formation of connective tissue septa and hence the

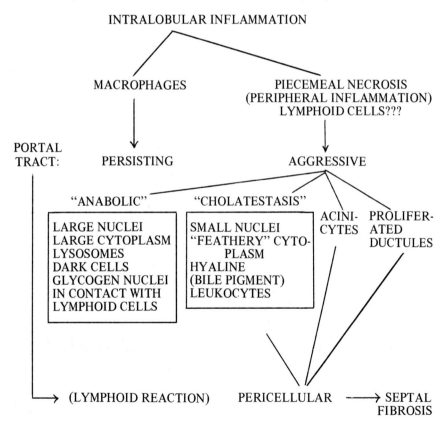

Fig. 7. Cellular reactions in chronic hepatitis.

CHRONIC NON-SUPPURATIVE CHOLANGITIS

DESTRUCTIVE (PRIMARY BILIARY CIRRHOSIS)		NONDESTRUCTIVE (SCLEROSING)
LATE IRREGULAR MAINLY PERIPHERAL CHOLESTASIS		EARLY CENTROLOBULAR REGULAR CHOLESTASIS
TRANSIENT GRANULOMAS		
MANY	PLASMA CELLS	FEW
POSITIVE	ANTIMITOCHONDRIAL ANTIBODIES	NEGATIVE
OVERLAP WITH CHRONIC HEPATITIS		SYSTEMIC CONNECTIVE TISSUE DISEASE OR ULCERATIVE COLITIS

Fig. 8. Classification of chronic non-suppurative cholangitis.

transition into cirrhosis. Unfortunately, there is no good way to determining the development of septal fibrosis other than liver biopsy. But needle biopsy may not provide a representative sample of the liver as far as fibrosis is concerned, and a biochemical parameter, as for example the hypergammaglobulinaemia of the lymphoid reaction, has not been established for hepatic fibroplasia. It remains to be established to what degree the lymphoid reaction triggers the fibroblastic reaction in chronic aggressive hepatitis, as it does in other diseases, e.g. in rheumatoid arthritis.

PRIMARY BILIARY CIRRHOSIS

The diagnostic feature of this condition, chronic nonsuppurative destructive cholangitis, has been shown by Dr. Scheuer. I want to supplement this description with some of the immunofluorescent observations of Paronetto *et al.,* (1961). Firstly, immunoglobulins, mainly IgM macroglobulins, can be demonstrated in hepatic plasma cells. We originally thought that the presence of IgM in these cells was characteristic for primary biliary cirrhosis, but this is not so as we have now found it in other conditions. Secondly, the serum of patients with primary biliary cirrhosis contains antibodies that bind to biliary ductules in specimens of liver from patients with this disease. Thirdly, in three cases of early primary biliary cirrhosis Dr. Paronetto has demonstrated extracellular deposits around bile ducts containing both gammaglobulin and complement, suggesting that they are immune aggregates. This is the only liver disease so far in which he has demonstrated complement and antibody complexes with the exception of conditions with non-hepatic antigens such as schistosomiasis (Rubin *et al.,* 1961). The presence of immune aggregates strongly supports the thesis that primary biliary cirrhosis is an immune disorder of autoaggressive character.

In the second stage of primary biliary cirrhosis, a ductular reaction associated with a periportal inflammation, i.e. piecemeal necrosis can be found. But in this type the "cholate-static" reaction is in the foreground while the "anabolic" is almost missing. Periductular fibrosis is prominent and explains the conspicuous peripheral cholestasis which, though variable throughout the liver, is very prominent in some areas in this stage of the disease (Rubin *et al.* 1965). In primary biliary cirrhosis, cholestasis is usually both central and peripheral. We have observed centrilobular cholestasis alone, only when administration of a cholestatic drug, e.g. anabolic steroids, has induced or aggravated jaundice in the early stages of the disease.

We have recently been impressed by a group of cases which resemble primary biliary cirrhosis and which share with it a conspicuous portal inflammatory reaction particularly around bile ducts. In contrast, however, frank destruction of bile ducts is absent and only periductal inflammation and fibrosis are present. Moreover centrilobular cholestasis appears early. These cases we suggest have the hepatic manifestations of sclerosing cholangitis (Sherlock 1968) – a condition which may be associated with chronic ulcerative colitis but was not so in the majority of our cases. None of the cases of this group had antimitochondrial antibodies or Australia antigen.

So, chronic nonsuppurative cholangitis can be divided into two forms. The first is the more frequent and represents the classical picture of primary biliary cirrhosis. It is destructive in the early stages and if cholestasis appears, it is both peripheral and central. Transiently, granulomas may be present and plasma cells are frequent. Antimitochondrial antibodies are very common but there may be an overlap with chronic aggressive hepatitis. In the second, the non-destructive fibrotic form, there is early centrilobular cholestasis but few plasma cells. Antimitochondrial antibodies are absent. This sclerosing cholangitis may be associated with generalized connective tissue diseases or with ulcerative colitis (Fig. 8).

Overlap with Chronic Aggressive Hepatitis

In returning to this question to which Dr. Scheuer referred and which Doniach *et al.* (1970) presented so well in their recent review, I would like to draw attention to a common observation which I cannot explain. In almost all cases in which there was morphological overlap, and in which there were high titres of both smooth muscle and antimitochondrial antibodies, the clinical features of primary biliary cirrhosis were not found. Hypercholesterolemia and pruritus were absent and sometimes neither jaundice nor high levels of alkaline phosphatase were seen despite a classical picture of bile duct destruction presumably encouraging regurgitation of bile. The clinical manifestations and the evolution of such cases are that of chronic aggressive hepatitis. I would be grateful if somebody were to explain this paradoxical and to me disturbing situation.

CONCLUSIONS

Let me close by summarizing the two main points I wanted to make. First, I have to concede that we created more confusion than clarification by introducing the term "piecemeal necrosis" for clinico-pathological correlation. The observations presented here were obtained by classical techniques, i.e. haematoxylin-eosin staining. That means that they should have been made years ago and confirms the old saying that we only see what we want to see and what we know. Anyway, piecemeal necrosis should now be resolved into a lymphoid phenomenon, which is important diagnostically and may be significant pathogenetically, and a fibroplastic component related to "cholate-static" cells, cells in acini, and proliferated bile ductules – this latter component may be more important prognostically than the lymphoid reaction.

Finally I want to subdivide chronic nonsuppurative cholangitis into a destructive form representing early primary biliary cirrhosis and a fibrosing form as the intrahepatic component of sclerosing cholangitis.

ACKNOWLEDGEMENT

This work was supported by U.S. Public Health Service Grant AM 03846 and U.S. Army Medical Research and Development Command Contract DA-49-193-MD-2822.

REFERENCES

Doniach, D., Walker, J. G., Roitt, I. M. and Berg, P. (1970), New Eng. J. Med. 282, 86–89.
Edmondson, H. A., Peters, R. L., Reynolds, T. B. and Kuzuna, O. T. (1963), Amer. J. Int. Med. 59, 646.
Gall, E. A. and Dabrogorski, O. (1964), Amer. J. Clin. Path. 41, 126–139.
Hutterer, F., Bacchin, P. G., Raisfeld, I. H., Schenkman, J. B., Schaffner, F. and Popper, H. (1970), Proc. Soc. Exp. Biol. Med. 133, 702–717.
Hutterer, F., Denk, H., Bacchin, P. G., Schenkman, J. B., Schaffner, F. and Popper, H. (1970), Life Sci. 9, 877–887.
Paronetto, F. and Popper, H. (1966), Amer. J. Path. 49, 1087–1101.
Paronetto, F., Schaffner, F. and Popper, H. (1967), J. Lab. Clin. Med. 69, 979–988.
Popper, H., Barka, T., Goldfarb, S., Hutterer, F., Paronetto, F., Rubin, E., Schaffner, F., Singer, E. J. and Zak, F. G. (1962a), J. Mt. Sinai Hosp. 29, 152.
Popper, H. and Orr, W. (1970), Scand. J. Gastroent. 6, 203–222.
Popper, H., Rubin, E. and Schaffner, F. (1962b), Am. J. Med. 33, 807.
Rubin, E., Hutterer, F., Gall, E. Cs. and Popper, H. (1961), Nature, 192, 886.
Rubin, E., Schaffner, F. and Popper, H. (1965), Amer. J. Path. 46, 387.
Schaffner, F. (1964),Tijdschr. Gastroenterol., 76, 31–38.
Sherlock, S. (1968), Brit. Med. J. 2, 515–521.
Tobias, H., Safran, A. P. and Schaffner, F. (1967) Lancet 1, 193–195..

DISCUSSION
Chairman: Dr. Roger Williams

WEINBREN

I would accept much of your discussion with regard to the various types of cholangitic lesion in primary biliary cirrhosis. But in your analysis of piecemeal necrosis, I think I am a little too old to join you in this revolution. I can accept that there is anabolism in the liver cells, but I have never heard of a liver cell transforming for the same reasons as lymphocyte does. We need more evidence before it can be said that liver cell transformation implies an immunological mechanism. There are other possible causes for anabolism in this situation: the liver cell could be making more protein or it could be responding to destruction of other liver cells.

The second point: you describe the cells inside the portal tracts as giving evidence of bile duct obstruction . . . .

POPPER

No — of bile acid retention.

WEINBREN

Bile acid retention? Well, I am not sure if I can accept that either. Did you measure measure the nuclei?

POPPER

The nuclei are smaller.

WEINBREN

But the point is this: There is a great variability in nuclei in the liver lobules, as you know better than I do. I do not know if all small nuclei are in one place, and all the other nuclei in another. Secondly, feathery degeneration is not a lesion that occurs diffusely when a bile duct is obstructed; it seems to occur in foci and unless you are postulating a mechanism which is similar to bile lake formation, then the evidence for retention of biliary secretion is not very sound. Furthermore, there is nothing to suggest that cells entrapped by lymphocytes, plasma cells and fibrous tissue would accumulate bile into them and then not let it get out. It is much more likely that with the subtle mechanisms of blood-flow, there would be less uptake into these cells.

Another point is that what you call "hepatobiliary" does not seem to me to be hepatobiliary! These are simply enlarged cells around a canaliculus. I refer to the cells of truly adenoid formation. They are liver cells not bile duct cells.

POPPER

No, no! They are biliary hepatocytes!

WEINBREN

And their central canal is not mucin-secreting, but a canaliculus. So those are liver cells and why you should call them "hepatobiliary" I do not know.

POPPER

I did not. I said biliary hepatocytes! (Laughter).

WEINBREN:

I do not like that either, and the last thing that you said was that there was much ductular proliferation. I think that until these cells are shown *not* to have the mitochondrial pattern of liver cells, and to have other characteristics of bile ductules, you should not refer to "biliary proliferation".

POPPER

Peculiarly enough, I agree with all your points except the one referring to the lack of biliary secretion. But I wanted to make it clear that instead of referring to "piecemeal necrosis" we must now subdivide it into the various morphological features. Some of these liver cells, we agree, are anabolic. It appears to me, and it is in no way proven, that this cell may be responding in a similar way to the transformed lymphocyte. I have in no way definitely equated the two. The proof that an immunological reaction takes place in these cells is not available, only the suggestion of it comes from the morphological analogy that I presented.

Regarding bile retention, the point which I wanted to bring out is this is an entirely different type of reaction from the anabolic one. The appearance of the cytoplasm of these cells is very similar whatever the cause of the cholestasis.

The third point — biliary hepatocytes. This happens to be a name coined by Steiner. These cells are undoubtedly hepatocytes, especially as they have the typical mitochondrial pattern. They are peculiar in that they are arranged four, five or six cells round a canaliculus instead of as two or three. This is the area where I feel I am on the safest ground. because this happens to be published by various other people.

WEINBREN

But that does not necessarily make it okay!

POPPER

Yes it does! (Laughter).

Now the last question you raise, is one of the oldest. Whether the bile ductules, actually are bile ductules or modified liver cells. It is clear, from the evidence of the electron microscope, that this type of cell has a basement membrane and very few mitochondria. I really feel there is no doubt, especially considering Gresham and Rubin's studies on tritiated thymidine uptake, that these are proliferated bile ductules.

WEINBREN

But the experimental proliferated bile ductule is a different sort of cell, morphologically, from what we see here. Again you may be correct but we ought to prove that they are in fact bile duct cells.

POPPER

Under the electron microscope, they have few mitochondria and relatively little endoplasmic reticulum.

WEINBREN

I accept this entirely, if you have got the evidence. In my hands, they do not seem to have deficient mitochondria, and in fact even under the light microscope there are plenty to be seen.

SCHEUER

I would like to ask about Dr. Paronetto's antiductular antibodies in primary biliary cirrhosis. Are these antibodies directed against the calibre of duct primarily involved in the disease?

POPPER

No – they react with any bile duct structure. It is an entirely non-specific antibody, seen in any type of hepatitis.

SCHEUER

I am sure you would agree that in piecemeal necrosis, the liver tissue gradually gets eaten away at the expense of the mesenchyme. Do you think that your "Anabolic" cell is going to become the "stasis" cell?

POPPER

It may be so although I do not know, because there are plenty of cases in which there is no evidence of this progression.

THE AUSTRALIA ANTIGEN IN AUTO-IMMUNE LIVER DISEASE
Ralph Wright

The discovery of the Australia (Au) antigen and the recognition of its close association with at least one of the infective agents responsible for viral hepatitis (Blumberg *et al.*, 1967) – probably serum hepatitis specifically – provides the opportunity to examine the possible relationship of infection with a hepatitis virus to a number of so-called auto-immune diseases of the liver. There are clearly a number of possibilities. One is that a hepatitis virus might in fact be responsible for the lesions and that the auto-immune phenomena and auto-antibodies which are observed might be secondary phenomena. The other possibility is that infection with an agent such as a hepatitis virus might trigger off a response which is then perpetuated by an auto-immune process.

INCIDENCE OF POSITIVE RESULTS

The most common method used for the detection of the Au antigen is immunodiffusion in one per cent agarose, with an antiserum usually obtained from patients who have been multiply transfused, such as patients with haemophilia, in the central well, and the test sera in the peripheral wells. In a study of the Au antigen in sera from patients with acute and chronic liver disease at Yale (Wright *et al.*, 1969) we used this method of detection. The coded test sera are placed in the peripheral wells and in each instance one looks for a reaction of identity with a standard antigen-containing serum. We confirmed the earlier observations of Blumberg *et al.* (1967) and Prince (1968) that there is a high incidence of Au antigen in the serum of patients with acute viral hepatitis (Table I). In addition, we noted that patients with prolonged hepatitis including unresolved classic hepatitis and subacute hepatic necrosis with progression to cirrhosis (a term used by Klatskin (1958) and which others would call "active chronic hepatitis" starting as acute viral hepatitis) had the Au antigen in their serum in a high proportion of cases. We also detected the antigen in 6 out of 24 patients with active chronic hepatitis of unknown aetiology with an insidious onset.

Table I

Australia Antigen in Biopsy-Documented Liver Disease

	No. of Patients		Positive Tests	
Acute viral hepatitis, < 4 months duration	88		52%	
Prolonged viral hepatitis, > 4 months duration	29		38%	
Unresolved classic hepatitis		14		50%
Subacute hepatic necrosis → posthepatitic cirrhosis		15		27%
Active chronic hepatitis, ? etiology	24		25%	
Other hepatic disease	248		1%	
Healthy controls	135		0%	

Of interest were the negative findings which have also been noted by others. None of 44 patients with primary biliary cirrhosis had the antigen in their serum and only 1 of 57 patients with Laennec's cirrhosis, and 1 of 26 patients with postnecrotic (cryptogenic) cirrhosis were positive. The patients with other hepatic diseases included a number with halothane hepatitis, and at least some of the conditions to which Professor Read has already referred, such as a patient with the CRST syndrome and primary biliary cirrhosis. It was significant that all three patients in this group in whom the antigen was detected had had multiple multiple blood transfusions within one week before the serum was tested, and we think that these positive reactions were due to passive transmission of the antigen.

RESULTS IN ACTIVE CHRONIC HEPATITIS

Table II summarizes the results to date in selected series of patients with active chronic hepatitis. In the most recent study from the Royal Free Hospital (Sherlock *et al.*, 1970) all but one of the 6 patients with the antigen in their

Table II

Incidence of Au Antigen in Chronic Active Hepatitis

Author	Number of Patients	Number with Au Antigen
Wright *et al.*, 1969	39	10 (25%)
Gitnick *et al.*, 1969	31	3 (10%)
Fox *et al.*, 1969	32	0 (0%)
Mathews & Mackay, 1970	53	2 (4%)
Krassnitzky *et al.*, 1970	15	9 (60%)
Sherlock *et al.*, 1970	74	6 (8%)
Vischer, 1970	85	19 (22%)

serum had come from abroad. It will be noted that there is a much lower incidence of the antigen in series from the United Kingdom (Fox *et al.*, 1969) and Australia (Mathews and Mackay, 1970) than from series in the United States (Wright *et al.*, 1969; Gitnick *et al.*, 1969), Austria (Krassnitzky *et al.*, 1970) and Switzerland (Vischer, 1970).

A number of possibilities have been suggested for the discrepancy in these results from different centres. The most likely explanation is that it is due to a different geographical distribution of the long incubation period, serum hepatitis virus in the apparently healthy population. It is unlikely that the differences are due to differences in technique since antisera were exchanged between various centres. The frequency with which the Au antigen is detected in patients with active chronic liver disease might therefore depend upon the prevalence of the serum hepatitis virus in the community, transmitted either by inoculation or by the faecal-oral route. This view is supported by the finding that 3 of the 4 patients with Au antigen in their serum in the Yale study, whose illness started acutely, had epidemiological evidence of serum hepatitis. Furthermore, of 20 patients with active chronic hepatitis examined at Oxford, only one has had the Au antigen in the serum, a finding in keeping with that of Fox and associates (1969) in this country.

TRANSMISSION OF Au ANTIGEN FROM MOTHER TO CHILD

That exceptional circumstances are necessary for the Au antigen to be associated with active chronic hepatitis is well illustrated by the only such case seen at Oxford (Wright *et al.,* 1970).

This patient was an infant who acquired acute viral hepatitis with a high transaminase and bilirubin from its mother, who had jaundice at the end of pregnancy and for one month after delivery. The Au antigen was present during the acute attack and throughout a period of eight months during the development of cirrhosis, which was present on surgical liver biopsy when the infant was aged one year. During this period the transaminase and bilirubin fluctuated. We did not have sera from cord blood or from the mother during the acute attack of hepatitis but when she returned for reexamination, at the time at which the infant developed acute viral hepatitis, we detected the antigen in her serum and this has continued to be present over a period of several months. The mother's liver biopsy showed no significant abnormality, apart from mild focal necrosis. The infant's biopsy showed a severe active cirrhosis with marked round-cell infiltration, piecemeal necrosis and multinucleated giant cells (Figs. 1 and 2).

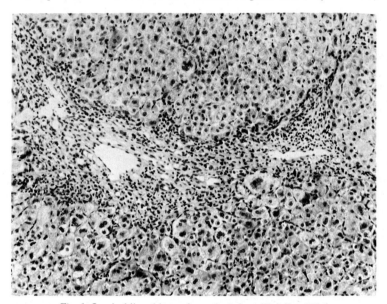

Fig. 1. Surgical liver biopsy from the infant. (H & E x 100.)

The Au antigen was detected repeatedly by immuno-diffusion and electron microscopy. An interesting feature was the presence of long tubular forms of the Au antigen in both the mother's serum and the infant's serum (Fig. 3). The infant's serum also contained large antigen particles, described by Dane and associates (1970) which they suggest is the parent virus. An unusual feature is that these large particles as well as the tubular forms, were present during the acute attack of hepatitis (Fig. 4) and this might conceivably have some prognostic significance. During the acute attack of hepatitis the infant showed a slight elevation in IgM levels, which then returned to normal. The IgG levels rose during the progression to cirrhosis (Fig. 5) and antibody to the Au antigen was later detected by immuno-diffusion and electron microscopy. Australia antigen positive acute viral hepatitis is uncommon in the Oxford area, which is in

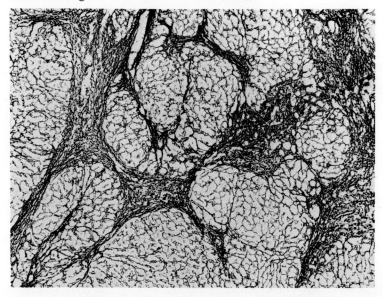

Fig. 2. Surgical liver biopsy from the infant. (Reticulin ×32.)

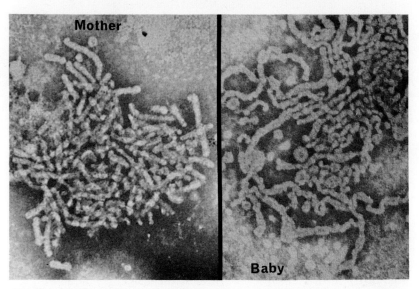

Fig. 3. Au antigen particles in serum from mother and baby (×80,000) to illustrate the predominance of long tubular forms.

keeping with the observation of Mosley *et al.* (1970), that rural or semi-rural infectious hepatitis is usually antigen negative. The special circumstances in this case became apparent when we learned from the patient's general practitioner that the mother had worked as a dental assistant until late in her pregnancy. Furthermore, the baby's scalp had been lacerated during surgical induction of

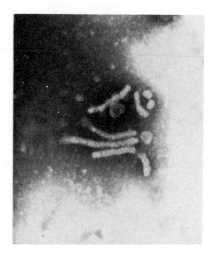

Fig. 4. Au antigen particles in the infant's serum during the acute attack (×100,000).

labour and the mother had had a perineal tear. It would seem that the transmission of Au antigen-positive hepatitis and the development of an antigen-positive chronic active hepatitis in areas where antigen-positive acute viral hepatitis is rare, only occurs under exceptional circumstances.

FACTORS DETERMINING FREQUENCY OF Au ANTIGEN IN ACTIVE CHRONIC HEPATITIS

Thus, although there is evidence to indicate that the Au antigen may be responsible for some cases of active chronic liver disease, the frequency will vary considerably. In certain areas such as Asia and Africa, where, as shown by Blumberg *et al.* (1968), the carrier state is common, Au antigen-positive chronic liver disease may be frequent. There is a ready opportunity for spread of the antigen by tribal customs of scarification and by insect vectors, and accidental inoculation in such communities can readily occur even if the faecal-oral route of transmission of the long incubation period hepatitis is not invoked.

The factors which determine whether the infective agent is eliminated from serum, persists in the carrier state or produces chronic active liver disease may be extremely complex, but the immunological response of the host is likely to be of paramount importance and it is likely that the age at which this infant was infected is highly relevant to this point. Similarly in tropical and subtropical areas, the modification of immunological responses by malnutrition and parasitic infection may be important in determining whether chronic liver disease develops.

What then is the role, if any, of the Au antigen in relation to the active chronic hepatitis which we see commonly in this country? In an attempt to answer this question, we have examined sera from patients with acute and chronic hepatitis for antibodies to rat smooth muscle, by indirect immuno-fluorescence, using a specific antihuman IgG conjugated with fluorescein-isothiocyanate. Positive reactions were regarded as "weak" or 1+ if present only at a serum dilution of 1 : 10, and "strong" or 2+ if present at a serum dilution of 1 : 20 or greater.

Table III shows the relationship of the smooth muscle antibody to the Au antigen in patients with acute viral hepatitis. As can be seen the smooth muscle antibody was present in 24 per cent of patients usually at low titre in both antigen-positive and antigen-negative sera (Wright, 1970a). Walker and Doniach (1970) and Farrow and associates (1970) have confirmed these findings and indeed a much higher incidence has been reported by the latter group. The significance of this finding is unclear. In the limited number of patients with serial specimens which we studied, we could not find any difference between early and late sera in terms of the incidence of the smooth muscle antibody, although recently Farrow *et al.,* (1970) have found that the antibody tends to disappear with recovery, suggesting that it is a consequence of hepatocellular damage.

Of much greater interest is the negative correlation which is observed between the smooth muscle antibody and the Au antigen in patients with active chronic hepatitis. Table IV shows the figures from Yale and Oxford combined. Of 12

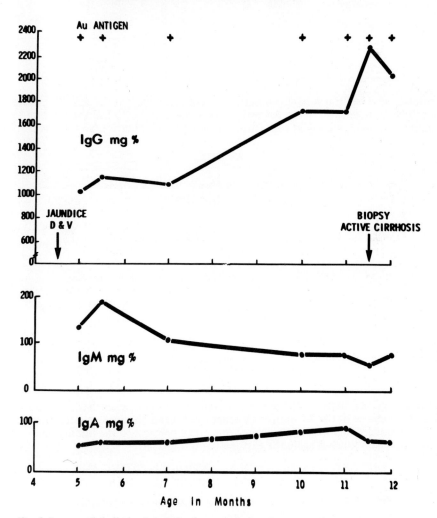

CHANGES IN IMMUNOGLOBULIN LEVELS
DURING THE DEVELOPMENT OF CIRRHOSIS FOLLOWING ACUTE VIRAL HEPATITIS
ASSOCIATED WITH A POSITIVE Au ANTIGEN

Fig. 5. Immunoglobulin levels in infant's serum during the progression to cirrhosis.

Table III

Relation of Smooth Muscle Antibody to Australia Antigen in Acute Viral Hepatitis
(< 4 months duration)

	Au Antigen Negative Smooth Muscle Antibody				Au Antigen Positive Smooth Muscle Antibody			
	Neg	+	++	Total	Neg	+	++	Total
Serum Hepatitis	17	1	2	20	12	4	2	18
Infectious Hepatitis	7	0	0	7	3	0	0	3
"Unknown Source"	2	1	4	7	18	4	1	23
Total	26	2	6	34	33	8	3	44
		24%				25%		

patients who had the Au antigen in their serum, only one had the smooth muscle antibody at high titre. In the Au antigen negative patients, 30 had the smooth muscle antibody, usually at high titre, whereas 17 were negative. So there is a

Table IV

Au Antigen and Smooth Muscle Antibody in Active Chronic Hepatitis

	No. of Patients	Smooth Muscle Antibody		Mean Serum Globulin g./100 ml.
		Positive	Negative	
Au Antigen Positive	12	1	11	3·8
Au Antigen Negative	47	30	17	4·8
	59	31	28	

clear dissociation between the presence of the smooth muscle antibody in serum and the presence of the Au antigen. Vischer (1970) and Sherlock et al. (1970) have obtained similar results, which are in marked contrast to the findings in acute viral hepatitis but again the explanation is not clear.

DIFFERENCES BETWEEN Au ANTIGEN POSITIVE AND NEGATIVE ACTIVE CHRONIC HEPATITIS

The main differences between these two groups which have been found to date are:—

1. Au antigen positive active chronic hepatitis occurs in males more commonly

than in females, whereas there is a striking female preponderance in the Au antigen-negative hepatitis;
2. Patients who have the antigen are often older than the antigen-negative group;
3. The serum globulin levels are higher in the antigen-positive than in the antigen-negative group;
4. Auto-antibodies such as smooth muscle antibody and antinuclear factor are rarely present in Au antigen-positive chronic active hepatitis, but are frequently positive in antigen-negative chronic active hepatitis;
5. The geographical distrubution of antigen-positive active chronic hepatitis appears to be very variable, whereas it is unlikely that there is much variation in the geographical distribution of antigen-negative active chronic hepatitis;
6. Another difference, which Sherlock and associates (1970) have emphasized, is the fact that the systemic manifestations, such as those described earlier by Professor Read, are much more likely to occur in the antigen-negative group than the antigen-positive group.

There therefore appears to be good evidence to indicate that the infective agent associated with the Au antigen is responsible for a syndrome which histologically does not differ from classical active chronic hepatitis although there are certain clinical and immunological differences.

AETIOLOGY OF Au ANTIGEN NEGATIVE ACTIVE CHRONIC HEPATITIS

What then is the aetiology of this group in which auto-antibodies are most commonly found? There are a number of possibilities:—
1. That free-circulating Au antigen is absent or not detectable;
2. Circulating antigen may be present in complex with antibody because of the nature of the immunological response of these patients, and therefore not detectable by immunodiffusion;
3. The antigen may be bound to hepatic cells;
4. The antigen may initiate the disease, which is then perpetuated by an auto-immune response;
5. It is possible that antigen-negative active chronic hepatitis is aetiologically distinct, either associated with a different infective agent, or truly auto-immune.

We have examined some of the possibilities. Electron microscopy of liver biopsy tissue for the Au antigen, such as had been reported by Nowoslawski and associates (1970) from Poland, were negative in the few cases that we examined, notably the mother and infant mentioned above. We have also attempted to detect the antigen using direct immunofluorescence with conjugates raised in guinea pigs or with human Au antibody, but we could not convince ourselves that we could see specific fluorescence in liver biopsy tissue, such as had been described by Coyne *et al.* (1970). Clearly both of these approaches require further investigation.

We have been interested in the possibility that the antigen may only be present transiently in the serum, or that it is bound with antibody and therefore might only be detected by a technique such as electron microscopy with negative staining. For example, one patient seen at Yale had the antigen in the serum early in the course of acute viral hepatitis, and subsequently, at the time of the development of cirrhosis, the Au antigen was absent from the serum and the smooth muscle antibody positive. We have therefore examined sera from patients with active chronic hepatitis, who were antigen-negative by immunodiffusion, for such complexes using electron microscopy, but the results have been negative (Wright, 1970b).

Uncomplexed particles of the Au antigen can be readily recognized by the presence of the characteristic tubular forms or the large particles described by Dane and associates (1970), but there are a variety of particles present in serum and one could quite readily fail to recognize small spherical Au antigen particles. We have attempted to detect such particles by immunising guinea pigs with sera from patients with active chronic hepatitis who are Au negative in the hope of producing an, antiserum to the Au antigen which could not be detected by other means. In one patient, a child of twelve, who developed active chronic hepatitis with a positive L.E. cell phenomenon as part of a small family outbreak of acute viral hepatitis in 1966, particles suggestive of small spherical Au antigen were present in the serum examined by electron microscopy. We used the acute serum to immunise guinea pigs and then absorbed the serum with a normal serum pool, a technique which Melartin and associates (1968) used initially when raising antisera in rabbits to the Au antigen. We then added this antiserum to the patient's serum and there was marked clumping of particles as observed by electron microscopy. When tested by immunodiffusion the sera, which had been absorbed with a normal serum pool, showed lines of identity with a reference Au antigen-positive serum. This raises the possibility that in some cases the antigen might be detectable in the serum by other means, in patients who would otherwise appear to have the classical form of active chronic hepatitis. However, the most cogent argument against this being a common phenomenon is the epidemiological one to which I referred earlier.

CONCLUSIONS

It therefore seems likely that in the majority of cases of classic active chronic hepatitis seen in this country and of primary biliary cirrhosis and other forms of auto-immune liver disease, the Au antigen does not appear to play a direct role in pathogenesis. Of interest in this respect, is the report by Zuckerman and associates (1970) of particles in serum with surface projections resembling corona or paramyxoviruses which they detected in a patient with Au antigen negative active chronic hepatitis. We too have observed similar particles, with surface projections (Fig. 6) in sera from patients with acute or chronic hepatitis, but carefully controlled objective studies are necessary before this agent can be identified as being responsible for antigen-negative active chronic hepatitis.

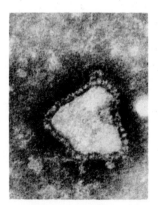

Fig. 6. Particle with surface projections resembling a corona or paramyxovirus in the serum of a patient with Au negative acute hepatitis (x200,000.)

REFERENCES

Blumberg, B. S., Gerstley, B. J. S., Hungerford, D. A., London, W. T., Sutnick, A. I. (1967) Ann. intern. Med. 66, 924.

Blumberg, B. S., Sutnick, A. I., London, W. T. (1968) Bull. N.Y. Acad. Med. 44, 1566.

Coyne, V. E., Millman, I., Cerda, J., Gerstley, B. J. S., London, W. T., Sutnick, A., Blumberg, B. S. (1970) J. exp. Med. 131, 307.

Dane, D. S., Cameron, C. H., Briggs, M. (1970) Lancet i, 695.

Farrow, L. J., Holborow, E. J., Johnson, G. D., Lamb, S. G., Stewart, J. S., Taylor, P. E., Zuckerman, A. J. (1970) Brit. med. J. 1, 693.

Fox, R. A., Niazi, S. P., Sherlock, S. (1969) Lancet ii, 609..

Gitnick, G. L., Gleich, G. J., Schoenfield, L. J., Baggenstoss, A. H., Sutnick, A. I., Blumberg, B. S., London, W. T., Summerskill, W. H. J. (1969) Lancet ii, 285.

Klatskin, G. (1958) Am. J. Med. 25, 333.

Krassnitzky, O., Pesendorfer, F., Wewalka, F. (1970) Deut. Med. Wschr. 95, 249.

Mathews, J. D., Mackay, I. R. (1970) Brit. med. J., i, 259.

Melartin, L., Blumberg, B. S. (1966) Nature (Lond.) 210, 1340.

Mosley, J. W., Barker, L. F., Shulman, N. R., Hatch, M. H. (1970) ibid, 225, 953.

Nowoslawski, A., Brøzosko, W. J., Madalinski, K., Krawczynski, K. (1970) Lancet i, 494.

Prince, A. M. (1968) Proc. nat. Acad. Sci., 60, 814.

Sherlock, S., Fox, R. A., Niazi, S. P., Scheuer, P. J. (1970) Lancet i, 1243.

Vischer, T. L. (1970) Brit. med. J., 1, 695.

Walker, J. G., Doniach, D. (1970) Immunology of Liver Disease Symposium, King's College Hospital.

Wright, R. (1970a) Lancet i, 521.

Wright, R. (1970b) Proc. Symposium on Virus Hepatitis Antigens and Antibodies. Intern. Soc. Bld. Transf., Karger, Bosch in press.

Wright, R., McCollum, R. W., Klatskin, G. (1969) Lancet ii, 117.

Wright, R., Perkins, J. R., Bower, B. D., Jerrome, D. W. (1970) Brit. med. J. in press.

Zuckerman, A. J., Taylor, P. E., Almeida, J. D. (1970) Brit. med. J., i, 262.

DISCUSSION

Chairman: Dr. Roger Williams

CHAIRMAN

Could you tell us where Micronesia is. Some of us are not so widely travelled as you!

WRIGHT

Micronesia is in the Pacific, northwest of New Zealand, near New Guinea.

SCHEUER

May I comment very briefly on the liver biopsy appearances of active chronic hepatitis in relation to Au antigen? It was initially thought that the biopsies in Au positive cases were going to show a rather mild chronic aggressive hepatitis, and that those in Au negative cases, were going to have the classical fullblown picture with rosettes. This turned out to be untrue as both appearances could be found in either group. Furthermore, it was not possible to predict the Au antigen status of the patients from the liver histology.

CHAIRMAN

The methods for detecting the antigen are all of different sensitivity — complement fixation and electron microscopy giving more positive results than immunodiffusion. How does radioimmunoassay compare with these other methods? These figures are meaningless unless you really know that you are detecting the antigen.

SAUNDERS

I have been told that radioimmunoassay is more sensitive.

POPPER

In our area relatively few cases of active chronic hepatitis are Au positive, and if they are positive they remain so. The situation is not like acute hepatitis where the antigen can disappear very rapidly. Complement fixation is more sensitive than gel diffusion but I have no information on radioimmunoassay.

VELASCO

In Chile we have looked for the antigen in 15 cases of active chronic hepatitis. In 39 samples taken during periods of activity or remission we have not found a single positive case. The prevalence of the antigen in Chile is 0·5%, much the same as in the United States or Europe, despite the fact that some parts of our country are tropical.

SCHAFFNER

Most of our cases of Au antigen positive chronic hepatitis come from abroad. We have three major sources from Latin America, — Peru, Mexico and Puerto Rico. Almost all of the cases from Mexico have been Au positive whereas the cases from the other two countries have been negative.

WRIGHT

Certainly, a few of the patients in the Yale series were from abroad and we did not appreciate the significance of this at the time. But some of them had never left the United States, notably patients who had had blood transfusions or were heroin addicts.

AUSTRALIA ANTIGEN IN THE CHILEAN POPULATION

Marta Velasco and Ricardo Katz

In the last few years a considerable amount of information about Australia antigen and its relationship to acute viral hepatitis has been obtained (Giles *et al.,* 1969; McCollum, 1969). Our purpose today is to present our findings in Chile and to compare these with the results from other countries.

Chile is the southernmost country of South America, by the Pacific Coast. Its population of 10,000,000 is homogeneous and entirely white, mainly resulting from the mixing of Spaniards with Indians. These half-breeds have been absorbed by a steady and peaceful immigration from several European countries. Germans and British first, then French, Yugoslavian and Italians and later Arabs, Jews and more Spaniards. The climate is cold in the South, getting warmer to the North, but in general it is mild. The Northern part of the country is a desert and the climate is also mild although it is located in the tropical area.

We have collected blood samples from the normal population in two places; (a) the north of the country in a small seaport called Mejillones, with a total population of 3,000 and (b) in Santiago, the capital with 3,000,000 inhabitants.

The Australia antigen was studied with the immuno-diffusion technique of Ouchterlony modified by Prince (1969). The human antisera used were kindly given by Dr. Alfred Prince of the New York Blood Centre and Dr. Robert W. McCollum of the Department of Epidemiology, Yale University.

INCIDENCE OF AUSTRALIA ANTIGEN IN DIFFERENT POPULATION GROUPS

The prevalence of the Australia antigen in the different groups is shown in Fig. 1. The variations from one group to another are small. In school children in Mejillones, the prevalence was 1·3% against 0% in adults. In Santiago the percentage positive was: 0·59% in the military cadets, 0·19% in the voluntary blood donors and 0% in a sample of the hospital staff, all of them blood handlers. All positive cases were still positive after six months.

In total, 7 positive sera were found in 1,272 cases studied, a prevalence of 0·5 per cent. All the positive cases were under thirty years of age. Of the 7 positive cases 3 were siblings. This finding led us to investigate the frequency of the Australia antigen through positives.

FAMILY STUDIES

Figure 2 shows the findings in four families examined in detail. In the first family are the three positive siblings already referred to. The mother was also positive; the father, a maternal aunt and two maternal cousins were negative. In the second family the brother of the propositus, the mother and a maternal aunt were positive, the remainder of the family being negative. Of considerable interest in this family, was the finding that two brothers of the propositus had died at the age of 14 and 16 years of confirmed primary carcinoma of the liver for this disease is very uncommon in Chile. In families number 3 and 4 we did not find any positive cases apart from the propositus.

The immunoglobulin levels were studied in the family members including the propositus. In eight cases with a positive antigen the level of IgG was high and the IgM low. In 16 cases with negative antigen the IgG level was almost normal but

39

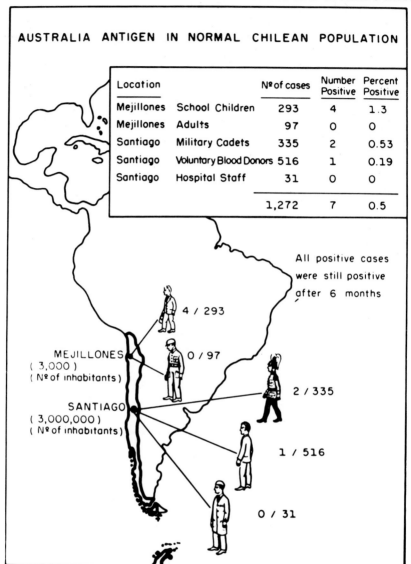

AUSTRALIA ANTIGEN IN NORMAL CHILEAN POPULATION

Location		Nº of cases	Number Positive	Percent Positive
Mejillones	School Children	293	4	1.3
Mejillones	Adults	97	0	0
Santiago	Military Cadets	335	2	0.53
Santiago	Voluntary Blood Donors	516	1	0.19
Santiago	Hospital Staff	31	0	0
		1,272	7	0.5

All positive cases were still positive after 6 months

4 / 293

MEJILLONES
(3,000)
(Nº of inhabitants)

0 / 97

SANTIAGO
(3,000,000)
(Nº of inhabitants)

2 / 335

1 / 516

0 / 31

Fig. 1.

the IgM was reduced to the same level as in the positive cases. The magnitude of the coefficient of variation does not allow us to draw any conclusions (Fig. 3).

INCIDENCE OF AUSTRALIA ANTIGEN IN ACUTE AND CHRONIC LIVER DISEASES

Before going into the results I want to describe the present situation concerning post-transfusion hepatitis in Chile. Since 1965 a prospective study has been performed in patients receiving blood transfusions at the Hospital del Salvador in Santiago. 1,905 patients have received 4,025 units of blood; 2,030 patients hospitalized in the same wards but not transfused served as controls.

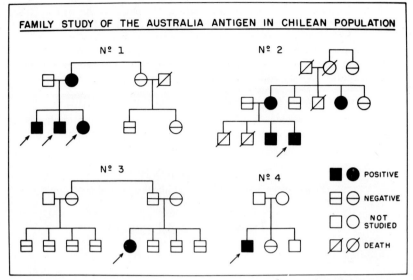

Fig. 2.

31 cases of acute hepatitis were observed in the transfused group an incidence of 1·5% as opposed to 0·2% in the control group. The difference is highly significant (Fig. 4).

The results of the Australia antigen determination in acute liver disease are illustrated in Fig. 5. In 39 cases of hepatitis of unknown type, with 53 determinations, only 4 cases were positive. In 9 cases of post-transfusion hepatitis with 68 determinations, who were part of the above mentioned prospective study, 4 were positive and all of them had a long incubation period. The Australia antigen was not found in 7 cases of drug hepatitis, 5 of which were related to contraceptive pills. Idiopathic jaundice of pregnancy is a very common disease in Chile. In 8 cases we have not found the antigen. 24 other cases of acute jaundice such as infectious mononucleosis, etc., were also negative.

AUSTRALIA ANTIGEN AND IMMUNOGLOBULINS LEVELS IN THE FAMILY STUDY

	No. of Cases	IgG mg. per 100 ml.	Coefficient of Variation	IgM mg. per 100 ml.	Coefficient of Variation
1 - Antigen Positive	8	1,900 ± 290	15·2%	99·2 ± 37	36·2%
2 - Antigen Negative	16	1,197 ± 347	28·9%	101 ± 34	33·6%
3 - Normal Levels		1,340 ± 160		150 ± 50	

Fig. 3.

In Fig. 6 a case of post-transfusion hepatitis is shown in order to emphasize the transient presence of the antigen. The results of the investigations in the patients with chronic liver disease are shown in Fig. 7. To-date we have not found any patient with a positive antigen. The patients with active chronic hepatitis have been studied prospectively, 39 samples having been collected during periods of activity and remission of the disease.

ANTIBODY TO AUSTRALIA ANTIGEN IN CHILE

The serum of 101 subjects has been investigated and the antibody has been found in only one case — a member of the Hospital Staff. No antibody was

POST-TRANSFUSION HEPATITIS
(Prospective Study: Clinical, Laboratory and Histological)
1965–1970

	Transfused	Not Transfused	
Number Patients Hospitalized	1,905	2,030	
Units of Blood Received	4,025	0	
Acute Hepatitis	31	5	
Percentage of Hepatitis ●	1·5%	0·2%	● $x^2 = 20\cdot487$ p $= 0\cdot00001$
per 1,000 units of blood	7·7		

Fig. 4.

AUSTRALIA ANTIGEN IN ACUTE LIVER DISEASE

Diagnosis	No. of Patients	No. of Tests	Antigen Positive
Infectious Hepatitis (Unknown type)	39	53	4
Post-Transfusion Hepatitis (Long incubation period) (Short incubation period)	9 8 1	68	4 4 0
Drug Hepatitis	7	16	0
Idiopathic Jaundice of Pregnancy	8	8	0
Others	24	24	0

Fig. 5.

AUSTRALIA ANTIGEN IN CHRONIC LIVER DISEASE

Diagnosis	No. of Patients	No. of Tests	Antigen Positive
Alcoholic Cirrhosis	15	16	0
Postnecrotic Cirrhosis	4	8	0
Active Chronic Hepatitis	15	39	0
Unresolved Hepatitis	7	15	0
	41	78	0

Fig. 6.

AUSTRALIA ANTIGEN IN A CASE OF POST TRANSFUSION HEPATITIS

Days After Transfusion	Total Serum Bilirubin mg. per 100 ml.	Serum S. G. P. T.	Australia Antigen
1	0·36	26	Negative
30	0·24	30	Negative
48	0·24	28	Negative
71	0·22	25	Negative
81	0·44	86	POSITIVE
93	2·60	806	POSITIVE
96	7·02	1,013	Negative
102	8·96	447	Negative
123	2·46	146	Negative
138	2·76	25	Negative
143	0·76	30	Negative

Fig. 7.

ANTIBODY TO AUSTRALIA ANTIGEN IN CHILE

	No. of Subjects	Antibody Positive
Hospital Staff	34	1
Patients in Haemodyalisis Unit	7	0
Multiply Transfused Patients	32	0
Acute Hepatitis	18	0
Active Chronic Hepatitis	10	0
	101	1

Fig. 8.

detected in the other groups comprising 7 patients on chronic haemodialysis; 32 multiply transfused patients (leukemias, hemophilia and aplastic anaemia); 18 patients with acute hepatitis and 10 patients with active chronic hepatitis (Fig. 8).

CONCLUSIONS

The prevalence of Australia antigen in the normal Chilean population is comparable with that obtained by other authors in normal North American and European populations. Shulman *et al.* (1970) in a recent publication gave a prevalence of 0·25%. The prevalence in our population was about the same in Mejillones and in Santiago, although the first place is located in the tropics, and Blumberg *et al.* (1968) have shown that up to 20% of people in tropical areas in other parts of the world may carry detectable antigen in their sera.

Our family study is still in progress and definitive conclusions have not been drawn. However, the results obtained in one of our families agree with Blumberg's hypothesis (1969) of a genetically determined susceptibility to this carrier state.

In Chile the Australia antigen is detected less often in acute hepatitis classified as unknown type than in other countries. Wright *et al.* (1969) reported a frequency of 47% of positive sera in this group. In active chronic hepatitis in spite of the numerous determinations performed, our results have been consistently negative in contrast to the results in other series (Gitnick, 1969). We cannot attribute these differences to the methods employed because the reagents have been the same as those used in some parts of the United States. It appears that a geographical difference exists as Mathews and MacKay (1970) and Fox *et al.* (1969) have suggested.

This geographical difference would also explain the low incidence of antibody against the Australia antigen found in our patients. In England, Australia and Chile the incidence is 1% and this is to be compared with the very much higher incidence of the antibody in the U.S.A., the figures in various series ranging from 17 to 28%.

REFERENCES

Blumberg, B. S., Sutnick, I. and London, W. T. (1968) Bull. New York Acad. Med. 44, 1566.
Blumberg, B. S., Friedlander, J. S., Woodside, A., Sutnick, A. I. and London, W. T. (1969) Proc. Nat. Acad. Sc. 62, 1108.
Fox, R. A., Niazi, S. P. and Sherlock, S. (1969) Lancet 2, 609.
Giles, J. P., McCollum, R. W., Berndtson, L. W. Jr. and Krugman, S. (1969) New Engl. J. Med. 2, 119.
Gitnick, G. L., Gleich, G. J., Schoenfield, L. J., Baggenstoss, A. H., Sutnick, A. I. Blumberg, B. S. London, W. T. and Summerskill, W. H. J. (1969) Lancet 2, 285.
Mathews, J. D. and Mackay, I. R. (1970) Brit. Med. J. 1, 259.
McCollum, R. W. (1969) J. Infect. Dis. 120, 641.
Prince, A. M. (1969) New Engl. J. Med. 281, 163.
Shulman, N. R., Hirschman, R. J. and Barker, L. F. (1970) Ann. Int. Med. 72, 257.
Wright, R., McCollum, R. W. and Klatskin, G. (1969) Lancet 2, 117.

DISCUSSION
Chairman: Dr. M. H. Lessof

FOX

I was very interested in the cases of primary liver cell cancer in your family study. Did they die before you were able to examine their serum?

VELASCO
 Yes, but I saw the liver histology which was definitely that of primary carcinoma of the liver.

FOX
 Did any patients who were antigen-carriers give a history of acute hepatitis?

VELASCO
 No, none of them.

FOX
 What about others in the same family who were not carriers? Did any of those have hepatitis?

VELASCO
 No. They were biochemically and serologically normal.

WILLIAMS
 And has the Au antigen persisted in those carriers?

VELASCO
 As most of this study has been done during the last year we do not know.

WILLOUGHBY
 Were all the families from the same ethnic group?

VELASCO
 Yes.

MacLAURIN
 Could I ask further about that family with the two tumour cases? The question arises whether the infection was transmitted via the placenta or whether it appeared later in life. In measles which may be transmitted through the placenta there is impaired cellular immunity. If the children who died of the liver cancer had contracted their virus infections in the intrauterine period, this would further support the view that impaired cellular immunity may increase the chances of tumour development later in life.

VELASCO
 I do not know.

MacLAURIN
 The incidence is so low everywhere else, that for that particular family to have two cases of liver cancer makes it seem very likely that this is virus related. The question is whether there could be an immunological basis for this? I was also interested in Dr. Fox's cases of hepatoma who were Au antigen positive.

FOX
 We tested 43 patients with primary liver-cell cancer and 6 were positive for the antigen. Delayed hypersensitivity responses in these positive patients were impaired.

EDDLESTON
 What results did you get in the ones who did not carry Au antigen?

FOX
 We did not study many.

EDDLESTON
 But does the anergy come as a result of the tumour or vice versa?

FOX

I do not know. Another case relevant to this point, that we have had, was that of a young man with massive necrosis of the liver who was found to be positive for the Au antigen. He recovered and still carries the antigen a year later. Now he has developed a cryptococcal meningitis and has, or appears to have, impaired hypersensitivity responses!

VELASCO

I wonder if you have measured the immunoglobulin levels in the Au antigen positive patients. There is a suggestion that the IgM levels in our patients were diminished.

FOX

IgG levels may be slightly increased in the Au positive hepatitis patients. We did not find a decrease in IgM levels in these patients although the level was somewhat raised in Au negative ones.

WRIGHT

We have seen very little Au antigen positive hepatitis or anicteric hepatitis in Oxford. The two positive patients have been West Indian, both of them had focal necrosis on biopsy and one had a primary carcinoma of the liver. I think your point about Chile being subtropical and yet not having a high incidence is important. Positivity is not related to the tropics *per se*, although there may well be some environmental factor. In many of the areas where the incidence is high, scarification is carried out either as a therapeutic or tribal custom. One knows that serum hepatitis can be transmitted in the most bizarre fashion: for example as in the Swedish long distance track runners. Was there anything unusual about this family?

VELASCO

Not at all.

FOX

Dr. Wright has brought up the question of transmission of antigen positive hepatitis. There is good evidence in the literature that we do not need scarification or blood to transmit serum hepatitis; urine is probably infective and faeces certainly are in some transmission studies. Also, there is still some doubt as to whether antigen positive hepatitis correlates with serum hepatitis.

ELECTRON MICROSCOPIC OBSERVATIONS ON SH ANTIGEN USING POSITIVE STAINING

P. T. Jokelainen, Kai Krohn, A. M. Prince, and N. D. C. Finlayson

Serum hepatitis (SH) antigen, identical with the Australia (Au) antigen has been observed in the serum in acute and chronic liver diseases (Prince, 1968; Wright *et al.,* 1969). Electron microscopy has shown that this antigen is located on a 200 Å spherical structure (Bayer *et al.,* 1968). Recently, a 420–430 Å particle was described containing the SH antigen and the substructure of this larger particle, with outer and inner membranes and a central core, suggested that this particle might be a virus (Dane *et al.,* 1970). Our electron microscopic observations, based on differences in staining properties, indicate that only the larger of these particles may contain nucleic acid, which supports this view.

Serum samples from a case of acute serum hepatitis, a case of chronic SH-antigenemia and a case of SH positive active chronic hepatitis were used. Preliminary EM study, using negative staining with phosphotungstic acid (Almeida and Waterson, 1969), showed that these sera contained large 430 Å particles, as well as smaller 200 Å particles and rods with 200 Å diameter. Pretreatment of the sera with SH-antiserum caused all these particles to clump (Fig. 1), indicating antigenic similarity.

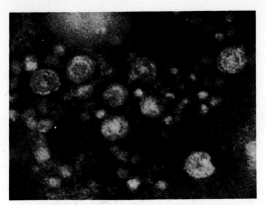

Fig. 1. Aggregated SH antigen particles (large spheres, small spheres and rods) after SH antiserum treatment (×180,000).

POSITIVE STAINING TECHNIQUE

An attempt was then made to stain the particles positively. They were separated from the serum by centrifugation (Almeida and Waterson, 1969), fixed for 1 hour with 2·5% glutaraldehyde, recentrifuged and suspended in phosphate buffered saline (PBS). A drop of suspension was placed on a 400 mesh carbon-formvar coated grid for one minute and excess PBS removed with filterpaper without further drying. Each grid was then stained either with 5% uranyl acetate, (pH 5·0), potassium-permanganate (Luft's fixative – Luft,1956),

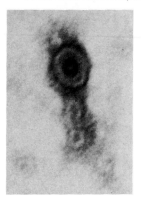

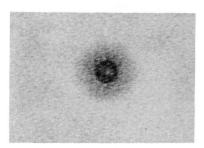

Fig. 2. Large and small spherical particles and a rod stained with uranyl acetate (no washing). All show central staining (x250,000).

Fig. 3. Retained uranyl acetate staining of central core of large spheres after prolonged washing (x300,000).

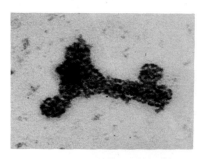

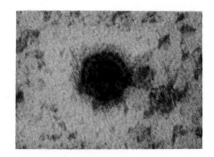

Fig. 4. Potassium permanganate staining of small spheres and rods (x300,000).

Fig. 5. Potassium permanganate staining of outer and inner membranes of large spherical particle (x300,000).

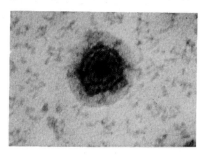

Fig. 6. Staining of large spherical particle with potassium permanganate (outer and inner membranes) and uranyl acetate (core). (x300,000).

or both. After treatment with stain, the grids were either examined without further washing, after gentle, or after vigorous washing. It was noticed that the degree of washing greatly affected the staining of different particles.

DEMONSTRATION OF THREE COMPONENTS IN LARGER PARTICLES

Uranyl acetate treatment for 10 minutes without further washing stained all the three types of particle negatively (Fig. 2). Some of the 200 Å particles and rods revealed central staining in unwashed preparations (Fig. 2). However, this was removed readily by gentle washing. In the large (430 Å) particles, three components were seen; a 70 Å thick outer membrane, a 20 Å thick inner membrane, and a central core (Fig. 2). The central core, measuring 180 Å, was most intensely stained. After vigorous washing only the central core remained stained, and this was most intense peripherally (Fig. 3). Potassium permanganate staining for 10 minutes resulted in positive staining of all the three types of particle (Figs. 4 and 5). Washing, even vigorously, did not affect this staining. The outer membrane of the large particles as well as the membrane of the 200 Å particles and rods seem to be composed of 30–40 Å globular subunits which were 30–40 Å apart (Figs. 4 and 5). The inner membrane of the 430 Å particle was often stained, but no staining of the central core was observed. Post staining the potassium permanganate stained grids with uranyl acetate as described above, followed by vigorous washing, resulted in staining of the central core of the 430 Å particle with uranyl acetate, while the potassium permanganate staining of the outer and inner membranes (Fig. 6), as well as the 200 Å particle membranes remained unaffected.

CONCLUSIONS

The results of these experiments indicate that the outer membrane of the 430 Å particles is similar to the membrane of the 200 Å particle, both in staining characteristics and morphology. Furthermore, as only the central core of the large particle stains positively with uranyl acetate, only this form of SH containing particle can contain nucleic acid and possibly be a virus.

ACKNOWLEDGEMENT

This work will be published in full in the Journal of Virology and we are indebted to that journal for permission to reproduce the figures.

REFERENCES

Almeida, J. D. and Waterson, A. P. (1969) Lancet 2, 983.
Bayer, M. E., Blumberg, B. S. and Werner, B. (1968) Nature (London) 218, 1057.
Dane, D. S., Cameron, C. H. and Briggs, M. (1970) Lancet 1, 695.
Luft, J. H. (1956) J. Biophys. Biochem. 9, 799.
Prince, A. M. (1968) Proc. Nat. Acad. Sci. U.S.A. 60, 814.
Wright, R., McCollum, R. W., and Klatskin, G. (1969) Lancet 2, 117.

ROUND TABLE DISCUSSION ON CLINICAL, MORPHOLOGICAL AND VIROLOGICAL ASPECTS
Chairman Dr. Roger Williams

DONIACH

Do the "anabolic" cells in the liver resemble the Ashkenazi cells found in auto-immune thyroid disease?

POPPER

They are not quite the same but similar. I do not know the electron microscopic appearances of Ashkenazi cells. The "anabolic" cells have increased amounts of rough endoplasmic reticulum and also of lysosomes. Do the Ashkenazi cells have increased lysosomes?

DONIACH

No, they have increased mitochondria and large nuclei.

POPPER

Another difference is that these "anabolic" cells with increased rough endoplasmic reticulum are blue – whereas the Ashkenazi cell is red.

ROITT

In experimental thyroiditis, you see exactly the same thing, hyperplastic cells close to regions of inflammatory response. This hyperplasia is not related to TSH and certainly seems to be a local response. All sorts of materials appear to be released from activated lymphoid cells which can do everything from stimulating mitosis to inhibiting it.

POPPER

Whether the anabolic reaction in the liver is related to an attack by the lymphocytes, I would not care to say.

CHAIRMAN

Have you, Professor Popper, seen the Au antigen in the liver tissue from any of these patients?

POPPER

Not yet.

FOX

It would seem that active chronic hepatitis is a disease of multifactorial aetiology. Dr Wright's finding with respect to the smooth muscle antibody is important, because it is now possible to separate a subgroup of these cases that are positive for the antigen and negative for the smooth muscle antibody. Dr. Wright's figures also suggest that antigen positive acute hepatitis is more likely to go on to subacute hepatic necrosis and to chronic disease – not necessarily active chronic.

WRIGHT

One interesting finding that requires confirmation concerns the size and shape of particles in acute hepatitis in relation to prognosis. In the Yale sera, small antigen particles were found in the cases that resolved very rapidly. However, in two or three other cases including the Oxford baby, where long tubular forms and large particles were seen early on, the disease has pursued a chronic course.

CHAIRMAN

Does this fit in with the finding of antigen in patients with a hepatoma? This must indicate long persistence.

FOX

I cannot answer that as we have not followed these patients for a long time — we now have six antigen positive patients with a hepatoma.

TROWELL

It seems that in this country there are only a few patients with chronic hepatitis who have Au antigen in the serum at any stage of their illness. Surely any discussion of the possible role of infective agents causing or triggering chronic disease is not realistic, until we have some marker similar to Au antigen which we can apply to infective as opposed to serum hepatitis.

WRIGHT

One hopes that the particles with surface projections might prove such a marker, but they appear to occur in both Au positive and Au negative cases. A fascinating thought is that they might not be viruses at all but bits of mitochondria floating around, because some of them certainly show resemblances to mitochondrial membranes.

GLYNN

Could I revert to the question of the nature of the proliferating bile ducts? Has Professor Popper ever applied Paronetto's fluorescent antibody to see whether these are bile ducts or not?

POPPER

They do react with them.

SCHAFFNER

A few years ago we presented to the American Society of Pathologists and Bacteriologists the electron microscopy of the bile ducts in primary biliary cirrhosis. The component cells are definitely not hepatocytes but are bile duct epithelial cells. They go through a rather interesting evolution. Early in the disease they contain numerous vacuoles with liquid crystals, probably consisting of mixed micelles of bile salts and lipid. This we considered good evidence for a reabsorptive function of the ductules at that time. As the disease progresses and there is more periductular fibrosis, these vacuoles disappear and the cytoplasm becomes more atrophic and even disconnected from the neighbouring structures.

A VOICE

Could Professor Read tell us why he thinks multiple organ involvement is a prerequisite of auto-immunity? After all, in auto-immune haemolytic anaemia no other organs are involved.

READ

I agree, it is not necessarily a prerequisite. However, without exception, the various diseases affecting other organs in association with active chronic hepatitis have all been considered to have an auto-immune basis when they occur on their own.

PART II
The Occurrence and Role of Antibodies

OCCURRENCE AND DISTRIBUTION OF TISSUE ANTIBODIES IN LIVER DISEASES

J. Geoffrey Walker and Deborah Doniach

We have heard today the conditions which must be fulfilled for a disease to be regarded as 'auto-immune' (see also Doniach, 1970). In the field of hepatic disease it must be stated that serum antibodies reacting specifically and consistently with the liver are yet to be described. The tissue antibodies discussed in the present communication are all of a non-organ-specific nature and cannot be held directly responsible for the hepatic lesions. It is possible, however, that they represent markers of an auto-immune process as is more fully discussed later.

ACUTE VIRAL HEPATITIS

The incidence and significance of tissue antibodies in acute viral hepatitis may be summarized first. We studied 45 unselected patients in whom this diagnosis was substantiated (Walker *et al.*, 1970a). Ten patients were positive for Australia (Au) antigen by gel diffusion and electron microscopy, while 30 were negative by these tests. The 5 remaining patients had infectious mononucleosis with liver involvement.

Figure 1 shows the overall incidence of tissue antibodies in these patients. Mitochondrial immunofluorescence remained negative in all cases despite repeated testing throughout the illness. The incidence and titres of thyroid, gastric and antinuclear antibodies was extremely low as might be expected in view of the young age group of these patients. Non-organ-specific complement

| | AUSTRALIA – ANTIGEN | | INFECTIOUS MONONUCLEOSIS |
| | POSITIVE | NEGATIVE | |
NUMBER OF CASES	10	30	5
SMOOTH MUSCLE	4	21	3
CFT (TISSUE HOMOGENATE)	4	13	2
MITOCHONDRIAL	0	0	0
ANTINUCLEAR	1	1	0
THYROID & GASTRIC	1	1	0

Fig. 1. Incidence of tissue antibodies in three varieties of acute viral hepatitis.

55

fixation tests performed with rat kidney homogenates were positive in
approximately 40% of all three types of acute viral liver damage, but the titres
generally remained low.

Smooth muscle fluorescence was remarkably common in these patients,
positive results occurring in about 60% of cases as has been recently described by
Farrow *et al.,* (1970) and Wright (1970). However, in 33% of all cases the titre
of smooth muscle fluorescence did not exceed 1 : 10, in 25% of the patients
they reached 1 : 20 while titres of 1 : 40 were unusual (Fig. 2). The sera were

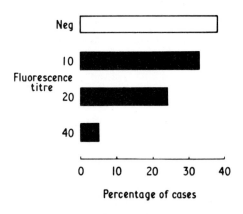

Fig. 2. Smooth muscle immunofluorescence titres in 45 patients with viral hepatitis.

titrated on rat stomach sections and results of less than 1:10 were considered as
negative.

The important features regarding the appearance of tissue auto-antibodies in
acute hepatitis may be briefly summarized. Their distribution is roughly equal in
all the three groups of viral infections, and they usually occur only in low titre.
Furthermore, the antibodies disappear from the serum on clinical recovery from
hepatitis in the great majority of patients. Thus the tissue antibodies in these
conditions may be comparable to the temporary auto-immunization seen in
animals following experimental liver damage induced with carbon tetrachloride
and other chemicals (Pinckard and Weir, 1966).

USE IN DIFFERENTIAL DIAGNOSIS

Figure 3 shows the application of the mitochondrial fluorescence test to the
differential diagnosis of cholestatic jaundice and depicts the combined results
obtained in five different laboratories. Although the test discriminates extremely
well between primary biliary cirrhosis and extrahepatic biliary obstruction, it is
sometimes positive in patients with drug jaundice, particularly in halothane
hypersensitivity. Rodriguez *et al.,* (1969) found weakly positive results in over
70% of patients with halothane jaundice and it was later shown (Paronetto and
Popper, 1970) that the appearance of these antibodies correlated to some extent
with the development of delayed hypersensitivity responses to halothane.
However, it appears possible that there may be some differences between the
'mitochondrial' antibodies detected in these patients with acute liver injury and
those associated with classical primary biliary cirrhosis. In addition to the low
titres and transient nature of these reactions in acute hepatic necrosis, it has

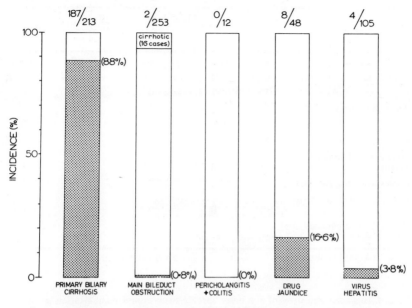

Fig. 3. Application of mitochondrial immunofluorescence test for the differential diagnosis of obstructive jaundice. Combined results from five laboratories.

been reported that the antibodies in halothane jaundice are labile on storage and are damaged upon freezing and thawing of the serum. These features again resemble the situation seen in animals treated with liver poisons.

PATTERN OF ANTIBODIES IN CHRONIC LIVER DISEASE

The non-organ-specific tissue complement fixation test (CFT) reflects a series of distinct auto-antibodies which cannot be easily separated from each other. Positive reactions occur in a variety of liver disorders, including viral infections, as mentioned above. However, high titres are confined almost exclusively to three chronic liver diseases: active chronic ("lupoid") hepatitis (ACH), primary biliary cirrhosis (PBC) and cases of cryptogenic cirrhosis, chiefly in middle-aged women (Fig. 4).

Application of immunofluorescent techniques has further strengthened the evidence for polarization of a number of tissue antibody reactions to the same three diseases. The incidence of antinuclear antibodies in liver disease is shown in Fig. 5. In the three major groups the results have been compared with those in age and sex matched, healthy controls. The group labelled "miscellaneous hepatocellular disease" includes patients with alcoholic cirrhosis, drug induced liver injury, viral hepatitis, Wilson's disease and haemochromatosis. Included under "cholestasis" are cases of main bile-duct obstruction, secondary biliary cirrhosis, cholestatic drug jaundice, and colitis with pericholangitis. The polarization of high titre ANA to the three chronic liver disorders already mentioned is apparent. In active chronic hepatitis there was a statistically significant correlation between serum γ-globulin levels and antinuclear antibody titres (Fig. 6). The fluorescent pattern seen in this condition was usually of the

Diagnosis	No. patients tested	Liver–kidney CFT titres*			Total positive
		1:4 to 1:8	1:16 to 1:32	1:64 to 1:4000	
Active chronic hepatitis	43	0	4	9	13 (30%)
Primary biliary cirrhosis	41	1	7	27	35 (85%)
Cryptogenic cirrhosis	32	1	0	9	10 (31%)
Alcoholic cirrhosis	14	0	0	0	0
Extrahepatic obstruction	28	0	0	0	0
Infective hepatitis	25	2	0	0	2 (8%)
Drug-induced hepatic necrosis	5	·0	2	0	2
Cholestatic drug jaundice	7	1	0	0	1
Cholestasis and ulcerative colitis	5	0	0	0	0
Mixed thyroid patients (control for CFT)	850				26 (3%)

*The CFT detects antibodies to mitochondria and other cell constituents.

Fig. 4. Incidence and titres of non-organ specific tissue complement fixation in liver diseases. (From Doniach *et al.*, 1966).

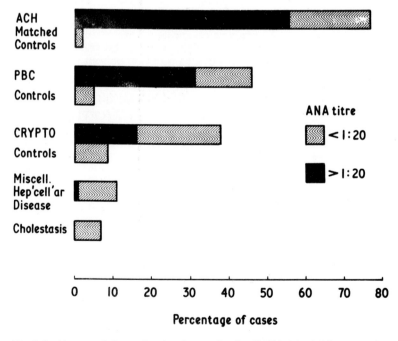

Fig. 5. Incidence and titres of antinuclear antibodies (ANA) detected by immunofluorescence in 200 patients with various liver disorders and healthy controls matched for age and sex.

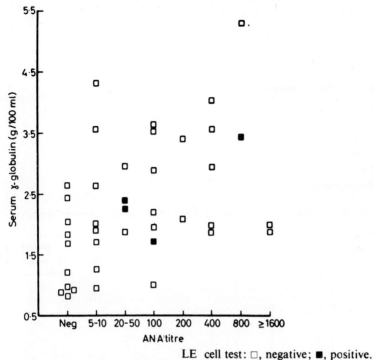

LE cell test: □, negative; ■, positive.

Fig. 6. Correlation of serum γ-globulin and antinuclear antibody titre in active chronic (lupoid) hepatitis. (From Doniach *et al.*, 1966).

"diffuse" variety and of IgG class, while in the other two diseases, "speckled" ANA was more frequently seen. Very few of these patients however, had a positive LE cell test. Correlation between activity of the liver disease and antibody titres could not be demonstrated. Smooth muscle fluorescence of high titre (1 : 200 – 1 : 800) is seen predominately in active chronic hepatitis but occasionally also in primary biliary and cryptogenic cirrhosis.

Mitochondrial Fluorescence

The incidence of mitochondrial fluorescence in different liver diseases is illustrated in Fig. 7. The very high incidence in primary biliary cirrhosis has been confirmed in many centres and the minor variations can be attributed to differences in technique. In this disease the titre of mitochondrial fluorescence bears no relation to the duration of symptoms (Fig. 8). Primary biliary cirrhosis cases with negative mitochondrial fluorescence cannot be distinguished clinically or histologically from strongly positive reactors (Hadziyannis *et al.*, 1970). Treatment with azathioprine or corticosteroid drugs does not appear to influence the "M" antibodies (Fischer and Schmid, 1967) but liver transplantation led to a significant decrease (from 1 : 2,000 to 1 : 100) in one patient who survived the operation for five weeks (Williams, 1970).

MITOCHONDRIAL ANTIBODIES WITHOUT OVERT LIVER DISEASE

Mitochondrial antibodies are occasionally seen in other diseases (Fig. 9) and in order to understand their significance with regard to liver disease, we studied a group of patients who had persistent significant titres of mitochondrial

DIAGNOSIS	NUMBER TESTED	PERCENTAGE POSITIVE
Primary Biliary Cirrhosis	139	93
Active Chronic Hepatitis	102	24
Cryptogenic Cirrhosis	84	26
Extrahepatic Biliary Obstruction	81	5
Viral Hepatitis	79	4
Alcoholic Cirrhosis	34	0
Haemochromatosis	26	0
Chlorpromazine Jaundice	17	(1/17)
Halothane Jaundice	3	(2/3)
Hyperbilirubinaemias	29	(1/29)

Fig. 7. Incidence of positive mitochondrial immunofluorescence in various liver disorders.

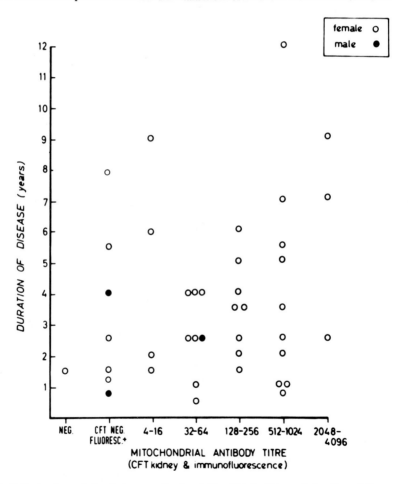

Fig. 8. Lack of correlation between mitochondrial antibody titres and duration of disease in 41 patients with primary biliary cirrhosis. (From Doniach *et al.*, 1966).

DIAGNOSIS	NUMBER TESTED	PERCENTAGE POSITIVE
Lupus Erythematosus	59	7
Other "Collagen" Disorders	153	8
Rheumatoid Arthritis	331	1·5
Pernicious Anaemia	142	0·7
Auto-immune Thyroiditis	296	0·7
Graves' Disease	183	2
Addison's Disease	29	3
Myasthenia Gravis	17	0
Colloid Goitre	91	0
Other Diseases	746	0·8

Fig. 9. Incidence of positive mitochondrial immunofluorescence in various non-hepatic disorders.

CLINICAL DIAGNOSIS	NUMBER OF CASES
Systemic Lupus Erythematosus	2
Rheumatoid Arthritis	5 (2 with LE cells)
Polyarteritis Nodosa	1
Sjogren's Syndrome	1
Fibrosing Alveolitis	1
Raynaud's Phenomenon	1
Polyarthralgia	9
Thyroid and Gastric Auto-immune Disorders	10
Relatives of PBC and SLE	2
Other Diseases	3

Fig. 10. Principal clinical diagnosis in 35 patients with mitochondrial antibodies, some of whom also proved to have subclinical liver disease. (From Walker *et al.*, 1970).

antibodies but did not have overt liver involvement. Among some 10,000 sera tested there were 77 such cases and of these 35 were available for detailed investigation and follow-up (Walker *et al.*, 1970b). The majority of these 35 patients suffered from a collagen disorder or an organ-specific auto-immune disease (Fig. 10). Only three patients appeared to have conditions unrelated to auto-immunity and of these, one has since developed myxoedema, three years after mitochondrial antibodies were first detected at her initial presentation with dysphagia. The liver edge was just palpable in four cases and three admitted to some pruritus upon questioning, but none showed clinical jaundice, skin stigmata of chronic liver disease or splenomegaly.

Biochemical tests of liver function were abnormal in nine of the 35 cases. The serum bilirubin was slightly raised in one case and the serum glutamic pyruvic transaminase to a minor extent in four (Fig. 11). BSP retention was abnormal in seven of these patients, values at 45 minutes ranging between 8 and 34%. The most striking feature was the elevation of serum alkaline phosphatase, found in

LIVER FUNCTION TEST	NUMBER OF PATIENTS ABNORMAL	RANGE OF ABNORMAL VALUES
Serum Bilirubin	1	1·1 mg/100 ml.
SGPT	4	37–71 u/ml.
Alkaline Phosphatase	8	20–90 KA u/100 ml.
Bromsulphthalein Retention	7	8–34% at 45 mins.
Liver Biopsies*	8/8	

*One patient SLE with normal biochemical tests

Fig. 11. Abnormalities of biochemical liver function tests and hepatic histology in 10 out of 35 patients with mitochondrial antibodies. (From Walker *et al.*, 1970).

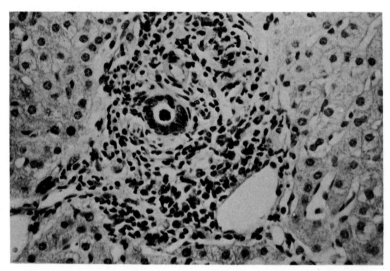

Fig. 12. Liver biopsy from patient with mitochondrial antibodies and subclinical liver disease showing portal tract with circumscribed lymphoid infiltration.

eight of the nine cases. In seven of these patients liver biopsies were obtained and were abnormal in each case. Furthermore, in one patient with normal liver function tests the liver histology was also abnormal. In none of the biopsies was there an established cirrhosis although "spotty" necrosis was seen in all the specimens together with portal infiltration by inflammatory and mononuclear cells. In some the infiltration was confined to the portal tract (Fig. 12), but in other instances there were more extensive lesions with "piece-meal" necrosis and erosion of the lobular limiting cellplates (Fig. 13). In two biopsies, small histiocytic granulomas were found (Fig. 14). Although bile duct proliferation was seen in half the biopsies, the bile ductular necrosis characteristic of primary biliary cirrhosis was not observed. When the extent of hepatic injury was compared with impairment of biochemical tests of liver function there was a remarkably good correlation (Fig. 15).

A variety of circulating auto-antibodies were found in the 35 patients. Apart from the mitochondrial fluorescence for which they were selected, three-quarters of the patients also fixed complement with rat liver mitochondria, sometimes to

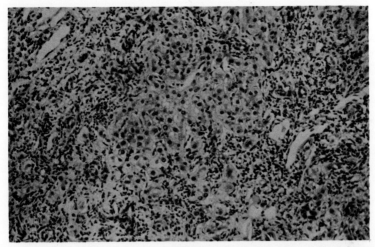

Fig. 13. Liver biopsy from male patient with four years' arthralgia and positive mitochondrial immunofluorescence, showing extensive lymphoid infiltration of portal tract with break-up of lobular limiting cell plate.

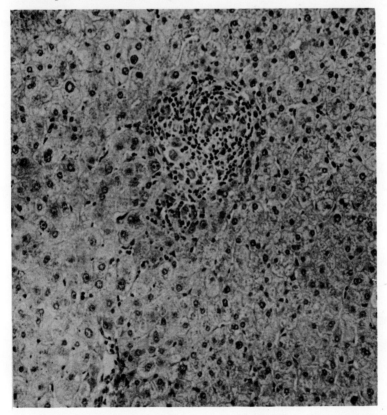

Fig. 14. Liver biopsy from patient with rheumatoid arthritis and positive mitochondrial fluorescence tests, showing a small histiocytic granuloma.

DIAGNOSIS	HISTOLOGICAL FEATURES				LIVER FUNCTION TESTS		
	Portal infiltration	Spotty necrosis	Bileduct proliferation	Breakup of limiting plate	Alkaline phosphatase KA u/100ml	SGPT u/ml	BSP % retention 45 mins.
RHEUMATOID ARTHRITIS WITH LE CELLS	+*	+	0	0	56	57	3
SLE	+	+	0	0	6	19	< 5
SLE, MYXOEDEMA	+	+	0	0	29	15	5
RHEUMATOID ARTHRITIS WITH LE CELLS	+	++	0	0	52	71	20
POLYMYALGIA RHEUMATICA	+	+	+	+	90	22	26
OSTEOARTHRITIS, CURED THYROTOXICOSIS	+	+	+	++	40	44	25
POLYARTHRALGIA	+*	+	+	++	20	50	34
POLYARTHRALGIA	+	++	++	++	54	52	13

*granulomas present

Fig. 15. Correlation of histological and biochemical hepatic abnormalities in eight patients having positive mitochondrial fluorescence and no overt liver disease.

ANTIBODY	NUMBER PATIENTS POSITIVE
MITOCHONDRIAL FLUORESCENCE	35
CFT RAT LIVER MITOCHONDRIA	27
CFT RAT KIDNEY HOMOGENATE	33
ANTI-NUCLEAR (ANF) (Titre 1:40–1:400)	21 (10)
SMOOTH MUSCLE FLUORESCENCE	7
LATEX FII ⩾ 1:40	11
SCAT ⩾1:16	6
WR or VDRL (BFP)	6
RAISED SERUM IMMUNOGLOBULINS IgG	10/34
IgA	5/34
IgM	16/34

Fig. 16. Auto-immune serology in 35 patients selected on the basis of positive mitochondrial fluorescence, ten of whom also showed subclinical liver disease.

a higher titre than expected from the results obtained with immunofluorescence. Over half had ANA in titres ranging from 1 : 10 to 1 : 400 and smooth muscle fluorescence of low titre was found in seven instances. Perhaps the most unusual finding was the occurrence of false positive reactions for syphilis (BFP) in six instances. Serum immunoglobulin levels were raised in some patients, IgM elevation being the most prominent (Fig. 16). A similar study has since been reported by Whaley *et al.*, (1970) who also found subclinical histological hepatic lesions in patients with mitochondrial antibodies and Sjögren's syndrome or rheumatoid arthiritis.

Some of these patients with mitochondrial antibodies and subclinical hepatitis have been followed for periods up to eight years. The majority have not developed signs of overt clinical liver disease despite persistence of the serum antibodies, but it is of interest that three of the ten patients with demonstrable hepatic abnormalities have now progressed in this direction. In one man the liver biopsy appearances have progressed towards classical primary biliary disease and two female patients developed severe pruritus and hepatic decompensation respectively.

UNIFIED CONCEPT OF AUTO-IMMUNE LIVER DISEASE

The polarization of tissue antibodies to the three chronic liver syndromes, with their known clinical and histological overlap, discussed today by Dr. Scheuer, together with the finding of subclinical hepatic lesions in patients with other diseases characterized by immunological disturbances, led us to propose the concept of a common underlying pathogenetic process under these varied circumstances (Doniach and Walker, 1969). We do not think that the antibodies themselves cause tissue damage directly, but that they are markers of an underlying auto-immunizing process associated with continuing injury to the liver. This process may remain silent, may show progression either towards active chronic hepatitis or primary biliary cirrhosis, or more commonly, to cryptogenic cirrhosis. The patients with mitochondrial antibodies in the absence of overt liver disease may be analogous to the symptomless relatives of Hashimoto patients who have subclinical thyroiditis on biopsy and organ-specific auto-antibodies in the serum. It is now known that asymptomatic relatives of primary biliary cirrhosis patients have an increased incidence of mitochondrial and other tissue auto-antibodies in the serum (Feizi *et al.*, 1970). We have also encountered a family in which two sisters had primary biliary cirrhosis and cryptogenic cirrhosis respectively, with mitochondrial antibodies, while two healthy male siblings also had these antibodies in significant titres.

The role of viruses in the initiation and progression of chronic liver diseases is still uncertain but the recent studies of Krohn *et al.*, (1970) suggest that silent viral infections may be as important as the genetic predisposition to auto-immunity in the aetiology of these disorders.

REFERENCES

Doniach, D., Roitt, I. M., Walker, J. G. and Sherlock, S. (1966) Clin. exp. Immunol. 1, 237.

Doniach, D. (1970) Proc. Roy. Soc. Med. 63, 527.

Doniach, D. and Walker, J. G. (1969) Lancet 1, 813.

Farrow, L. J., Holborow, E. J., Johnson, G. D., Lamb, S. G., Stewart, J. S., Taylor, P. E. and Zuckerman, A. J. (1970) Brit. Med. J. ii, 693.

Feizi, T., Naccarato, R., Doniach, D. and Sherlock, S. (1970) In preparation.

Fischer, J. A. and Schmid, M. (1967) Lancet i, 421.

Goudie, R. B., Macsween, R. N. M. and Goldberg, D. M. (1966) J. Clin. Path. 19, 527.

Hadziyannis, S., Scheuer, P. J., Feizi, T., Naccarato, R., Doniach, D. and Sherlock, S. (1970) J. Clin. Path. 23, 95.

Kantor, F. S. and Klatskin, G. (1967) Trans. Ass. Amer. Physcns. 80, 267.
Krohn, K., Finlayson, N. D. C., Jokelainen, P. T., Anderson, K. E. and Prince, A. M. (1970)
     Lancet ii, 379.
Paronetto, F., Schaffner, F. and Popper, H. (1967) J. Lab. Clin. Med. 69, 979.
Paronetto, F. and Popper, H. (1970) New Eng. J. Med. 283, 277.
Pinckard, R. N. and Weir, D. M. (1966) Clin. exp. Immunol. 1, 33.
Rodriguez, M., Paronetto, F., Schaffner, F. and Popper, H. (1969) J. Amer. Med. Assn.
     208, 148.
Walker, J. G., Doniach, D., Roitt, I. M. and Sherlock, S. (1967) In The Liver, Colston
     papers vol. XIX. Ed. A. E. Read, pp. 83. Butterworths, London.
Walker, J. G., Doniach, D., Willette, M., Cameron, C. H. and Dane, D. S. (1970a) Gut 11, 369.
Walker, J. G., Doniach, D. and Doniach, I. (1970b) Quart. J. Med. 39, 31.
Whaley, K., Goudie, R. B., Williamson, J., Nuki, G., Dick, W. C. and Buchanan, W. W.
     (1970) Lancet i, 861.
Whittingham, S., Irwin, J., Mackay, I. R. and Smalley, M. (1966) Gastroenterology 51, 499.
Williams, R. (1970) Brit. med. J. i, 585.
Wright, R. (1970) Lancet i, 521.

DISCUSSION
Chairman: Professor I. M. Roitt

BOYES
Did any of the patients whom you labelled as "Miscellaneous" have biliary atresia?

WALKER
We have studied patients with bilary atresia and they are included under the heading "Cholestasis". They did not have mitochondrial antibodies.

BOYES
We studied a series of young children with biliary atresia and in 3 of 6 with extrahepatic atresia and 6 of 12 with intrahepatic atresia we found smooth muscle antibody. But we did not find mitochondrial antibody in any of these patients.

FOX
In your unified hypothesis, should you not have an arrow going from "silent hepatitis" over to "primary biliary cirrhosis"? We have had 4 asymptomatic patients who were detected by the finding of a positive mitochondrial antibody test and subsequently shown to have the histological features of primary biliary cirrhosis. One of these has been followed for over a year and has now developed symptoms.

WALKER
Yes, I would agree with you. In fact two of our patients with silent hepatitis later developed pruritus and in one, the liver biopsy appearances progressed towards a primary biliary cirrhosis-like picture.

WILLIAMS
Are these antibodies directed specifically against antigens in liver cells — mitochondria, nuclei and so on?

WALKER
The antibodies react with mitochondria, nuclei and smooth muscle present in all tissues and thus there is no evidence for an organ-specific component.

WILLIAMS
How do they develop? There must have been some release of antigen initially.

WALKER

They are produced as a result of antigenic stimulation but whether this is due to cell damage with subsequent release of hidden components, whether it is due to reaction with altered cell components, or whether it is cross-reaction with some agent, perhaps a virus, I do not know.

CHAIRMAN

That is even further back than the problem of what is causing the tissue damage.

VELASCO

Have you found any patients with antiglomerular antibodies?

WALKER

Antiglomerular antibody has been described by Whittingham as a useful test in active chronic hepatitis but we have not investigated this specifically.

VELASCO

In our studies on chronic hepatitis we have found antiglomerular antibody more frequently than smooth muscle antibody.

WALKER

Smooth muscle antibody has been described as occurring in quite high percentages both by our own group and by the group at Taplow, but I am interested to hear that antiglomerular antibody may be found so frequently.

GLYNN

In a short communication on anti-smooth muscle antibody we also described antibodies against the glomerular basement membrane. We found, as far as I can recall, that the incidence was similar for each antibody. However, our series was a small one and the findings in other parts of the world might be different.

CHAIRMAN

Would you tell us, Dr. Velasco, the percentage positive for glomerular staining?

VELASCO

We studied 15 patients with chronic active hepatitis and 11 cases were positive for antiglomerular antibody. We did not find the antibody in any of 30 patients with other diseases or in 25 normal controls.

WRIGHT

I would agree entirely with that. I always look for glomerular antibody to rat kidney and these figures tie in very well with the high titres we have found in acute and chronic hepatitis.

CHAIRMAN

Do you see this Dr. Doniach?

DONIACH

We have seen positive fluorescence on the glomeruli. However, to be sure of a specific reaction it is necessary to use fluorescent conjugates with a very low background.

WILLIAMS

Dr. Walker, are you implying that only in some cases of halothane hepatitis is there an immunological reaction?

WALKER

I wanted to make the point that although some patients with halothane hepatitis develop mitochondrial antibodies, these may differ from those found in classical primary biliary cirrhosis. It has been reported that the antibodies are labile and do not store well. I am not suggesting that the mitochondrial antibodies cause the halothane liver damage.

POPPER

It is only certain drug reactions which are associated with mitochondrial antibodies. With halothane, we have found a fairly high incidence, as Dr. Schaffner will report tomorrow. With chlorpromazine, the incidence is much lower, and we have never seen them with methyl dopa or indomethacin.

WALKER

We have seen them occasionally with chlorpromazine and in other cholestatic drug reactions.

ANTIBODIES RELATED TO MITOCHONDRIA: MULTIPLE SPECIFICITIES AND CLINICAL ASSOCIATIONS

Deborah Doniach and Peter A. Berg

The close relationship of mitochondrial antibodies with primary biliary cirrhosis (PBC) has been discussed this morning, and was recently reviewed (Doniach, 1970). A further study from Professor Sherlock's Unit is now in progress on the implications of these antibodies in patients with "cryptogenic" cirrhosis, where the incidence of mitochondrial ("M") fluorescence is about 25%. Results in a group of forty-nine Australia—SH antigen negative cases suggest that mitochondrial antibodies occur mostly in females and can be correlated with certain histological features including granulomas, portal lymphoid infiltrates and piecemeal necrosis reminiscent of PBC, although the characteristic bile duct lesions could not be demonstrated. Cryptogenic cirrhosis patients with mitochondrial antibodies also tended to have associated thyroid auto-immune diseases and raised serum IgM levels as found in PBC (Ross *et al.*, 1971).

In the present communication an attempt will be made to summarize what is known of the nature of the "M" antigen and to assess it in the light of recent studies on cardiolipin antibodies and other mitochondria-related systems.

LOCALIZATION OF MITOCHONDRIAL ANTIGEN

Purification of the mitochondrial antigen reacting with PBC sera was achieved by using a serum with high activity as a standard in a quantitative complement fixation test (CFT) (Rapport & Graf, 1957) so that an arbitrary antigen unit could be established (Berg *et al.*, 1967). Mitochondria were then separated from rat liver homogenates by ultracentrifugation and submitted to various treatments known to break them up into smaller fragments. Fig. 1 shows a subcellular fractionation and it can be seen that the heavy mitochondria contain most of the antigen, although neighbouring fractions are contaminated. By combining osmotic swelling and ultrasonication with differential centrifugation, the mitochondria were separated into their outer and inner membranes (Parsons *et al.*, 1966) (Figs. 2 and 3) and it could be shown that the auto-antigen was entirely in the inner membranes (Berg *et al.*, 1969a). By combining these methods with separation on discontinuous sucrose gradients, it was possible to increase antigen concentration in the submitochondrial fragments from 20 units per mg. of protein to values between 500 and 1,300 units in different experiments, i.e. a 50-fold purification (Fig. 4) (Berg *et al.*, 1969b). These highly purified subfractions still had a micellar or membranous appearance on electron microscopy and were composed of phospholipids and proteins. Although the phospholipids themselves, including cardiolipin, are inactive when tested against PBC sera, their removal destroys the antigenic activity of the mitochondrial fragments. Since these are also inactivated on treatment with proteolytic enzymes such as trypsin, it is thought that the "M" antigen is a protein which is kept in a reactive configuration by phospholipids (Berg *et al.*, 1969c).

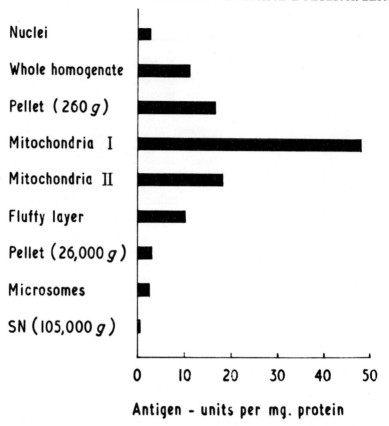

Fig. 1. Specific activity of "M" antigen in subcellular liver fractions obtained by differential centrifugation. (Reproduced from Berg *et al.*, 1967).

IMMUNOFLUORESCENT STUDIES ON VARIOUS TISSUES

Further information on the nature of this antigen was obtained by comparing the immunofluorescence patterns obtained in different organs with a PBC serum directly conjugated with fluorescein isothiocyanate. The most intense fluorescence was found in mitochondria of cells engaged in high energy transactions: continuous contraction in heart or flight muscle, "red" fibres in voluntary muscles (Fig. 5), ion transport in parotid ducts (Fig. 6), distal renal tubules, gastric parietal cells producing hydrochloric acid, lactating breast and brown fat of newborn animals. In all these tissues the mitochondria are known to utilize metabolic pathways involving fatty acids in preference to carbohydrate. By contrast, cells engaged in protein synthesis such as liver, thyroid, gastric chief cells or pancreas and salivary glandular epithelium show only a faint granular fluorescence with "M" antibodies and the mitochondria extracted from them have a much lower specific activity for "M" antigen (Table 1). Recent work on mitochondria suggests that the "cristal" part of the inner membranes (Fig. 7) contains most of the electron transfer chains of respiratory enzymes. Although the mitochondria richest in "M" antigen also have large and closely packed cristae to do their heavy work, it seems that this relationship is an indirect one since all the known electron transfer enzymes were totally inactive against PBC sera. It is more likely that

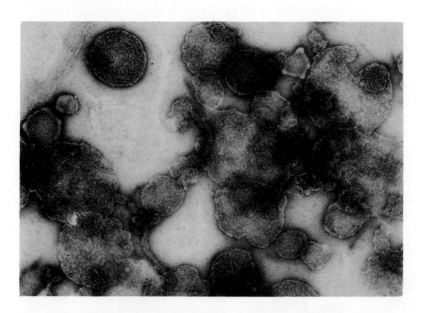

Fig. 2. Electron micrograph of outer mitochondrial membranes consisting mainly of vesicles with a smooth surface. × 32,000.

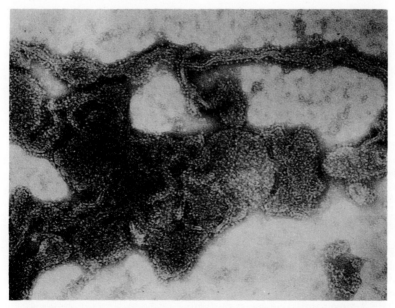

Fig. 3. Electron microscope appearance of inner mitochondrial membranes showing cristae with characteristic 90Å projections where oxidative phosphorylation takes place.

PURIFICATION OF CF-ANTIGEN IN SUBMITOCHONDRIAL
FRACTION BY DISCONTINUOUS DENSITY GRADIENT
CENTRIFUGATION

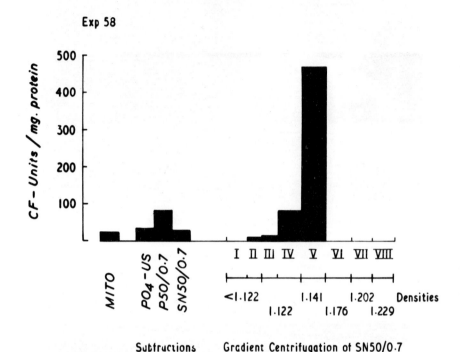

Fig 4. Purification of CF antigen in sub-mitochondrial fractions by moving zone
centrifugation. The fragmented mitochondria treated with hypotonic phosphate
buffer and ultrasound (PO_4 + US) were spun at 50,000 rev/min. for 40 minutes
(P50/0·7) and the corresponding supernatant (SN50/0·7) was layered on the
sucrose gradient and centrifuged at 25,000 rev/min. for 14 hours.
(Reproduced from Berg *et al.*, 1969b)

the antigen is on the "limiting membrane", the part between the cristae which is
thought to be concerned with the active transport of substrates and other
essential compounds into the inner space where they are utilized for synthetic
pathways within the cristae.

MITOCHONDRIA ASSOCIATED ANTIBODIES IN SYPHILIS AND FALSE
POSITIVE REACTORS

Further promising clues have arisen from the study of patients with active
syphilis (Wright *et al.*, 1970) and a number of unusual cases of auto-immune
disorders with associated chronic "biologic false positive" (BFP) reactions for
syphilis (Doniach *et al.*, 1970). The classical "Wasserman reagins" are known to
include complement-fixing and agglutinating antibodies to cardiolipins, a
family of diphospholipids extracted from beef heart and localized to the inner
membranes of the mitochondria. Although the basic structure of cardiolipins

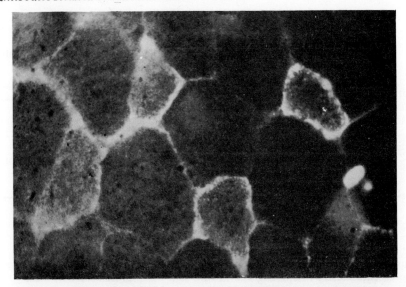

Fig. 5. "M" fluorescence. Transverse section of rat quadriceps muscle stained with a direct fluorescent conjugate of primary biliary cirrhosis serum. The mitochondria in the smaller "red" fibres show a much brighter fluorescence than those of "white" fibres. White blob on right is an artefact.

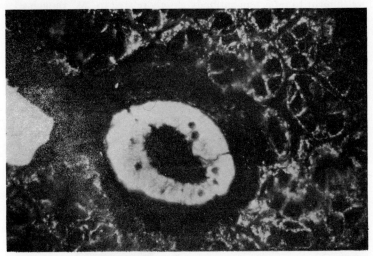

Fig. 6. "M" fluorescence. Section of rat parotid gland treated as in Fig. 5 showing intense staining of salivary duct epithelium.

is not complex, in biological membranes they are present as a subtle mixture of lipid species with a variety of fatty acids and different types of polar groups (Gulik-Drzywicki *et al.*, 1969). Since cardiolipins account for 20% of the total phospholipids in mitochondria, it is not surprising that syphilitics with a positive WR react in CFT with rat liver mitochondria to the same titre as with purified cardiolipin (Fig. 8). The agglutination test with "veneral diseases research laboratory" (VDRL) antigen is more sensitive and also correlates well with the mitochondrial CFT in syphilis. However, when patients with BFP reactions are

COMPARISON OF ANTIGENIC ACTIVITY IN DIFFERENT
ORGANS WITH RESPECT TO CELL FUNCTION

	Rat liver	Pigeon breast-muscle	Rat heart	kidney	Newborn Rabbit brown fat
Total CF-antigen					
Units/g. tissue	2,150	5,380	5,100	4,800	3,456
Units/mg. protein	11	28	25	26	55
Major Cell Function	Protein-synthesis detoxification	Contraction		Ion-transport	Heat generation

Table 1. The antigen reacting with PBC sera is present in greater concentration in mitochondria of cells engaged in high energy activity. The highest specific activity (units/mg. protein) is found in brown fat where mitochondria transform fat directly into heat.

considered, the situation is more complicated as seen in Fig. 9. A tissue immuno-fluorescence closely resembling that of PBC sera was found in some of these cases, particularly those with systemic diseases related to the collagenoses. Unlike PBC, the tissue fluorescence was always of low titre, not exceeding 1:40 and the antibodies were mostly of the IgM class. The fluorescence could not be abolished by prior absorption of the serum with cardiolipin and is therefore thought to reflect an antibody closely related to "M" though all the BFP reactors investigated had normal liver function tests.

When immunofluorescence was applied to syphilis, it was found that the serum of patients in the infective secondary stage of the disease gave a mitochondrial fluorescence (Figs. 10 and 11) which had a similar distribution among different tissues as that of "M" antibodies (Fig. 12). The essential difference was that the reaction could be abolished by absorption with

MITOCHONDRIAL   STRUCTURE

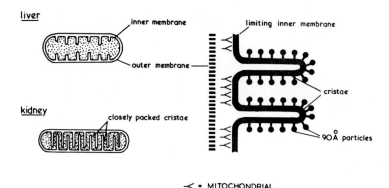

-◁ = MITOCHONDRIAL ANTIBODIES

Fig. 7. Diagrammatic representation of mitochondrial membranes. It is thought that the 'M' antibodies in PBC serum react with a lipoprotein on the limiting inner membranes situated between the cristal projections.

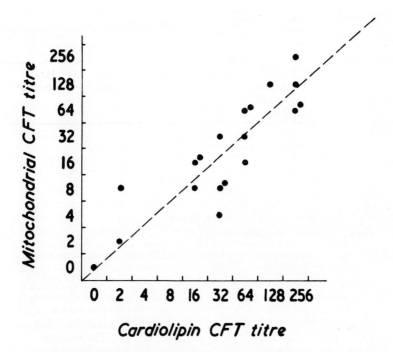

Correlation of Mitochondrial and Cardiolipin CFT titres in syphilis

Cardiolipin CFT titre

Fig. 8. With syphlitic sera the quantitative Wassermann reaction (cardiolipin CFT) gives the same titre as CFT with rat liver mitochondria as these particles have a high content of the diphospholipid(from Wright *et al.*, 1970).

cardiolipin. The "cardiolipin fluorescent" antibody (CLF) is thought to be distinct from classical WR antibodies as it disappears from the serum within a few weeks after penicillin treatment and is absent in late syphilis when the WR is still positive. Fig. 13 summarizes the differences between "M" and "CLF" antibodies.

THE RELATION BETWEEN "M" AND CARDIOLIPIN ANTIBODIES

Two connections appear important in relation to liver diseases: if the fluorescence produced by "M" and "CLF" antibodies is strongest on the same type of mitochondria, i.e. the two antigens are associated with high energy work and metabolic pathways utilizing fatty acids, it implies that the particular cardiolipin which is antigenic, is linked possibly in the same part of the mitochondrial inner membrane with the protein or enzyme which represents the "M" antigen. This may shed light on the nature of tissue antigenicity in human disease. Secondly, if *Treponema pallidum* can provoke antibodies to cardiolipin, perhaps a micro-organism could be responsible for the auto-immunization to "M". If the recent claim (Krohn *et al.*, 1970) can be substantiated that PBC patients have Aust.—SH antigen or a closely related viral product in their serum, it could be visualized that such an organism could invade the mitochondria of

CORRELATION OF MITOCHONDRIAL CFT WITH VDRL TITRES IN 41 PATIENTS WITH CHRONIC BFP REACTIONS

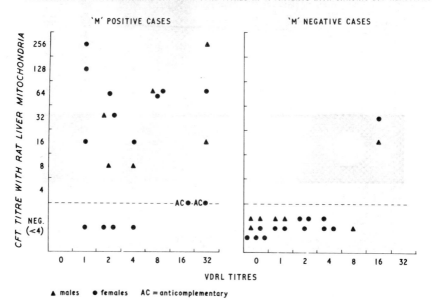

Fig. 9. The "venereal diseases research laboratory" (VDRL) agglutination test measures
Wasserman antibodies. In the absence of other antibodies VDRL of 1:8 or greater
usually corresponds with a positive CFT with mitochondria (cf. "M" negative
cases). Patients with chronic false positive tests for syphilis (BFP) sometimes have
"M" fluorescence of low titre (cf. "M" positive cases) and some have CFT titres with
mitochondria that are out of proportion with both the fluorescence and the VDRL
titres, suggesting the existence of a separate (4th) antibody related to mitochondria (from Doniach et al., 1970).

bile ducts and modify an enzyme slightly so as to make it antigenic. Perhaps a
special form of viral cholangitis is responsible for the necrosis of bile ducts and
also provokes the exceptionally chronic and intense auto-immunization to
mitochondria seen in primary biliary cirrhosis.

A FURTHER MITOCHONDRIAL ANTIBODY

Finally, the question may be considered as to whether there is yet another, a
fourth mitochondrial antibody. If WR antibodies and "CLF" are separate reactions
to cardiolipin, it is possible that the "M" system may also include two types of
antibody, one fluorescent and the other complement fixing only. Contrary to
initial findings in primary biliary cirrhosis, where the titres in the two tests
corresponded fairly closely, some categories of patients with obscure "collagen
disorders" show unexplained discrepancies when their sera are titrated by
immunofluorescence on kidney sections and in the conventional CFT using rat
liver mitochondria as antigen. Our previous studies on chronic BFP reactors
already presented such discrepancies. Some of the cases in Fig. 9, gave "M"
fluorescence to titres between 1:5 and 1:40 while their CFT went up to 1:256
a difference not always attributable to the simultaneous presence of WR antibodies,
since these were often of very low titre. We have now obtained similar results
in a selection of sera from patients with "auto-immune" disorders and a negative
WR. Furthermore, some of the fluorescent reactions failed to fix complement

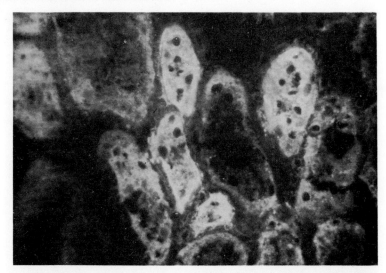

Fig. 10. Cardiolipin fluorescent antibody. Human kidney treated with serum from patient with secondary syphilis followed by anti-IgG conjugate. Distal tubules are brightly stained while proximal tubules show a faint fluorescence.

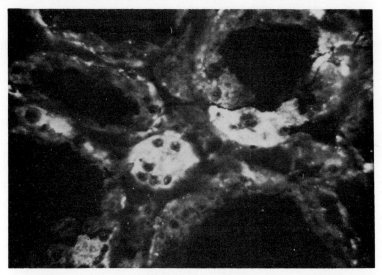

Fig. 11. Cardiolipin fluorescent antibody. Thyrotoxic thyroid gland treated as in Fig. 10. Cells with hypertrophied mitochondria (oxyphil cells) are uniformly bright. Normal thyroid epithelium shows hardly any fluorescence. The fluorescence is less "compact" and less granular than that obtained with primary biliary cirrhosis sera, and can be completely abolished with cardiolipin.

when tested with anti-β_{1C} conjugates, which further suggests that the antibodies might be distinct from those fixing complement in liquid media, and present in the same serum. Studies with the quantitative CFT and submitochondrial fractions are in progress to see if these sera react with purified "M" antigen, or whether the reactive protein is in a separate mitochondrial fraction.

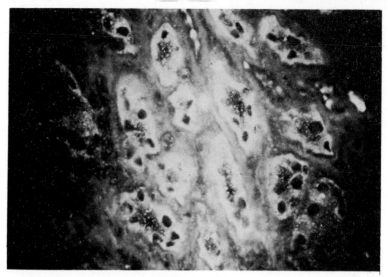

Fig. 12. "M" fluorescence. Section of human kidney treated with primary biliary cirrhosis serum followed by anti-human Ig conjugate, showing a brightly stained group of distal tubules. The connective tissue fibres between tubules had a blue auto-fluorescence which, in UV light, cannot be confused with the apple green colour of the specific immunofluorescence.

MITOCHONDRIAL FLUORESCENT ANTIBODIES

Antibody	Clinical Associations	Mitochondrial Immunofluorescence	Absorption with Cardiolipin (CL)
"M"	Auto-immune liver disease:		
	PBC, ACH, Crypto.cirrhosis	+	−
	Subclinical hepatitis	+	−
	Some BFP reactors	+	−
"CLF"	Active syphilis	+	+
	Occasional BFP reactors	+	+

Fig. 13. Comparison of the two mitochondria-associated fluorescent antibodies. The main difference is that the syphilitic fluorescence can be absorbed out with cardiolipin whereas the primary biliary cirrhosis fluorescence is unaffected.

CONCLUSIONS

The relationships of the four mitochondria-associated immune reactivities described in this paper are summarized in Fig. 14. The two types of cardiolipin antibodies may be directed against hydrophobic and hydrophilic aspects of the phospholipid which is anatomically and functionally close to the "M" lipoprotein. Two types of antibodies are now postulated for this system as well. "M" antibodies are almost confined to three chronic liver syndromes and cardiolipin antibodies when detectable for prolonged periods are uncommon outside syphilis. There is, however, a mixed territory in atypical cases of collagen diseases and in rare patients with Waldenström's macroglobulinaemia where

MITOCHONDRIA-ASSOCIATED ANTIBODIES

Antibody	Clinical associations	Rat Liver Mitochondria		Cardiolipin
		CFT	fluoresc.	CFT
"M"	Liver disease some BFP reactors	+	+	−
Wasserman Antibody	All syphilitic All BFP reactors	+	−	+
"CLF"	Active syphilis Occasional BFP	+	+	+
4th Mito AB	Miscellaneous Collagenoses	+	−	−

Fig. 14. Summary of the four mitochondria-related complement fixing reactions and the behaviour of the postulated distinct antibodies in immunofluorescence and on absorption of the sera with cardiolipin.

at least three mitochondria-associated antibodies are present at the same time. The particular area of the mitochondrial membrane carrying these auto-antigens must have some special significance in relation to auto-immunity and the loss of self tolerance.

REFERENCES

Berg, P. A., Doniach, D. and Roitt, I. M. (1967) J. Exp. Med. 126, 277.
Berg, P. A., Muscatello, U., Horne, R. W., Roitt, I. M. and Doniach, D. (1969a) Br. J. exp. Path. 50, 200.
Berg, P. A., Roitt, I. M., Doniach, D. and Horne, R. W. (1969b) Clin. exp. Immunol. 4, 511.
Berg, P. A., Roitt, I. M., Doniach, D. and Cooper, H. M. (1969c) Immunol. 17, 281.
Doniach, D. (1970) Proc. Roy. Soc. Med. 63, 527.
Doniach, D., Delhanty, J., Lindqvist, H. L. and Catterall, R. D. (1970) Clin. exp. Immunol. 6, 871.
Gulik-Kryzywicki, T., Schechter, E., Luzzati, V. and Faure, M. (1969) Nature, 223, 1116.
Krohn, K., Finlayson, N. D. C., Jokelainen, P. T., Anderson, K. E. and Prince, A. M. (1970) Lancet, ii, 370.
Parsons, D. F., Williams, G. and Chance, B. (1966) Ann. N.Y. Acad. Sci. 137, 2, 643.
Rapport, M. M. and Graf, L. (1957) Ann. N.Y. Acad. Sci. 69, 608.
Ross, A., Doniach, D., Scheuer, P., and Sherlock, S. (1971) Cryptogenic cirrhosis: A search for aetiological factors. In preparation.
Wright, D. J. M., Doniach, D., Lessoff, M. H., Turk, J. L., Grimble, A. S. and Catterall, R. D. (1970) Lancet i, 740.

DISCUSSION
Chairman: Professor I. M. Roitt

WRIGHT
Have you been able to raise any antisera reacting in the immunofluorescent test to the inner mitochondrial membrane, which show the same reaction that one sees in the patients with primary biliary cirrhosis?

DONIACH
Dr. Berg injected some rats with liver mitochondria and obtained a complement-fixing antiserum, without fluorescent properties. However, in another mitochondria-related system, sera from animals immunized with treponemes show a tissue fluorescence similar to that obtained with human syphilitic sera, which can be absorbed out with cardiolipin.

MacSWEEN

Have you tried to absorb "M" fluorescence out with plant mitochondria?

DONIACH

We have tried plant mitochondria in the complement fixation tests against cirrhosis sera and they were completely negative.

Meyer zum BUSCHENFELDE

I believe Dr. Berg was unable to show good fluorescence with rat liver or with liver from other species. Do you have any explanation for this phenomenon?

DONIACH

The antigen reacting with primary biliary cirrhosis sera is present in relatively small amounts in the liver and other organs mainly concerned with protein synthesis, such as normal thyroid, pancreas and salivary glandular epithelium. That is why PBC sera produce only a faint fluorescence on these organs.

Meyer zum BUSCHENFELDE

We have found it very difficult to do a complete blocking test. Have you had the same experience?

DONIACH

Yes, it is difficult to block the fluorescence obtained with a direct conjugate of PBC serum by first treating the section with unconjugated PBC serum. However, "M" fluorescent antibodies may be removed from PBC sera by absorbing them with an excess of rat liver mitochondria.

Meyer zum BUSCHENFELDE

We have tried to absorb the antibody with mitochondria obtained by ultracentrifugation. However, even after absoprtion a little fluorescence remains — have you seen that?

DONIACH

One has to absorb with a large excess of mitochondria. To get rid of all the fluorescence, we had to use 20 times the quantity of mitochondria and then to do two successive absorptions.

Meyer zum BUSCHENFELDE

We have had great difficulty in deciding what is specific and what is not.

DONIACH

To obtain really specific "M" fluorescence, it is necessary to use a direct conjugate of the patient's serum.

CHAIRMAN

What do you mean Dr. Meyer zum Buschenfelde, by having difficulty in showing that it is specific?

Meyer zum BUSCHENFELDE

I mean that we find nonspecific fluorescence, especially on the distal tubules of kidney. However, if we use gastric or thyroid tissue the nonspecific reaction is less marked. We have no explanation for this phenomenon.

DONIACH

This is because the intensity of the fluorescence varies between tissues — everything is much brighter on the kidney and, therefore, even non-specific reactions are more marked. But if you use a good conjugate, such as anti-IgG, for instance, there is no trouble.

Meyer zum BUSCHENFELDE

As a result of our difficulties we now use the complement-fixation test to study mitochondrial antibodies. We have found positive results in nearly 40 per cent of patients with active chronic hepatitis. I cannot say anything about primary biliary cirrhosis, because these patients are rare in Mainz. In several years we have seen only five patients.

DONIACH

Perhaps because they have not been diagnosed? They used to say that Hashimoto's disease did not exist in Spain, until somebody did an M.D. thesis on it, and then they found plenty of cases.

Meyer zum BUSCHENFELDE

I would like to know the incidence of primary biliary cirrhosis in other parts of Europe.

DONIACH

This will depend partly on diagnostic criteria used in different countries. It is no longer safe to use the complement fixation test in the diagnosis of primary biliary cirrhosis since high CFT titres may be associated with a negative immunofluorescence.

CHAIRMAN

I do not think we should let that discussion finish with the idea that the fluorescent test cannot be highly specific even on the kidney. Immunofluorescence is easy with the correct reagents.

McINTYRE

If you add antibody, are the mitochondria still metabolically active?

DONIACH

Yes.

McINTYRE

Have you looked to see whether you have destroyed any mitochondrial markers when you add the antibodies?

DONIACH

This has been done in Dr. Chappell's laboratory at Bristol. Unfortunately the mitochondria that are used for these enzyme tests have to be whole, with their outer membranes still on. The mitochondria can still respire normally after addition of PBC serum but perhaps the antibodies cannot penetrate intact mitochondria.

McINTYRE

And all the enzymes, as far as one can tell, are active, and you do not selectively destroy one of them?

DONIACH

Unfortunately, we are not far advanced enough to be able to show this.

CHAIRMAN

Certainly the respiratory chains are still intact.

Meyer zum BUSCHENFELDE

Have you studied antibodies against microsomal fractions in liver disease?

DONIACH

Yes. We have found two sera with possible antiribosomal antibodies and they give a very beautiful fluorescence on liver, much brighter than that seen with PBC sera. This is rather rare and we have only found it in once case of active chronic hepatitis.

ANTIBODIES TO BILE CANALICULI IN PATIENTS WITH CHRONIC ACTIVE LIVER DISEASE

H. Diederichsen, N. C. Linde and P. Møller Nielsen

In the sera from patients with chronic active liver disease Johnson *et al.*, found a serum factor which they thought was an auto-antibody against bile canaliculi. In a previous investigation, I found that sera from a few patients with chronic active liver disease reacted with bile canaliculi in bovine liver but not with bile canaliculi in human liver. This presentation deals with the results of further investigations which we have carried out on the occurrence of this bile canalicular antibody.

DEFINITION AND THE SERIES EXAMINED

We define "active chronic liver disease" as a disease lasting for more than six months. In this investigation the mean duration was 39 months; ranging from nine months to more than 10 years. The diagnosis was established on clinical and biochemical findings and verified by needle biopsy in 18 of the 24 patients.

The disease showed varying degrees of activity at the time of investigation although in most patients the disease was highly active. 13 patients had hyperbilirubinaemia and in 19 the serum aspartate aminotransferase level was more than twice the normal. In 11 the prothrombin index was below 50 per cent and in 12 the gamma globulin was more than 3 g. per cent. In 9 the alkaline phosphatase was twice the normal value. In 3 patients the disease was clinically inactive and the laboratory findings were almost normal. In one of these three patients liver biopsy showed the histological appearances of cryptogenic cirrhosis and in another chronic persistent hepatitis; in the third patient the biopsy failed.

As shown in Table 1 there were 18 females and 6 males in the group. The mean age for women was 58 years ranging from 15—79 years and the mean age for the men was 45 years ranging from 12—61 years. Five patients had other systemic manifestations of auto-immune disease, these were pernicious anemia, rheumatoid arthritis, myxoedema, ulcerative colitis and psoriasis respectively.

We also investigated patients with other forms of liver disease (Table 1), which included acute hepatitis, liver disease in alcohol consumers (>23g. of alcohol

Table 1

Diagnosis, Age and Sex in 103 Patients with Liver Diseases

Diagnosis	No. Patients Tested	Females		Males	
		No.	Mean Age (Range)	No.	Mean Age (Range)
Chronic active liver disease	24	18	58 (15—79)	6	45 (12—61)
Acute hepatitis	20	14	38 (7—72)	8	34 (14—76)
Liver disease in alcohol consumers	15	2	48 (44—51)	14	45 (31—66)
Main bile duct obstruction	23	13	68 (34—83)	10	65 (51—82)
Cholecystitis	21	18	54 (33—81)	3	62 (49—71)

Table 2

Diagnosis, Age and Sex in 697 Patients with Various Diseases

Diagnosis	No. Patients Tested	Females		Males	
		No.	Mean Age (Range)	No.	Mean Age (Range)
Systemic lupus erythematosus	12	11	58 (8−75)	1	26
Mixed hospital patients	446	241	54 (5−90)	205	51 (9−87)
Thyroid diseases with CF antibodies	9	9	47 (22−63)	0	
Pernicious anaemia	18	13	77 (60−88)	5	62 (52−69)
Infectious mononucleosis	19	11	17 (8−24)	8	20 (14−28)
Blood donors	193	74	52 (18−75)	119	53 (18−74)

per day), extrahepatic biliary obstruction and lastly cholecystitis. Table 2 lists 697 patients with various other diseases that we investigated for bile canalicular antibody. The groups were not matched for sex and age. The blood donors had been used as controls in a previous study.

DEMONSTRATION OF BILE CANALICULAR ANTIBODY

All sera were investigated for bile canalicular antibody with the indirect immunofluorescent technique. The antigen was fresh bovine liver frozen in liquid oxygen and stored until use. Unfixed cryostat sections of this liver were incubated first with serum, and thereafter with commercially obtained fluorescein conjugated antihuman globulin. The sections were examined for immunofluorescent staining of bile canaliculi and liver cell nuclei and cytoplasm. Sera producing a granular cytoplasmic fluorescence were considered to contain mitochondrial antibodies. All sera were investigated both diluted 1/10 and undiluted.

Figure 1 illustrates bile canaliculi stained by Burstone's method for acid

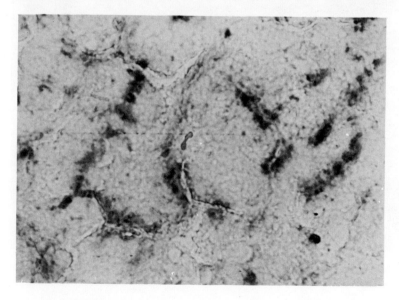

Fig. 1. Bile canaliculi stained by Burstone's method for acid phosphatase.

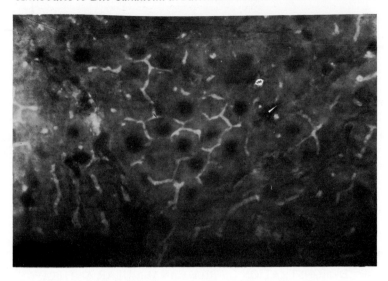

Fig. 2. Immunofluorescent staining of bile canaliculi in fresh bovine liver treated with inactivated serum from a patient with active chronic liver disease and fluorescein conjugated antihuman globulin. Original magnification ×330 (from Diederichsen, 1969).

Fig. 3. Showing a negative reaction for bile canaliculi after using inactivated normal human serum.

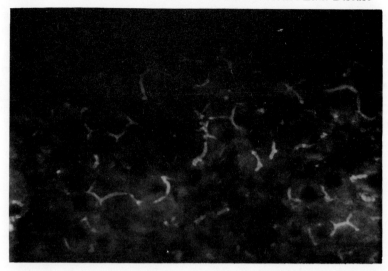

Fig. 4. Another example of a positive reaction for bile canaliculi (Original magnification ×330).

Table 3

Reactions of Sera in Various Diseases Against Bovine Liver

Diagnosis	No. Patients Tested	Sera Reacting With		
		Bile Canaliculi	Nuclei	Mitochondria
Liver diseases	103	19 (18%)	21 (20%)	4 (4%)
Systemic lupus erythematosus	12	1 (8%)	11 (91%)	0
Mixed hospital patients	446	2 (0, 4%)	81 (18%)	9 (2%)
Thyroid diseases with CF antibody	9	0	0	0
Pernicious anaemia	18	0	0	0
Infectious mononucleosis	19	0	0	1 (5%)
Blood donors	193	0	14 (7%)	6 (3%)

Serum dilution 1:10

phosphatase. The bile canalicular staining shown in Fig. 2 was produced by using sera containing bile canalicular antibody. This should be compared with Fig. 3 in which a negative reaction, using sera not containing bile canalicular antibody is shown. Another positive reaction for bile canalicular antibody is shown in Fig. 4 this time using sera which did not also contain mitochondrial antibodies.

INCIDENCE OF THE BILE CANALICULAR ANTIBODY

The results of examination for bile canalicular antibody in the various diseases are shown in Table 3. In all, 103 patients with liver disease were studied and of these 18 per cent gave a positive reaction for bile canalicular antibody. In the other diseases investigated, there was one positive reaction from a patient with systemic lupus erythematosus and two positive reactions from a group of mixed hospital patients. The patient with systemic lupus erythematosus refused liver biopsy, but the other two patients had normal liver histology. One of these had Sjögren's syndrome and the other had an undiagnosed disease with a high erythrocyte sedimentation rate, periods of fever and arthralgia. Also shown in Table 3 are the reactions against nuclei and mitochondria. The sera from twenty per cent of the patients with liver disease were positive for antinuclear factor and four per cent for mitochondrial antibodies.

Of the positive reactions against bile canaliculi, 16 were seen in patients with chronic active liver disease (Table 4). Only one of these patients subsequently

Table 4

Reactions of Sera in Liver Diseases Against Bovine Liver

Diagnosis	No. Patients Tested	Sera Reacting With		
		Bile Canaliculi	Nuclei	Mitochondria
Chronic active liver disease	24	16 (66%)	12 (50%)	2 (8%)
Acute hepatitis	20	2 (10%)	3 (15%)	2 (10%)
Liver disease in alcohol consumers	15	0	1 (6%)	0
Main bile duct obstruction	23	0	4 (17%)	0
Cholecystitis	21	1 (5%)	1 (5%)	0

Serum dilution 1:10

gave a negative reaction. We have made no systematic investigation to find out why the positive reaction for bile canalicular antibody persists in these patients. The duration of the chronic liver disease, prior to the first examination for bile canalicular antibody, varied from less than one month to more that 10 years with a mean of 33 months. Sera from only two patients with chronic active liver disease showed a positive reaction against bovine liver mitochondria. Five of the patients had a positive reaction against the tubules in mouse kidney. Only one of these five reacted with liver mitochondria.

Two of the 20 patients with acute hepatitis gave a positive reaction against bile canaliculi and in each case the reaction became negative as the disease subsided. Bile canalicular antibody was also found in one patient with cholecystitis — unfortunately investigation for possible co-existing chronic liver disease in this patient was inadequate, and no liver biopsy was obtained.

RELATION TO SERUM ANTIBODIES, BIOCHEMICAL AND CLINICAL CHANGES

All sera containing bile canalicular antibody were titrated against bovine liver. The titres for this antibody and also for antinuclear factor are shown in Fig. 5. The hatched areas in each column represent the dilutions at which the reactions were positive and the open areas, dilutions at which the test was negative. The highest titre for bile canalicular antibody was 1:256. In only four cases was there a positive reaction in undiluted sera. The remainder showed positive reactions only in diluted sera. As a rule, the titre for antinuclear factor was higher than for bile canicular antibody, although seven patients with the latter had no antinuclear factor.

Figure 6 concerns those sera which contained mitochondrial antibodies. The respective titres of mitochondrial antibody, antinuclear factor and bile canalicular antibody are illustrated. The small horizontal lines indicate that the mitochondrial antibody titre was 1. Serum from one patient only contained more mitochondrial antibody than bile canalicular antibody and antinuclear factor. All the other sera had low titres of mitochondrial antibody. In one of the 7 sera with mitochondrial antibody there was no bile canalicular antibody.

To find out to which immunoglobulin class the bile canalicular antibody belonged, we examined cryostat sections of bovine liver, previously incubated with serum containing bile canalicular antibody, after incubation with FITC labelled anti-IgG, anti-IgA and anti-IgM. All the sera from patients with chronic active liver disease gave a reaction only with anti-IgG, as did one of the two patients with acute hepatitis. The serum from the other patient with acute hepatitis gave a doubtful positive reaction with anti-IgM.

To-date we have found no correlation between clinical or biochemical findings and the presence of bile canalicular antibody. Six patients had normal or almost normal serum gamma globulin levels and in two patients the disease was inactive despite bile canalicular antibody being found in the serum. Neither was there a correlation between any particular histological type of chronic liver disease and serological findings in this small series (Table 5). The histological diagnosis was based on one liver biopsy only, in the majority of cases. Bile canalicular antibody was detected in some of the sera from all three histologial groups.

Table 5

Correlation of Histological and Serological Findings in 18 Patients

Diagnosis	No. of Positive Reactions	Bile Canalicular Antibody	ANF	Mitochondrial Antibody
Chronic aggressive hepatitis	5	+	+	–
(13 patients)	4	+	–	–
	1	–	+	–
Chronic persistent hepatitis	1	+	+	–
(2 patients)				
Cryptogenic cirrhosis	1	+	+	–
(3 patients)				

Serum dilution 1:10

Table 6

24 Sera Tested for Bile Canalicular Antibody Against Bovine and Human Liver

No. Sera	Bovine Liver	Human Liver	
		E	S
3	+	+	+
3	+	+	–
4	+	–	+
14	+	–	–

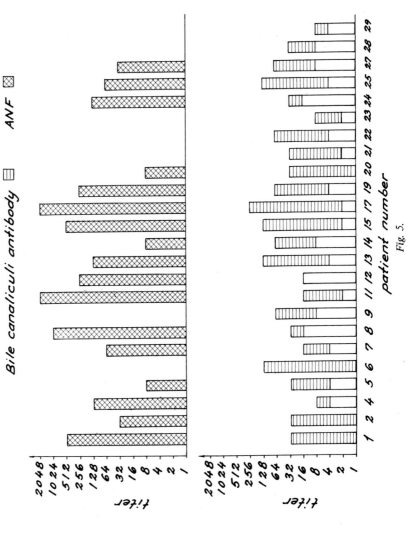

TITER OF BILE CANALICULI ANTIBODY AND ANF.

Bile canaliculi antibody   ANF

Fig. 5.

ANTIBODY TITERS IN SERA
WITH MITOCHONDRIAL ANTIBODY

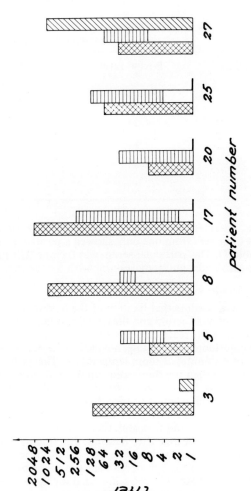

Fig. 6.

EXAMINATION FOR BILE CANALICULAR ANTIBODY
WITH HUMAN LIVER

All sera containing bile canalicular antibody reacting with bovine liver were examined for reactivity with cryostat sections of two normal human livers, E and S (Table 6). Ten of the sera reacted with one or both of the two human livers, whereas 14 of the sera only reacted with bovine liver. In 14 cases autologous

Table 7

*14 Sera Tested for Bile Canalicular Antibody Against Bovine,
Human and "Own" Liver*

No. Sera	Bovine Liver	Human Liver		"Own" Liver
		E	S	
1	+	+	+	+
2	+	+	+	−
2	+	+	−	−
2	+	−	+	−
7	+	−	−	−

liver, obtained by needle biopsy, was available for use as the antigen. Of these cases, the sera from one only showed a positive reaction to autologous liver (Table 7). This particular serum was the one that had given the highest titre for bile canalicular antibody reacting with bovine liver.

Relation to Fixation Procedure

It was possible that fixation of the bovine or human liver sections before applications of serum and fluorescein conjugated antihuman globulin had influenced the reaction between sera and bile canaliculi. Therefore, before the immunofluorescent testing, bovine liver sections were put into different fixatives for three minutes at room temperature. Thereafter, first the positive reacting serum and then the fluorescein conjugated antihuman globulin were applied to the sections. In the acetone-fixed section there was bright fluorescence of the bile canaliculi, whereas in the ethyl alcohol-fixed section there was only slight fluorescence. In the sections fixed with Lillie's fixative, Carnoy's solution or methyl alcohol and formalin, there was no reaction at all, that is to say, the reaction disappeared after fixation. The finding that sera with bile canalicular antibody reacting with bovine liver did not react with autologous liver, could be explained if the appropriate antigen in the human liver sections was soluble in the phosphate buffered saline used for the washing procedures. Therefore two sera which reacted with bovine liver but not with autologous unfixed liver were re-examined using sections of autologous liver fixed in various ways. However in no case did a negative reaction become positive.

CONCLUSION

We have demonstrated in the sera from many patients with chronic active liver disease an antibody reacting with bile canaliculi in bovine liver. In nearly half of the cases this antibody reacted with normal human liver but in only one of 14 sera did it react with autologous liver. As a rule the bile canalicular antibody was found together with antinuclear factor. It was seldom found together with mitochondrial antibody. Further investigation will be necessary to assess the role of this serum factor I today referred to as bile canalicular antibody.

This work is reported in greater detail in: H. Diederichsen (1969) Acta Med Scand 186, 299.

The reference to Johnson *et al.,* is as follows: Johnson, G. D., Holborrow, E. J., Glynn, L. E. (1966). Lancet: 2, 416.

DISCUSSION
Chairman: Professor I. M. Roitt

CHAIRMAN

Does the antibody fix complement if you use immunofluorescence?

DIEDERICHSEN

All the sera were inactivated.

DONIACH

Have you tried rat liver?

DIEDERICHSEN

No, because Johnson's studies were with rat liver.

CHAIRMAN

Dr. Glynn, have you any comments on the species reactivity, and what this might mean?

GLYNN

The incidence of what we thought was bile canalicular antibody in active chronic hepatitis was less than half the incidence of smooth muscle antibody. However I am not convinced that we were studying bile canalicular antibody because I have seen some preparations stained for bile canaliculi by Professor Sulitzeanu from Jerusalem which were quite different from our preparations. I must admit that his looked more like bile canaliculi although I am not sure how they were stained.

CHAIRMAN

Are you convinced that Dr. Diederichsen is staining bile canaliculi?

GLYNN

Well, his look more like ours! (LAUGHTER)

CHAIRMAN

What do you think yours might have been?

GLYNN

I don't know.

DONIACH

Is it at all possible that this has something to do with blood groups?

DIEDERICHSEN

We have not investigated that.

CHAIRMAN

But you have studied a number of other bovine tissues and if it was a blood group like antigen you would probably have detected fluorescence elsewhere.

DONIACH

We often see the intercellular ground substance staining in the thyroid — does this happen with bovine liver?

DIEDERICHSEN

One of the reasons that we used both diluted and undiluted sera was to avoid non-specific fluorescence, although the latter appears, to me at least, quite different from the fluorescence of bile canaliculi.

MacSWEEN

Have you in fact used other bovine tissues in your tests?

DIEDERICHSEN

No.

WALKER

In view of this argument about the canaliculus, have you used any special liver cell preparations? For instance, teased out cells or a suspension?

DIEDERICHSEN

No.

POPPER

What does formalin do to the fluorescence?

DIEDERICHSEN

It destroys it and therefore the reaction cannot be with acid phosphatase, as this would not be destroyed by formalin.

CHAIRMAN

This point about other bovine tissues could be an important one; I thought you had used them in your test — but now it seems that it might be something specifically antibovine.

DIEDERICHSEN

Yes, One of the two people with acute hepatitis had heterophile antibodies, although the other did not.

SERUM TOTAL HAEMOLYTIC COMPLEMENT IN LIVER DISEASE

A. P. Pagaltsos, M. G. M. Smith, A. L. W. F. Eddleston and Roger Williams

Recent developments in immunology have led to increased awareness of the biological importance of antibodies but at the same time it has become apparent that antibodies themselves are largely ineffective unless aided by certain effector systems. Complement constitutes the main immunologically relevant effector system that is present in serum.

THE COMPLEMENT SYSTEM AND PREVIOUS STUDIES IN LIVER DISEASE

Complement consists of nine components made up from 11 distinct serum proteins. These components exist in the serum in the form of precursors and are converted to the active form after interaction with immune complexes. The actual order of activation of the complement components in immunological haemolysis is shown in Fig. 1. Disorders of this system have been recognized in

COMPLEMENT COMPONENTS IN ORDER OF ACTION

$C'1$	$C'4$ $C'2$ $C'3$ $C'5$ $C'6$ $C'7$ $C'8$ $C'9$
$C'1q$ $C'1r$ $C'1s$	

Fig. 1.

human pathology for many years but despite its importance in immunological reactions the behaviour of this system in liver disease has been little studied. So far as I am aware, there have been only two studies of total haemolytic complement in liver disease in the last ten years.

Asherson (1960) found variable levels of total haemolytic complement in the serum of patients with disorders of the liver but his diagnoses were made on clinical grounds and without examination of liver histology. Townes (1967) in a more limited study found reduced complement levels in 6 of 7 patients with lupoid hepatitis but he did not examine patients with comparable liver damage due to other causes. In three other studies reduced levels of $\beta1C$ globulin, the third component of complement, have been reported in patients with active chronic hepatitis (MacLachlan *et al.,* 1965; Zlotnick and Rodnan, 1965; Mackay *et al.,* 1965).

TOTAL HAEMOLYTIC COMPLEMENT LEVELS IN PRESENT SERIES

We have used the method of Roulier (1950) to measure the total serum haemolytic complement. Sera were obtained from 108 patients admitted to the

Table 1

Diagnosis in the 108 Patients Studied

Diagnosis	Number of Cases	Diagnosis	Number of Cases
Cholangitis	4	Alcoholic Cirrhosis	13
Hepatic Abscess	5	Cryptogenic Cirrhosis	7
Primary Hepatoma Secondary Tumours	20	Haemochromatosis	14
Infective Hepatitis	13	Active Chronic Hepatitis	14
Acute Hepatic Necrosis	6	Primary Biliary Cirrhosis	10
Acute Budd Chiari Syndrome	2		

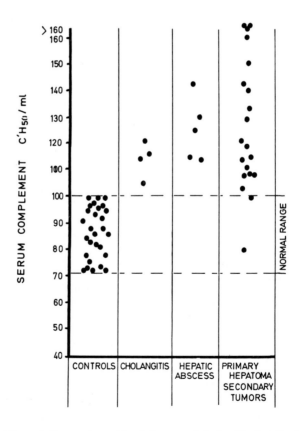

Fig. 2. Total haemolytic complement levels in cases of cholangitis, hepatic abscess and hepatic tumour.

Liver Unit of King's College Hospital. All diagnoses were confirmed histologically by percutaneous liver biopsy or at autopsy and the number of patients in each group is given in Table 1. The patients included in the group "active chronic hepatitis" had the clinical features of this condition with the histological appearances on biopsy of chronic aggressive hepatitis or active cirrhosis.

In general there were clear-cut differences in the various groups of patients with liver diseases. It is known that complement levels are elevated in presence of infection and the finding of elevated levels in our patient with cholangitis or hepatic abscess was not unexpected (Fig. 2). Others have described increased complement levels in patients with neoplasms, and again not unexpectedly, we found increased serum complement levels with a primary hepatoma or secondary hepatic deposits – this occurred in 18 of the 20 patients in this group. The elevation of complement levels in this condition is very likely to reflect an increase in production of complement proteins.

We have also found increased complement levels in infective hepatitis (Fig. 3). These were cases of moderate severity and all recovered to normal. In contrast, patients with acute hepatic necrosis showed extremely low complement levels. This was likely to be due to failure of production rather than increased utilization in an immune reaction. Two cases with the acute Budd Chiari syndrome, in whom one would not expect immunological reactions to be of prime importance, also had very low complement levels.

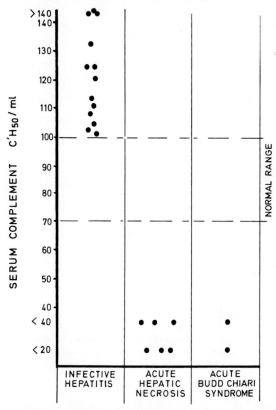

Fig. 3. Total haemolytic complement levels in cases of infective hepatitis, acute hepatic necrosis and acute Budd Chiari syndrome.

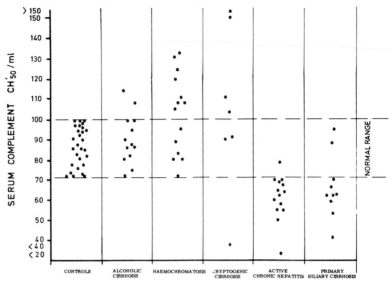

Fig. 4. Total haemolytic complement levels in case of cirrhosis.

Table 2
Possible Mechanisms of Alteration in Serum Complement
A ALTERATION IN SYNTHESIS OF C′ COMPONENTS B INCREASE OR DECREASE OF INHIBITORS C PASSIVE LOSS OR DESTRUCTION D ACTIVATION OR FIXATION *IN VIVO*

In cirrhosis there were distinct differences between the various subgroups (Fig. 4). In 12 of the 14 patients with alcoholic cirrhosis and in 6 of the 14 with idiopathic haemochromatosis the complement level was normal, high levels being found in the remaining patients in these two groups. In cryptogenic cirrhosis, some were normal and others increased and one was low. In contrast, the majority of the patients with active chronic hepatitis had low complement levels and 8 of 10 cases with primary biliary cirrhosis also showed low complement levels. As the degree of liver damage in these two groups appeared comparable to that in cryptogenic and alcoholic cirrhosis it is unlikely that the low complement level was simply due to a failure of synthesis. It is interesting that we found low complement levels in these two diseases in which there is most evidence of an auto-immune aetiology, and an increased utilization of complement may be the cause of the reduced level in these patients.

POSSIBLE MECHANISMS INVOLVED

Interpretation of the results is difficult because of the many different factors which can influence the complement levels in the serum (Table 2). The possible mechanisms leading to change in serum complement level are:—

(a) Alteration in synthesis of complement components.
(b) Alteration in concentration or activity of complement inhibitors.
(c) Passive loss or destruction of complement.
(d) Activation or fixation of complement *in vivo*; and there may be a combination of these mechanisms.

It is thought that some of the complement components are synthesized in the reticulo-endothelial system and some, particularly C′3, by the liver (Thorbecke *et al.*, 1965; Chester *et al.*, 1969). Failure of hepatic production might therefore be an explanation for the very low complement levels found in our cases with severe liver damage, i.e., acute hepatic necrosis and acute Budd Chiari syndrome. The increased levels of complement found in certain of the groups is likely to represent increased synthesis for many of the complement component proteins are known to behave as acute phase reactants. High levels in cirrhosis may also reflect increased activity of reticulo-endothelial system in these patients (Chiandussi *et al.*, 1963).

There are naturally occurring inhibitors of complement in the serum and it is possible for alteration in complement levels to be secondary to a change in concentration or activity of a complement inhibitor. This has been proved in hereditary or angioneurotic oedema in which the inhibitor of the first component is deficient or defective (Donalson and Evans, 1963). But the significance of alterations of complement inhibitors in liver disease is not known. Passive loss of complement may occur in situations in which increased protein loss occurs, such as in the nephrotic syndrome but this is unlikely to be of importance in patients with liver disease.

INCREASED UTILIZATION IN AUTO-IMMUNE LIVER DISEASE

Because of the many factors which may affect complement levels, it is difficult to pick out those cases where complement is involved in immunological reactions. However, by exclusion of other factors, it is possible that increased utilization of complement is the reason for the decreased serum levels in patients with active chronic hepatitis and primary biliary cirrhosis. On the other hand, although auto-antibodies are found in the serum of most of these patients, we were unable to demonstrate any quantitative relationship between titres of serum auto-antibodies and complement levels.

There was also no correlation between low serum complement levels and the high serum IgG levels in patients with active chronic hepatitis (Fig. 5). It is interesting that there was some suggestion of a quantitative relationship between levels of complement and of IgM in serum of patients with primary biliary cirrhosis (Fig. 6).

CONCLUSION AND FINDINGS AFTER LIVER TRANSPLANTATION

We would interpret the changes in the complement system in liver diseases in the following way (Table 3). Elevation of complement levels in cases of cholangitis or with primary or secondary hepatic tumour and in some cases of cirrhosis may be due to increased synthesis of complement. This is thought to occur with infections or inflammation in other sites. Decrease in synthesis of complement is the explanation for the very low levels in acute hepatic necrosis. Finally, increased utilization of complement through fixation by circulating or trapped immune complexes, or through fixation by antibody to cell or tissue antigens, may account for the low levels in active chronic hepatitis and primary biliary cirrhosis.

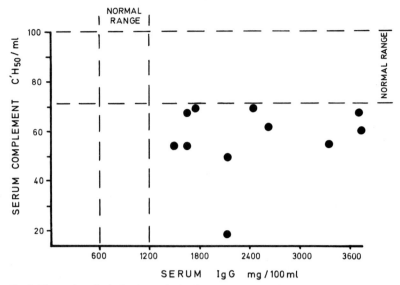

Fig. 5. Illustrating the lack of correlation between serum IgG levels and total haemolytic complement levels in cases with active chronic hepatitis.

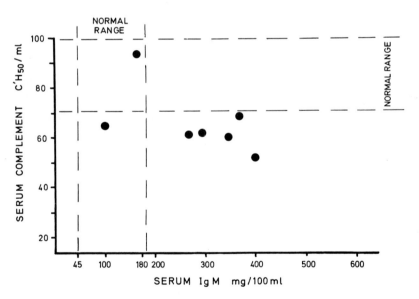

Fig. 6. Comparing total haemolytic complement levels with serum IgM levels in patients with primary biliary cirrhosis.

The main problem in studies of this kind is to differentiate between increased consumption of complement and decreased synthesis. This problem is well illustrated by Fig. 7. This shows serum total complement levels in one patient after liver transplantation. This patient had severe hepatocellular damage and on the 20th day after the transplantation the serum aspartate aminotransferase levels were more than 1,000 u/ml. At this stage total haemolytic complement

Table 3

Explanation for Changes in Complement Observed in Patients with Liver Disease

Increased C' Synthesis	Decreased C' Synthesis	Increased C' Utilization
Infections	Extensive Liver Damage	A – Fixation of C' by circulating or trapped antigen antibody complexes
Inflammatory States		
Tumours		B – Fixation of C' by antibody to cell or tissue antigens

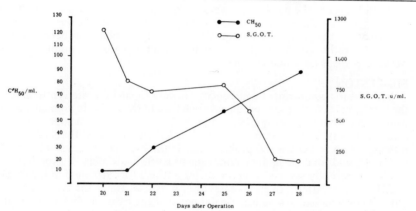

Fig. 7. Serial data in one patient after liver transplantation.

was very low. During the next 8 days liver function steadily improved and during the same period serum total complement gradually rose to normal levels. One might well say that this was due to recovery of the synthetic capacity of the liver. But on the other hand the prothrombin time was normal even on the 20th day suggesting that the synthetic capacity of the liver, at least with regard to the clotting factors, was not impaired. This would support the alternative explanation that there was increased consumption rather than decreased synthesis.

This distinction will only be possible when methods are available for studying the metabolism of individual components of serum complement. Such techniques are being developed and these should lead to a better understanding of the role of the complement system in the pathogenesis of auto-immune liver disease.

REFERENCES

Alper, C. A., Johnson, A. M., Birtch, A. G. and Moore, F. D. (1969) Science 163, 286.
Asherson, G. L. (1960) Australian Ann. Med. 9, 57.
Chiandussi, L., Greco, F., Cesaro, L., Murator, F., Vaccoino, A. and Corradi, C. (1963) J. Lab. Clin. Med. 62, 968.
Donalson, H. V. and Evans, R. R. (1963) Am. J. Med. 35, 37.
Mackay, I. R., Weiden, S. and Hasker, J. (1965) Ann. N.Y. Acad. Sci. 124, 767.

MacLachlan, M., Rodnam, G. P., Cooper, W. H. and Fennell, R. H. (1965) Ann. Int. Med.
      62, 425.
Roulier, P. (1950) Sur une reaction quantitative de fixation du complement titre and 50%
      d'hemalyse. These (de Pharmacie), Montpellier.
Thorbecke, G. J., Hochwald, G. M., Van Furth, R., Müller Eberhard, H. J. and Jacobson,
      E. B. (1965) In: Wolstenholme, G. E. W. and Knight, J. (EAS): Complement. Ciba
      Foundation Symposium. Boston, Little, Brown, p. 99.
Townes, A. S. (1967) Bull. Johns. Hopk. Hosp. 120, 337.
Zlotnick, A. and Rodnam, G. P. (1962) Proc. Soc. Exp. Biol. Med. 109, 742.

DISCUSSION
Chairman: Dr. M. H. Lessof

CHAIRMAN
At this stage of the meeting we were hoping to have Dr. Finlayson of New
York to talk about his work on Australia antigen. I believe that he was also to tell us
of his work in the complement field. Unfortunately his plane has been grounded.
However, I gather Dr. Adrian Eddleston has recently heard the complement
work, so perhaps he would comment.

EDDLESTON
Some of the complement components, mainly C_3 and C_4, are synthesized in
the liver, whereas others are produced elsewhere in the body. In animals the only
component definitely not synthesized in the liver is C1Q, which appears to be
made in the gut. There is some evidence that C1Q in man is synthesized in the
terminal ileum and colon and probably not in the liver. Dr. Finlayson has studied
C_3 and C_4 and total haemolytic complement levels in a variety of liver diseases
and he has recently succeeded in producing antisera for future use in the study
of C1Q concentrations. In all his cases of cirrhosis, whatever the aetiology, he
found some who had low values. He did not find the clear-cut distinction that
Dr. Pagaltsos has found. Examining his cases in more detail, he went on to plot
the levels of C_3, C_4 or total haemolytic complement against serum albumin
levels or the prothrombin time, the latter being taken as measures of synthetic
liver function. He found that all cases with low complement levels had low serum
albumin, and increased prothrombin times, whereas in patients with normal or
increased levels of complement these values were normal. Although some of his
cases of active chronic hepatitis had low complement levels, he felt this was
more likely to be due to the diminished synthesis of hepatocellular damage
rather than to increased consumption in an immunological reaction.
The answer to this problem should become clear from examination of C1Q
levels — the component of complement not made in the liver. He believes that
there is no good evidence as yet for increased consumption of complement in
any chronic liver disease but he also acknowledges the great difficulty of
deciding whether decreased synthesis or increased consumption is predominant.

WILLIAMS
Dr. Finlayson's patients with primary biliary cirrhosis and low complement
levels were all in advanced liver-cell failure, consistent with the concept of a
synthetic defect. But in Dr. Pagaltsos's series, these cases were not necessarily in
advanced liver-cell failure; they represented the whole spectrum of primary
biliary cirrhosis and yet all of them had low complement levels.

DYKES
Dr. Wentworth and I have studied complement levels after experimental
radiation hepatitis. Biochemical evidence of liver disease after radiation did not

appear for some weeks. However, as early as seven days after radiation there was a significant reduction in complement. At this time auto-antibodies were appearing in the serum several weeks before the rise in transaminase values or a reduction in albumin levels. Have you measured complement levels serially in relation to immuno-suppressive treatment?

PAGALTSOS

Unfortunately we have not carried out serial studies in our patients, nor have we related complement levels to immuno-suppressive therapy.

TUGHILL

Was there any significant difference in the serum complement levels between those with primary tumours of the liver and those with secondary tumours? Is there any evidence that primary hepatocellular tumours can synthesize complement?

PAGALTSOS

We found no difference between these two groups. Some of our primary hepatomas gave very high levels of complement, but not all.

FOX

I have measured the third component of complement in 25 patients with primary biliary cirrhosis and have not found any low levels to date. Some of the cases with active chronic hepatitis and one with cryptogenic cirrhosis had low levels. The most striking finding is in the patients with massive necrosis, who have consistently low values whatever the aetiology. One interesting lady was deeply comatose with a flat EEG as a result of massive necrosis of the liver. She was treated by pig liver perfusion and both during this time, and for a week afterwards her complement levels were very low. However, as her serum albumin rose so her complement levels returned to normal; this would support the idea of diminished synthesis in this situation.

PAGALTSOS

And did she recover?

FOX

Yes, she is now quite well with normal complement levels.

RAKE

There is a notable increase in consumption of proteins in acute hepatic necrosis, particularly of fibrinogen, so could there not also have been an increased consumption of complement?

FOX

I have no evidence on that.

DONIACH

We often notice very high anticomplementary effects in the serum during complement-fixation studies in active chronic hepatitis. I have attributed this to the presence of soluble complexes. Is that likely do you think?

PAGALTSOS

I cannot answer this. In some of our cases with low complement levels I have tried unsuccessfully to find anticomplementary substances.

Meyer zum BUSCHENFELDE

We, too, have seen anticomplementary activity in these patients and it occurred to us that another cause might be gamma globulin aggregates. Anticomplementary activity seems to be common in patients with high gamma globulin levels and such activity can be abolished by adding albumin to the serum as described by Wigand and by Schierz. Provided that the gamma globulin fraction is less than 30% of the total protein then little anticomplementary activity is found.

VELASCO

We have also found very low complement levels in fulminant hepatitis in Chile. The levels in active chronic hepatitis have varied according to the activity of the disease. In two of these cases as the activity of the disease increased so the complement levels fell.

EDDLESTON

Dr. Finlayson has measured complement serially in three patients and made the opposite point. He correlated complement levels not with disease activity *per se*, but with synthetic liver function and again found a close relationship with albumin levels and prolongation of prothrombin time.

PROPERTIES OF ANTIBODIES REACTING WITH HOMOLOGOUS AND HETEROLOGOUS LIVER MITOCHONDRIAL FRACTIONS

Gy. Dobias, Erzsebet Palasti, Marta Vegh and Gy. Szecsey

It is well known that antibodies reacting with human liver mitochondrial fraction (MF) may appear in the serum of patients suffering from various liver diseases. The production of antibodies reacting with MF has been demonstrated in animal experiments involving active immunization with homologous and heterologous liver and kidney mitochondrial fractions (Asherson and Dumonde, 1962; Dobias and Balazs, 1967a). The immune sera so produced gave rise to various pathological changes during 70-day passive immunization experiments (Dobias and Balazs, 1967b). In the present study we analyse the mechanisms by which the humoral antibodies reacting with mitochondrial fractions may induce pathological changes.

METHODS AND TECHNIQUES

Preparation of Mitochondrial Fractions

After removal, the livers from rats or rabbits were placed into chilled TMSK solution (see below) and then passed through a wire mesh. The resulting suspension was diluted 1:10 W/V with TMSK solution, homogenized in a Potter-Elvehjem homogenizer and centrifuged for 10 minutes at 700 g. The supernatant was set aside and the sediment was washed once with TMSK solution. The sediment obtained after the second centrifugation is subsequently referred to as the *nuclear fraction*. The pooled supernatants from preceding centrifugations were centrifuged at 8000 g. for 10 minutes. The sediment was washed once with TMSK solution and twice with 1 % NaCl solution. The sediment obtained after the last washing, the *mitochondrial fraction* (MF) was diluted with an equal volume of physiological NaCl solution; 100 U./ml. penicillin and 1 mg. ml. streptomycin were added as preservatives, and the material was stored at $-20°C$ until used. Each step of the subcellular fractionation was carried out at $+4°C$. The renal mitochondrial fraction was prepared by a similar procedure.

The TMSK solution was constituted as follows:— 10 ml. of 0·5 M $MgCl_2$ $6H_2O$, 20 ml. of 0·25 M KCl, 100 ml. of 0·2 M TRIS pH 7·4 and 85 g. of Sucrose made up to 1 litre with distilled water.

Prior to the immunization and *in vitro* tests, the MF was thawed and used either without centrifugation, or after further centrifugation, separating the supernatant of MF (MF SUP) and its sediment (MF SED). By freezing and thawing, the mitochondria were destroyed and their soluble antigens and some of the enzymes they contained were liberated into the supernatant.

Immunization procedures

Active immunization was induced in male rabbits weighing 2000 to 2500 g. in groups of four animals. Antigen admixed with equal parts of incomplete Freunds adjuvant (Difco), was administered intramuscularly on four occasions at intervals of 3 weeks. Each rabbit received 80 to 100 mg. of protein antigen per inoculation. The rabbits were exsanguinated 2 weeks after the last inoculation and the antisera so obtained were used in the subsequent experiments.

103

Passive immunization was carried out as follows: male rats weighing 150 to 170 g. were inoculated in groups of 5 animals with immune rabbit sera. The antisera were administered intravenously on 14 occasions at intervals of 3 to 4 days.

Complement fixation test

First, the maximum amount of MF which did not inactivate complement was determined. This corresponded to an MF dilution containing 3·0 mg. protein/ml. To facilitate comparisons, the sera were also diluted to as to contain 3·0 mg. protein/ml. In each test 0·2 ml. of diluted serum, 0·3 ml. of antigen, 0·5 ml. of complement (2·5 HU complement) were used. This mixture was incubated at 37°C for 30 minutes, then, after the addition of 0·25 ml. of a 4 % sensitized sheep erythrocyte suspension, it was allowed to stand for a further 30 minutes at 37°C. The serum titre was considered to be the first serum dilution which showed complete haemolysis.

Estimation of O_2 consumption

1 ml. volumes of the rat or rabbit liver MF were added to Warburg vessels, followed by the addition of 2·0 ml. of 100% glucose containing Krebs-Ringer phosphate solution (pH 7·4) and 1·0 ml. of rabbit immune serum or control serum. The CO_2 produced was adsorbed by 0·2 ml. of a 20 % KOH solution. The gaseous phase was air. The temperature of the mixture was adjusted to 37·5°C and, after 5 minutes of preincubation, the assay was started. Readings were taken at 10-minute intervals for 75 minutes. O_2 consumption was expressed as ul./mg. dry weight of MF. The test was done in triplicate and the mean taken.

Assay of Enzyme activity in MF (SUP)

Changes in enzyme activity were calculated from the activities of the following mixtures.
(a)   0·5 ml. of the diluted immune or control serum + 0·5 ml. of physiological saline.
(b)   0·5 ml. of MF SUP + 0·5 ml. of physiological saline.
(c)   0·5 ml. of the diluted immune or control serum + 0·5 ml. of MF SUP.
The mixtures were incubated for 30 minutes at 37°C, and aliquots were then assayed for enzyme activity. The results for (a) and (b) were summated and inhibition of enzyme activity by antisera was considered to have occurred when the value for (c) was at least 20% lower than that of (a) + (b). Stimulation of enzyme activity is spoken of when the former exceeded the latter by at least 20%.

Lymphocyte cytotoxicity reaction

The macro method of Engelfreit (1966) was used. 3 drops of test serum, 1 drop of leucocyte suspension in unheated AB serum (cell count 8000 per mm^3) and 1 drop of rat or rabbit complement were incubated for 1 hour at 37°C. 1 drop of a 1% trypan blue solution dissolved in distilled water was then added to the mixture. The ratio of killed cells to normal cells in expressed as a percentage.

RESULTS

The mitochondrial fractions used for the immunization studies were characterized microscopically and on the basis of their enzyme spectrum. The fraction was seen to contain small and large mitochondria, small amounts of lysosomes, parts of the endoplasmic reticulum and ribosomes. In the MF

SUP we could demonstrate not only aspartate aminotransferase isoenzymes of mitochondrial origin (pH optimum 6·0) but also lysosomal and endoplasmic reticulum enzymes — beta glucuronidase, acid phosphatase, and alkaline phosphatase.

Complement fixation test

In Table 1 the complement fixing titres of sera from rabbits immunized with homologous and heterologous antigens are presented. The frozen and thawed uncentrifuged mitochondrial fraction, containing both soluble and

Table 1

Complement Fixing Titres of the Immune Sera

Rabbit immune serum	No. of immu- nized rabbits	Antigens (3000μg. protein/ml.)			
		Rat MF	Rat serum	Rabbit MF	Rabbit serum
Anti-rat MF	4	1:40–1:80	<1:5	<1:5	<1:5
Anti-rat MF SUP	1	1:40	<1:5	<1:5	<1:5
Anti-rat MF SED	1	1:20	<1:5	<1:20	<1:5
Anti-rat serum	4	1:40–1:80	1:10–1:20	<1:5	<1:5
Anti-rabbit MF	4	1:10–1:20	<1:5	1:10–1:20	<1:5
Anti-rabbit serum	4	.1:5	<1:5	<1:5	<1:5

corpuscular antigens were used in each test. In some cases, sera from non-immunized rabbits reacted in low titres (<1:5) with both the rat and the rabbit mitochondria, as has been reported by Weir *et al.,* (1966). Therefore all immune sera were tested at dilutions of 1:5 or greater.

After immunization with *heterologous* (rat) MF, in addition to anti-rat MF antibodies, complement fixing auto-antibodies reacting with the rabbits' own antigens may be produced — presumably as a result of antigen cross reactivity (Asherson and Dumonde, 1964; Dobias and Balazs, 1967a). In an earlier experimental series, such auto-antibodies were produced following immunization with MF containing both soluble and corpuscular antigens. In the present series, however, complement fixing auto-antibodies cross-reacting with rat MF were only obtained by immunization with *MF sediment,* containing mainly corpuscular antigens.

No complement fixing antibodies reacting with rat or rabbit serum were formed, in spite of the fact that serum protein antigens could be demonstrated in the MF by means of antisera from rabbits immunized with pooled rat sera.

When homologous (rabbit) liver MF was used as the immunizing antigen, antibodies reacting with homologous liver were produced at much lower titres than following immunization with heterologous MF. Furthermore the antibodies could not be demonstrated in every rabbit. When they did occur these antibodies cross-reacted with the heterologous (rat) liver MF.

GEL diffusion studies

After immunization with heterologous (rat) liver MF, precipitating auto-antibodies reacting with soluble antigens of the homologous liver MF, were found. This provided another example of immunization with heterologous organ antigens stimulating auto-antibody production. However, unlike the complement fixing antibodies, the immune sera also cross-reacted with the serum proteins of both rats and rabbits, (Table 2). In the rabbit anti-rat MF serum at least 7 antibodies were detected by comparative gel diffusion analysis (Oakley and Fulthorpe, 1953) that reacted with the soluble antigens of the rat liver MF, but not with the serum proteins (Table 3).

Table 2

Minimum Number of Antigen-antibody Systems Demonstrable by Linear Double Gel Diffusion Technique

Rabbit immune serum	No. of immu-nized rabbits	Antigens			
		Rat NF SUP	Rat serum	Rabbit MF SUP	Rabbit serum
Anti-rat MF	1	10	5	2	0
	2	6	5	1	0
	3	6	4	0	0
Anti-rat MF SUP	4	6	–	–	–
Anti-rat MF SED	5	3	–	–	–
Anti-rat serum	6	6	22	0	1
	7	7	22	0	1
Anti-rabbit MF	9	0	0	2	1
	10	1	0	1	0
	11	0	0	0	0
	12	0	0	0	0
Anti-rabbit serum	13	0	0	0	0

Table 3

Comparative Gel Diffusion Studies

(Cross reaction between rabbit antibodies and rat antigens)

Rabbit immune serum	Antibodies not reacting with rat serum proteins	Antibodies reacting with rat serum proteins
Anti-rat MF	7*	4
Anti-rat MF SUP	4	2
Anti-rat serum	0	14
Anti-rabbit MF	1	1
Anti-rabbit serum	0	0

Antigens: Rat MF SUP
             Normal rat serum

* Number of the precipitation bands.

Serum proteins could be demonstrated in the rat MF both by the complement fixation and gel diffusion methods. The type and amounts of serum proteins present, were studied by antigen dilution (semiquantitative) immuno-electrophoresis (Jako, 1967). Using rabbit antisera to pooled rat sera, albumin, beta lipoprotein, transferrin and two unidentified beta globulins were detected in rat MF. After measurement of the distance of the precipitation bands of individual serum proteins from the antibody well, the values were compared with calibration curves plotted for individual serum proteins versus different dilutions of pooled rat serum. The results suggest that the concentration of albumin and transferrin in rat MF corresponded to that in normal serum diluted 1:35. However, the supernatant of the original liver homogenate was diluted about 8000 fold during preparation of MF! At such a dilution immuno-electro-phoresis would not detect the presence of serum proteins. Their presence in the MF could be due either to absorption onto the surface of the subcellular organelles or to contamination with endoplasmic reticulum, in which albumin and transferrin are synthesized.

Of the 4 rabbits immunized with homologous liver MF, the sera from 2 contained no antibodies to rabbit liver MF. In the two sera that did react many fewer precipitins were found as compared to the results of immunization with heterologous MF. In one case cross reaction with rat MF was observed (Table 2).

Studies of cytotoxic antibodies

It is known that iso, and species specific histocompatibility antigens are mainly found on the surface membranes of nucleated cells or on the membranes of subcellular organelles. The antibodies to these antigens may be demonstrated by lymphocyte cytotoxicity testing. We have designed our experiments to show whether such antibodies would appear in serum in response to immunization with MF.

Sera from rabbits immunized with heterologous (rat) MF were cytotoxic for rat lymphocytes at dilutions up to 1:16, whereas the sera from rabbits immunized with rat serum or rabbit mitochondria had no such effect on the rat lymphocytes. It should be emphasized that rabbit sera may contain natural antibodies capable of reacting with rat lymphocytes, therefore the cytotoxicity test with serum diluted 1:1 was only considered positive when the dead cell count exceeded 20%.

Sera from rabbits immunised with homologous mitochondria did not react with rabbit lymphocytes (Table 4). Ehrlich and Halbert (1968) have reported similar findings: duck anti-adult rabbit lens sera produced striking cytotoxicity against rabbit lens epithelium in tissue culture, whereas homologous antisera to rabbit lens did not produce cytotoxic effects *in vitro*.

Enzyme activity studies

By gel diffusion analysis, circulating antibodies reacting with soluble anti-gens in MF SUP that were not serum proteins, were found in sera from rabbits immunized with MF or MF SUP. As various enzymes can be demonstrated in substantial amounts in the MF SUP, it seemed worthwhile to investigate whether these immune sera contained antibodies capable of blocking or enhancing enzyme activity. In the literature, antibodies enhancing enzyme activity have been reported with respect to maltosidase, penicillinase (Pollock, 1964) and to ribonuclease (Cinader, 1966). According to Cinader, most enzymes contain more than one antigenic determinant group. The binding of antibody to these determinants may alter the form of the enzyme so that, as a result of steric inhibition, the substrate may not gain access to the active site. On the other hand different antibodies may make the active site more accessible for the substrate, leading to an increase of enzyme activity. Different individuals of the same species may produce these antibodies in varying amounts and although either inhibitory or stimulating antibodies may occur, a mixture of them is likely to be present in the immune serum. On adding enzyme to such a serum, the activity measured will be resultant of the two opposing antibody effects. Cinader (1964) immunized five rabbits with chemically modified ribonuclease and demonstrated the presence of

Table 4

Cytotoxicity Reaction with Sera from Rabbits Immunized with

Heterologous and Homologous MF

Rabbit immune serum	No. of immu-nized rabbits	Test cells			
		Rat lymphocytes** Serum dilution		Rabbit lymphocytes*** Serum dilution	
		1:1	1:16	1:1	1:16
Anti-rat MF	1	95*	44	1	2
	2	81	17	1	0
	3	58	2	2	2
Anti-rat serum	6	12	1	2	1
	7	12	0	0	1
	8	14	0	1	0
Anti-rabbit MF	9	4	1	0	1
	10	13	0	0	1
	11	6	1	1	0
	12	8	1	0	0
Anti-rabbit serum	13	8	0	0	0
	16	4	0	0	2
Control (Serum from unimmunized rabbit)		13	1	2	0

* The numbers represent the percentage of dead (blue) cells.
** Rat complement was used in the test.
*** Rabbit complement was used in the test.

"inhibitory" antibodies in the sera from 4 and of "stimulating" antibody in the serum from 1 rabbit.

Respiratory Enzymes – In this experiment, confirming our previous report (Szecsey *et al.*, 1966), pooled sera from rabbits immunized with heterologous (rat) liver MF, significantly inhibited the O_2 consumption by rat liver MF, although they increased the consumption by rabbit liver MF. Pooled sera from rabbits immunized with rat serum were used as the controls (Fig. 1).

Pooled sera from two rabbits (Nos. 9 and 10) immunized with homologous liver MF likewise inhibited the O_2 consumption of the rabbit liver, MF but to a lesser extent than the heterologous antiserum with rat MF. Pooled sera from rabbits immunized with rabbit serum were used as the controls (Fig. 2).

Other Enzymes – The antiserum to heterologous (rat) liver MF SUP reduced the aspartate aminotransferase activity (pH 7·4) of rat MF SUP by 50%, (Fig. 3). For aspartate aminotransferase (pH 6·0), alanine aminotransferase and; acid phosphatase the activity did not change significantly (see Methods) but in the case of beta glucuronidase (measured according to Szasz, 1963) the "c" value was 27% higher than "a + b" and therefore a slight increase of activity had been demonstrated. The sera from rabbits immunized with rat serum neither inhibited nor enhanced the activity of the above enzymes.

Of the sera from 4 rabbits immunized with heterologous (rat) liver MF, one contained antibody inhibiting aspartate aminotransferase (pH 7·4) activity

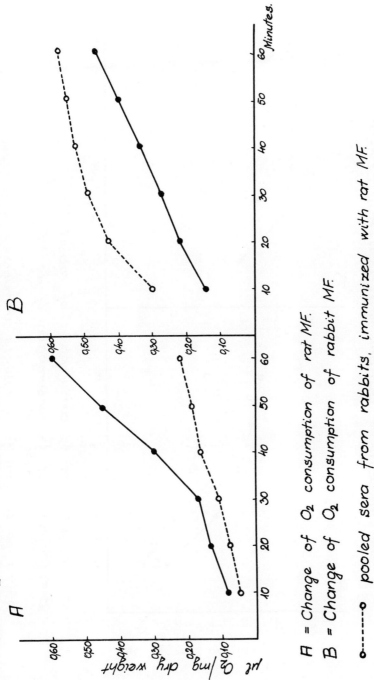

CHANGE OF O₂ CONSUMPTION OF MF-S BY RABBIT ANTI-RAT-MF SERUM AND CONTROL SERUM.

A = Change of O₂ consumption of rat MF.
B = Change of O₂ consumption of rabbit MF.

o----o pooled sera from rabbits, immunized with rat MF.
●——● pooled sera from rabbits, immunized with rat serum

Figure 1

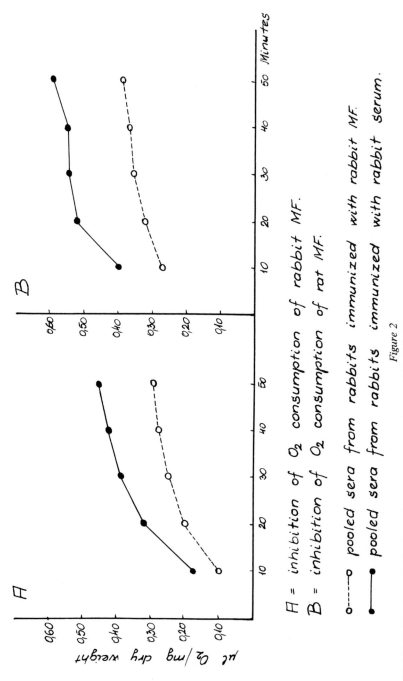

INHIBITION OF O₂ CONSUMPTION OF MF S by RABBIT
ANTI-RABBIT MF SERUM AND CONTROL SERUM

A = inhibition of O_2 consumption of rabbit MF.
B = inhibition of O_2 consumption of rat MF.

o------o pooled sera from rabbits immunized with rabbit MF.
●———● pooled sera from rabbits immunized with rabbit serum.

Figure 2

INHIBITION OF GOT ACTIVITY OF MF SUP BY RABBIT ANTI-RAT-MF SUP SERUM.

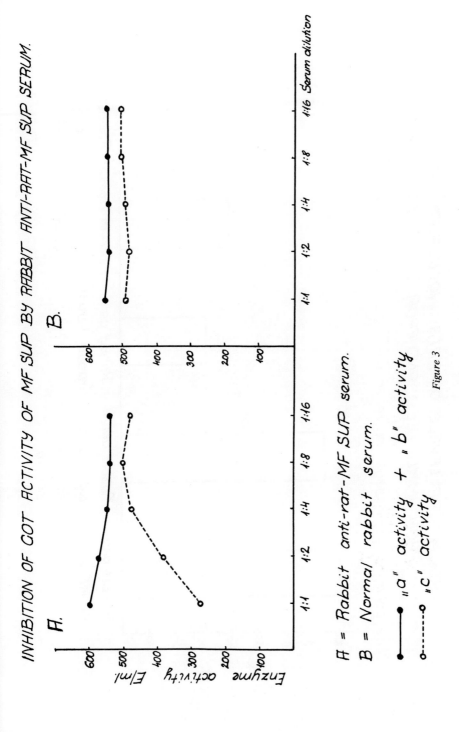

A = Rabbit anti-rat-MF SUP serum.
B = Normal rabbit serum.

●———● "a" activity + "b" activity
○----○ "c" activity

Figure 3

SERUM GPT LEVELS OF RATS INOCULATED WITH SERA FROM IMMUNIZED AND FROM UNTREATED RABBITS.

(The columns represent the mean GPT activity of sera from 5 rats each.)

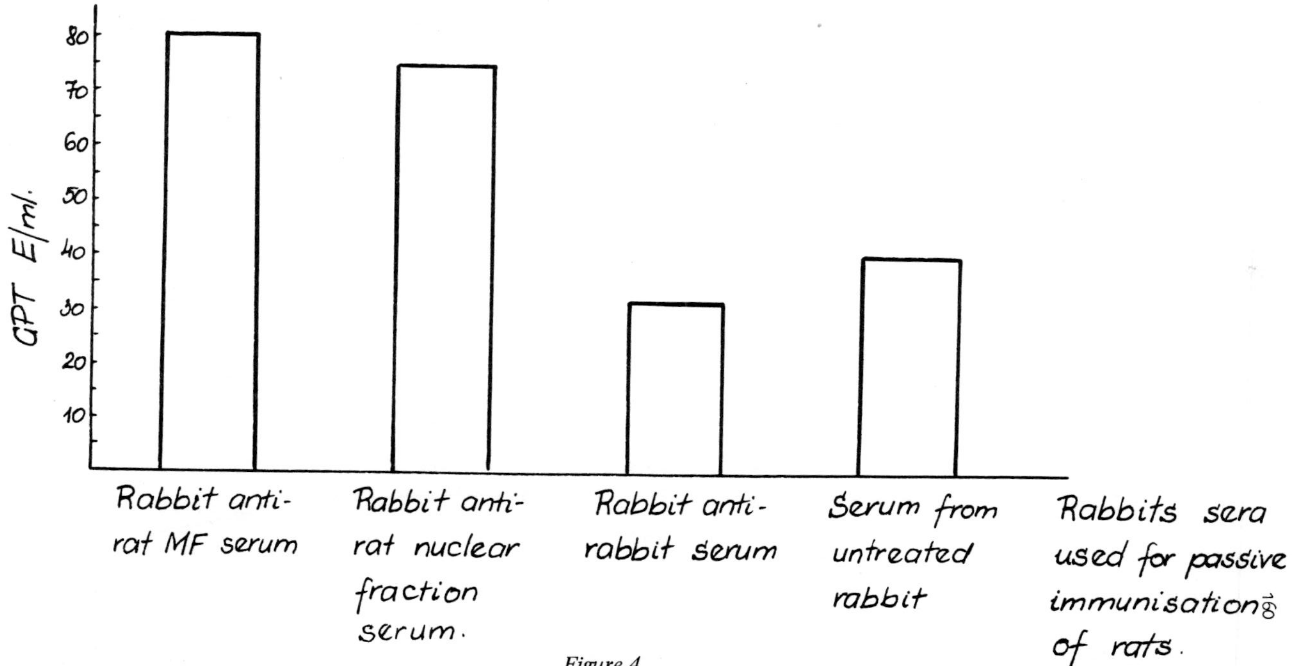

Figure 4

in rat MF SUP. This serum did not inhibit the alanine aminotransferase and beta glucuronidase activity of the rat MF SUP nor the aspartate aminotransferase activity (pH 7·4) of rabbit MF SUP.

In the present series, sera from rabbits immunized with homologous MF had no effect on the aspartate aminotransferase isoenzymes, alanine aminotransferase or beta glucuronidase activities. However in a previous study the serum from one of 3 rabbits immunized with this antigen did reduce alanine aminotransferase acitivity.

Passive immunization studies

In previous experiments (Dobias and Balazs, 1967a; Dobias and Balazs, 1967b) 4 rabbits had been immunized with rat liver MF and 5 with rat kidney MF. Batches of 5 rats were inoculated with the pooled sera from either group. Two weeks after the last inoculation, the % bromsulphthalein retention was determined at 45 mins. in each rat. The results were compared with those obtained from a control group of rats inoculated with sera from non-immunized rabbits. The % retention of bromsulphthalein in animals treated with antiserum to liver MF was nearly three times that found in the other two groups.

In the present investigation rats were inoculated with individual sera from untreated rabbits and from rabbits inoculated with rat liver MF, rat liver nuclear fractions, or pooled rat sera respectively. Fourteen days after the last inoculation, the serum alanine aminotransferase levels were determined. Levels in rats treated with immune sera reacting with the liver fractions were about double those found in the control group (Fig. 4).

DISCUSSION

It is known that humoral antibodies against autologous and less frequently isologous or heterologous antigens may have pathogenic significance in certain diseases. Examples that can be quoted include: the antibodies to red blood cells in auto-immune haemolytic anaemia; those reacting with the parietal cells of the gastric mucosa and with intrinsic factor in pernicious anaemia; the humoral antibodies reacting with transplantation antigens in homograft rejection and antibodies reacting with animal insulins in certain cases of insulin-resistant diabetes.

Recently, Hausaman *et al.*, (1969) have offered convincing proof as to the pathogenetic role of humoral antibodies in tissue reactions. In their experiments rabbits were immunized with guinea pig gastric and colonic mucosal antigens. Subsequently guinea pigs were inoculated with the immune sera. In response to the active immunization, the rabbits produced auto-antibodies as well as antibodies to guinea pig antigens. In the rabbits with auto-antibody to gastric mucosa as well as in the guinea pigs passively immunized with this serum, DNA synthesis by the gastric mucosal cells was significantly inhibited. Furthermore, pathological changes developed in the stomach of guinea pigs. In the guinea pigs inoculated with sera containing colonic mucosal antibodies, the synthesis of DNA was inhibited in the cells of the colonic mucosa, while in the rabbits with auto-antibodies to this tissue, the activity of DNA increased in the cells of the colonic mucosa. The cause of the latter phenomenon is unknown, although it is tempting to speculate that enhancing antibodies were involved. Choudhuri (1968) passively immunized dogs with antisera to dog liver raised in rabbits; following treatment, moderate increases were noted in the serum enzyme and cholesterol levels, as well as in bromsulphthalein retention.

Our aim was to determine what antibodies of biological importance were produced by active immunization with MF and to confirm the tissue damaging effect of humoral antibodies by means of passive immunization studies with heterologous immune sera. We had chosen passive rather than active immunization because the latter produces a delayed hypersensitivity response as well as a humoral response, and the relative roles of each in the production of tissue damage cannot then be assessed. We treated our animals with heterologous rather than homologous immune sera because we and others (Richter *et al.*, 1966) have found that under identical experimental conditions, immunization with heterologous antigens leads to the production of antibodies active on many more antigenic determinants.

In our experiments the serum alanine aminotransferase levels and bromusulphthalein retention levels in rats inoculated with antiserum to rat liver MF, were two or three times higher than the control values. We believe that under certain conditions humoral antibodies reacting with cells or cellular organelles can both initiate and exacerbate pathological processes. It is likely that in these experiments several antibodies, differing in site of action, are responsible for the pathogenic effect of the immune sera. In producing tissue damage the antibodies involved are presumably

(1) Cytotoxic antibodies reacting with the organ iso-, or species specific receptors of the cell membrane. These antibodies may, in the presence of complement, profoundly affect the integrity of the cell membrane. Thereby serious disorders in cell permeability and ionic equilibrium are produced making it possible for other antibodies to enter the cell.

(2) Antibodies reacting with intracellular antigens, inhibiting or occasionally enhancing enzyme activity. These may interfere with the fine mechanism of intermediate metabolism and may increase the severity of the cellular lesion outlined above.

It is also important that the individual animals differed considerably, both quantitatively and qualitatively, in response to immunization with the same antigens. There were differences in the number of precipitation bands, in the cytotoxic antibody titres and in the appearance of antibodies inhibiting enzyme activity from rabbit to rabbit; some rabbits produced neither complement fixing antigens nor precipitins in response to immunization with homologous MF, and so on. The cause of this heterogeneity is probably that MF contains many antigenic groups, and the formation of antibodies in a given case will depend on antigenic competition as well as on differences in individual reactivity.

May the results of these experiments be relied upon in human pathology? A generalization seems unwarranted in view of the following considerations.

(1) In animal experiments the best results were obtained using heterologous antigens, whereas in human pathology auto-antibodies play the most important role. This difference is not final because the antigen-antibody reaction is always specific. An antibody must react exclusively with its corresponding antigen and the end result is uninfluenced whether the production of the antibody was initiated by an autologous, isologous or heterologous antigen. The only important thing is with which structure the antibodies combine, and what biological processes they can inhibit. It seems most likely that some human auto-immune disease is initiated by bacterial or viral antigens cross reacting with tissue components (Perlmann, 1969; East, 1969).

(2) In some human disease auto-antibodies appear more readily than the homologous antibodies in experimental conditions. In human liver disease, for example, antibodies reacting with mitochondria are produced, as we and others have shown (Doniach and Walker, 1969; Widermann and Doerner, 1964) unlike some of the rabbits immunised with homologous MF in our experiments. The above mentioned antibodies are bound to the inner membrane of mitochondria

(Berg *et al.*, 1969a; Berg *et al.*, 1969b) at the site where the enzymes of the electron transport chain are situated. It seems highly likely that at least some of these antibodies are active against enzymes. By immunization with mito-chondrial or microsomal fractions, several authors have induced the formation of enzyme inhibiting auto-antibodies experimentally (Dobias and Bollet, 1962; Dobias and Balazs, 1967a). Of course, in human liver disease antibodies may also be produced to other intracellular components. The question is, whether or not these antibodies get inside the cells. Using ferritin-labelled antibodies, Goldberg (1963) demonstrated that they are able to invade intact cells by pinocytosis. An increase of cell permeability or destruction of the membrane would make antibody entry much easier. However, to our knowledge, the presence of cytotoxic humoral antibodies reacting with the cell membrane, has not yet been demonstrated in human liver disease.

The cell membrane, however, may be destroyed not only by cytotoxic humoral antibodies; such destruction may also result from delayed hyper-sensitivity reactions. It is known that on contact with the specific antigen, non-specific, biologically active cytotoxic substances may be released from sensitized lymphocytes. This was substantiated by Ruddle and Waksman (1968), who cultured lymphocytes from tuberculin sensitive animals with PPD *in vitro*. The supernatant of the mixture produced destructive changes in embryonic monolayer fibrolast culture. According to Roitt *et al.*, (1962) in auto-immune thyroiditis the cells of the thyroid are injured, the lesion being initiated by specifically sensitised lymphocytes. In the second step cyto-pathogenic humoral antibodies may penetrate the cell.

The evidence outlined above suggests that humoral antibodies may cause damage to cells in human liver disease. Further investigation is clearly necessary; it should be determined whether such antibodies do occur and attempts should be made to find out in individual cases how many kinds of antibody are produced, to which antigens they are directed, and whether they are persistent. These features are likely to vary from disease to disease, as well as from individual to individual.

REFERENCES

Asherson, G. L., Dumonde, D. C. (1962) Brit. J. Exp. Path. 43, 12.
Asherson, G. L., Dumonde, D. C. (1964) Immunology, 7, 1.
Berg, P. A., Roitt, I. M., Doniach, D., Horne, R. W. (1969) Clin. exp. Immunol., 4, 511.
Berg, P. A., Muscatello, U., Horne, R. W. (1969) Brit. J. Exp. Path. 50, 200.
Choudhuri, P. C. (1968) personal communication.
Cinader, B. In: Proceedings of the 2nd meeting of the Federation of European Biochemical Societies, Vienna 1965. Ed: B. Cinader, Pergamon Press, Oxford and New York. 1966. vol. 1. p. 85.
Davis, J. S., Bollet, A. J. (1962) J. Clin, Invest. 41, 2142.
Dobias, Gy., Marta Balazs (1967a) Immunology, 12, 373.
Dobias, Gy., Marta Balazs (1967b) Immunology, 12, 389.
Doniach, D., Walker, J. G. (1969) Lancet I, 813.
East, J. (1969) Vox Sang./Basel 16, 318.
Ehrlich, G., Halbert, S. P. (1968) Int. Arch. Allergy, 34, 428.
Engelfriet, C. P. (1966) In: Cytotoxic iso-Antibodies Against Leucocytes. Drukkerij Aemstelstad, Amsterdam, p. 45.
Goldberg, B. (1963) In: Immunopathology III Int. Symposium of Immunopathology, Schwabe, Base 1, p. 300.
Hauseman, T. W., Halcrow, D. A., Taylor K. B., (1969) Gastroenterology 56, 1053, 1062, 1071.
Jako, J. (1967), In Ungarische Wisenschaftliche Instrumente, Sonderausgabe, Metrimpex Budapest, p. 55.
Oakley, C. L., Fulthorpe, A. J. (1953), J. Path. Bact. 65, 49.
Perlmann, P. (1969), Vox Sang./Basel 16, 314.

Pollock, M. R. (1964), Immunology 7, 707.
Richter M., Sargent, A. U., Myers, J., Rose B. (1966), Immunology, 10, 211.
Roitt, I. M., Jones, H. E. H. Doniach, H. (1962), Immunopathology II-nd. Int. Symposium
    of Immunopathology Scwabe, Basel, Ed. Grabar, P. Miescher, P. A., p. 174.
Ruddle, N. H., Waksman, B. H. (1968), J. Exp. Med. 128, 1267.
Szasz, G., (1963), Orvosi Hetilap, 104, 1843.
Szecsey, Gy., Dobias, Gy., Marta Vegh, (1966), Z. Immun.–forsch. 331, 390.
Weir, D. M., Pinckard, R. N., Elson, C. J., Deirdre E. Suckling: (1966), Clin. Exp.
    Immunol. 1, 433.
Wiedermann G., Doerner, M., (1964). 94, 257.

ROUNDTABLE DISCUSSION ON THE OCCURRENCE AND ROLE OF ANTIBODIES

Chairman: Professor I. M. Roitt

CHAIRMAN

Perhaps I could start by trying to consider what might be causing the tissue damage. We have here antibodies which have not yet been convincingly shown to be directed specifically against the liver; therefore you have to postulate the existence of some agent which orientates the tissue-damaging effect against the liver. Now, supposing that you have one, you must ask the question: Could these antibodies which are directed against intracellular constituents in any way be responsible for tissue damage?

Theoretically you could argue a case that they might be, given some process which is causing a small amount of tissue damage, because you then release intracellular material. Subsequently immune complexes could be formed which can give rise to a wide variety of so-called nonspecific, immunological stimulation. These complexes can probably stimulate the macrophages; they can nonspecifically stimulate lymphocytes to divide and transform into blast cells, which in turn could produce a local inflammatory response that might be responsible for causing further tissue damage.

In experimental thyroiditis, we know that immunization with thyroglobulin in Freund's adjuvant produces a tissue lesion. Thyroglobulin is largly confined within the colloid space, and you might well ask how does the antibody or the sensitized cell manage to find the antigen to attack? The answer is that thyroglobulin is being released from the normal thyroid at a very low rate (at concentrations of 50 nanograms/ml.) and in the extra-acinar fluid there are very small amounts of thyroglobulin. Such molecules may provide the target for attack by the immunological agents. It is possible that even in the normal liver there are small amounts of intracellular materials which are being released from the cell. Alternatively, there may be some agent causing local trauma with release of intracellular antigens, which may then give rise to the immune complexes and cause further damage. Dr. Popper, would you like to say anything on that point?

POPPER

This question theoretically encompasses the entire problem. Obviously the first thing to say is that if intracellular material passes through the membrane, a simple explanation for cellular damage could be provided by the concept of a membrane combining protein as the important antigenic site.

CHAIRMAN

When you say "membrane combining" protein, are you now referring to the exterior of the cell?

POPPER

Yes.

CHAIRMAN

This of course would be easily accessible. The snag is that no antibodies directed against the outside of the cell have been detected.

Could Dr. Meyer Zum Büschenfelde tell us where his liver specific antigen is situated?

117

Meyer Zum BÜ SCHENFELDE
In Geneva we have used the isolated rat liver to study this problem. If the isolated liver is perfused over the course of 5 hours with an antibody to rat mitochondria, the antibody is not used up. Not only does it remain in the perfusate but also there is no consumption of complement. Therefore, we think that mitochondrial antibody cannot alone penetrate the cell. On the other hand, an antibody raised to a lipoprotein which we think is part of the cell membrane, is completely consumed during the first perfusion.

CHAIRMAN
And how do you demonstrate this membrane antibody?

Meyer Zum BÜSCHENFELDE
With immunofluorescence, but we have done too few electron microscopy studies to say exactly where it is found.

CHAIRMAN
Do you also say that there is an antibody to specific protein in some active chronic hepatitis sera?

Meyer Zum BÜSCHENFELDE
Yes. But, that is to a different protein from the one to which I have referred in describing experiments on the isolated rat liver. It is not a membrane protein, but a liver specific cytoplasmic protein, and antibodies to it are not consumed in the early stages of perfusion. However the longer the perfusion continues the more consumption of this antibody there is. Whereas the lipoprotein antibody fixes complement, this one does not. One other point about the lipoprotein antibody, I do not think it is the same as the antibody to the lipoprotein in mitochondria.

CHAIRMAN
Do you find antibodies to the surface of the liver cell in patients with active chronic hepatitis?

Meyer Zum BÜSCHENFELDE
On a few occasions I have found an antibody to the cytoplasmic protein in their serum after absorption with subcellular fractions of the liver — nuclei, mitochondria, lysosomes, etc.

CHAIRMAN
Have you found one against the membrane in those patients?

Meyer Zum BÜSCHENFELDE
No, not yet.

POPPER
What is the existing evidence for any circulating antibody or antigen-antibody complex playing a pathogenetic role in liver disease? Secondly, if they are pathogenetic would it not be necessary to demonstrate immune complexes in the liver? It is ironical that in patients with liver disease, we can demonstrate such complexes in the kidney, but not in the liver.

DONIACH
But you have shown complexes in the liver to us?

POPPER
In primary biliary cirrhosis only. And in that case I feel that they were a secondary effect. But in active chronic hepatitis, to my knowledge, nobody has ever demonstrated them.

WALKER

May I offer two indirect answers? Referring to our subclinical patients, who were selected on the basis of mitochondrial antibody alone, in only three was there no evidence of a disease process. In 32 a disease was found, usually one associated with auto-immunity. This surely is indirect evidence. Now, what about the alcoholic cirrhotic and the patient dying with massive hepatic necrosis? Why do they not become auto-immunized in the same way? We included in our miscellaneous group all grades of liver damage from inactive alcoholic cirrhosis to acute hepatic necrosis, and we did not find mitochondrial antibody. This requires explanation if we are to say that tissue antibodies simply arrive paripassu with liver damage.

WILLIAMS

Although there is a cellular immune attack during acute liver rejection, Dr. Doniach has been able to demonstrate very few antibodies, mitochondrial or other otherwise.

EDDLESTON

It is likely that after transplantation any antibody is mopped up by the graft as soon as it is formed. For example, in renal transplantation, they do not appear in the serum until after the grafted organ has been removed. If Dr. Meyer Zum Büschenfelde's antigen is readily available on the cell surface it is not surprising that his antibody is not found in the serum. This may not be the case for mitochondrial antibody as its antigen is sequestered and not easily accessible.

CHAIRMAN

You need a draining lymph node to culture *in vitro* to try and demonstrate antiliver antibodies.

EDDLESTON

Perhaps this grouping of patients with auto-immune disorders occurs because of a genetically inherited abnormality in their immune system, and the mitochondrial antibodies are a marker of that, rather than a marker of the disease process itself?

CHAIRMAN

But the mitochondrial antibody does seem to pick out one end of the spectrum. There is surely some considerable specificity related to the events going on in the liver.

EDDLESTON

Not all that much within auto-immune disease.

CHAIRMAN

Examining both ends of the spectrum, there is surely more than a little polarization.

EDDLESTON

In the patients with cryptogenic cirrhosis, did you try looking at the ones with smooth muscle antibody for resemblances to chronic aggressive hepatitis?

DONIACH

Yes. The ones that had high titres of smooth muscle antibody as a rule had piecemeal necrosis.

EDDLESTON

But this was also one of the features you used to determine whether they resembled primary biliary cirrhosis.

DONIACH

It was a separate feature, although it was included in the general assessment.

MacLAURIN

Can liver cells be used as a target monolayer in a system for studying mitochondrial antibody? To return to Professor Roitt's suggestion that something could be diffusing out of the cell, one could perhaps investigate this using the technique developed by the Kleins in Stockholm. Using the Birkett lymphoma cell they have shown antibody attachment both to cell membranes and intracellular structures. With this technique minute amounts of mitochondrial material diffusing to the surface could be detected in the living cell. Has this been tried?

DONIACH

Not yet.

CHAIRMAN

The problem with that is the high base line due to the continual leakage of intracellular content.

WRIGHT

Even if you find mitochondrial antibody early in the disease, the question is which is the cart and which is the horse? This was the point I was trying to make this morning in relation to the girl with a positive LE cell phenomenon whose mother had antinuclear factor in her serum. There was an outbreak of viral hepatitis in that family and this child, of all the children, went on to develop active chronic hepatitis.

CHAIRMAN

As Dr. Eddleston has suggested, I think that it is theoretically possible to have some cellular immunity against a liver-specific antigen and yet not see the humoral counterpart because it is mopped up by the large amount of liver antigen. Normally we would be unhappy to postulate cell-mediated immunity against a given antigen without humoral immunity; such situations are exceedingly rare. On the other hand, this would be one way of allowing it to exist and therefore it is obviously very pertinent for us to know how clearly you, Dr. Eddleston, or anyone else, has demonstrated cell-mediated immunity against liver specific antigen.

EDDLESTON

We have not yet shown a liver specific response.

Meyer Zum BÜSCHENFELDE

We have studied anti nuclear factors in various ways for some years and have found some anomalies. For instance LE cells are very rare in liver disease in comparison to systemic lupus erythematosus. On the other hand with complement-fixation tests and also the nonspecific gamma globulin consumption test there are very often high titres of antinuclear factor. We also find nonspecific phagocytosis in liver disease, but the results are very different from those in lupus erythematosus. Is this your experience?

DONIACH

Yes, very few lupus cells — but not all the antinuclear factors lead to the formation of lupus cells, only some of them do, and it seems that in these liver diseases most do not.

MacSWEEN

In view of the reports of antinucleolar factors as opposed to antinuclear factors in scleroderma, and of the possible associations between this condition and chronic hepatitis — what is the incidence of antinucleolar factor in liver disease?

DONIACH
I think they are uncommon in liver disease. We have found them in one or two cases of active chronic hepatitis and cryptogenic cirrhosis in our previous series. They are found mostly in scleroderma and dermatomyositis, sometimes in extremely high titres, up to 1 in 6,000 or more.

GLYNN
We have found no correlation between antinucleolar staining and scleroderma.

CHAIRMAN
So that contradicts the existing report in the literature.

WRIGHT
This sort of claim is comparable to the supposedly specific clinical connotation of speckled antinuclear factor. The same applied with the white cell-specific antinuclear factor in Felty's syndrome. Such reports seldom seem to hold up to critical examination later on.

DONIACH
It is the same with the canalicular antibody. If you look for it on rat liver sections, we do find the same as you have described but not necessarily in liver disease; we have also found it in patients with rheumatoid arthritis or other collagenoses.

SMITH
To return to the controversy concerning the role of sensitized cells and circulating antibody, it is worth remembering that Professor Good has described a patient with agammaglobulinemia whoch developed a chronic liver disease showing some features of active chronic hepatitis. There was some response to steroids intermittently, the patient dying after a ten month illness.

CHAIRMAN
We have heard this morning of two different types of active chronic hepatitis and we would like to know which of these types the patient had.

PART III
Cell Mediated Responses and Manifestations
of Immunological Damage

THEORETICAL BASIS OF THE LEUCOCYTE MIGRATION TEST
M. Søborg

Since the original work by Rich and Lewis (1932), antigen induced inhibition of the migration of immunocompetent cells *in vitro* has proved to be a reliable parameter of cellular hypersensitivity in animals. On the basis of the capillary tube migration system initiated by George and Vaughan (1962) and further elaborated by David *et al.,* (1964) in guinea pig experiments, Dr. Bendixen and I (1967) developed the leucocyte migration test using human peripheral leucocytes as the immuno-competent cells.

The leucocyte migration test (LMT) seems to give a reliable and reproducible expression of the degree of cellular hypersensitivity, as we and others have shown in various conditions (Søborg, 1967). So far the test has been applied in microbial hypersensitivity, auto-immune diseases, contact allergy, drug allergy, tumour immunity, and transplantation immunity. The principle of the test is by now well known; and I shall only describe the technical procedure in brief.

DETAILS OF TECHNIQUE AND SIGNIFICANCE OF INHIBITION

Heparinized blood is allowed to sediment spontaneously for 1 hour at 37°C. The supernatant, containing the leucocytes with a few contaminating erythrocytes, is harvested. After four cell-washings with Hanks balanced salt solution, the cell suspension is transferred to capillary tubes. The latter are centrifuged and then cut at the cell fluid interface and the cell packs put into tissue-culture chambers containing Tc199 and 10 per cent horse serum. The leucocytes are allowed to migrate from the capillary tubes onto the bottom of the chamber for 24 hours. At the start of the experiment, antigen is added to half of the chambers, the other half serving as controls. The action of antigen upon the cellular migration is expressed in the so-called "migration index". This is the average area of migration in the antigen-containing chambers divided by the average area in the non-antigen-containing chambers. Thus, if the value obtained is lower than 1·00, inhibition of cellular migration has occurred and if higher, stimulation. An example of the migration of peripheral leucocytes after 24 hours incubation without antigen is shown in Fig. 1a. Figure 1b. illustrates the inhibition of migration that is observed in the presence of antigen when the leucocyte donor was hypersensitive to the antigen.

The degree of inhibition has been shown to correlate well with the degree of cellular hypersensitivity of the cell donor (Søborg, 1967). In Brucella hypersensitivity a quantitative correlation can be demonstrated between inhibition of migration, as expressed by the migration index, and the induration of the delayed intracutaneous reaction to brucellin (Fig. 2). On the other hand, there is no correlation between the migration index and the titre of agglutinating antibodies (Fig. 3), indicating that the test does not reflect humoral hypersensitivity. A similar correlation between delayed intracutaneous reactions and inhibition of peripheral leucocyte migration has been demonstrated in tuberculin hypersensitivity, parasitic infection and organ-specific auto-immunity (Clausen, 1970, Nerup and Bendixen, 1969).

125

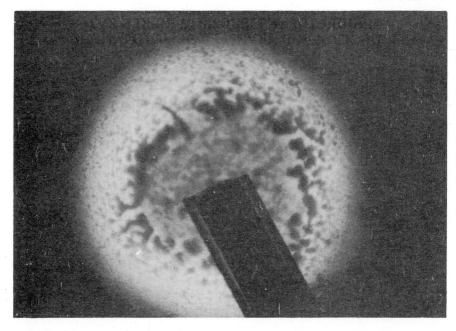

(a)

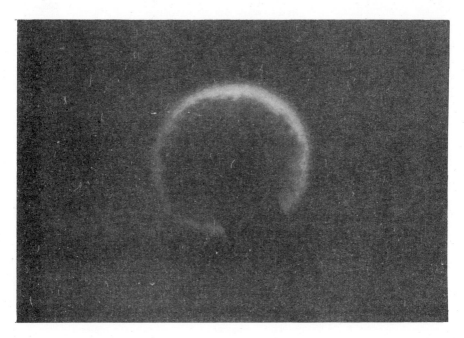

(b)

Fig. 1. The migration areas after 24 hours with (a) and without antigen.

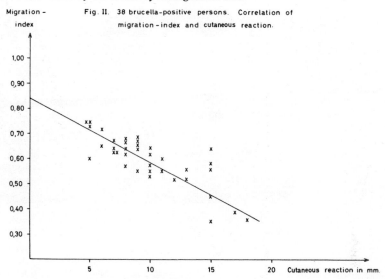

Fig. 2. Correlation of migration index and induration of delayed intracutaneous reaction to brucellin in subjects with brucellin hypersensitivity.

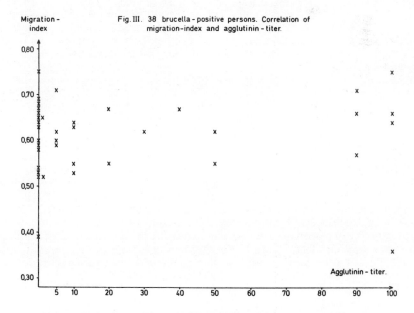

Fig. 3. Correlation between migration index and serum agglutination titre to brucellin bacteria in subjects with brucellin hypersensitivity.

MECHANISM OF MIGRATION AND INHIBITION

What, then, is the mechanism of the antigen-induced specific inhibition of the migration of peripheral leucocytes *in vitro*? At the moment we have some knowledge of the specific immunological processes which initiate the reaction but practically nothing is known about the processes involved in the inhibition of migration.

Two types of cell have been found to be essential in initiating the reaction. These are sensitized lymphocytes, and granulocytes which do not have to be sensitized (Søborg, 1969). When a pure population of sensitized lymphocytes is cultured with or without antigen, no inhibition of migration is found (Clausen, 1970). Similarly, there is no inhibition when pure sensitized granulocytes are used. However, when these pure cell types are mixed, the expected inhibition of migration occurs, implying that the cell-separation procedure in itself has not damaged the cells, and prevented the manifestation of inhibition (Clausen, 1970).

In several laboratories it has been demonstrated that pure sensitized human lymphocytes produce a substance called "migration-inhibitory factor" (MIF) on contact with antigen. MIF is able to inhibit the migration of non-sensitized guinea pig peritoneal macrophages. (Thor *et al.*, 1968, Dumonde *et al.*, 1969). In many experiments, animal cells have been used for migration studies because of the technical difficulties of obtaining a good human cell preparation. However, in preliminary experiments, we have demonstrated that MIF, produced by sensitized human lymphocytes, is able to inhibit the migration of human granulocytes. This active agent, has been characterized to some extent and shown to be non-dialysable, with a molecular weight of 70,000, and does not seem to be an ordinary immunoglobulin.

As I mentioned earlier, the migration of pure sensitized lymphocytes is not inhibited by the presence of antigen although these cells are presumably producing MIF. In this case, it is possible that the amount of MIF produced is insufficient to provoke inhibition. A simple explanation for the inhibition that may occur when a mixed cell population, granulocytes and lymphocytes, is used in this system, would be that MIF produces clumping of the granulocytes. This clumping mechanically hinders the otherwise unaffected migration of the lymphocytes. According to this theory the granulocytes would be acting as indicator cells, the net result being a visible inhibition of the migration of the total cell population.

STUDIES WITH DIFFERENT CELL PREPARATIONS

The following experiments indicate that the mechanism of inhibition is probably more complex. Two types of cell population were used. The first, consists of an average of 35 per cent lymphocytes, 63 per cent granulocytes and 2 per cent monocytes. This type of cell population, called L+G, was derived from either Brucella positive or Brucella negative donors. The second type of cell population consists of almost 100 per cent lymphocytes and is called "L". In the following experiments "L" was always derived from a Brucella positive donor. The various cell preparations were incubated either in separate culture chambers or in the same chamber. Figure 4 illustrates how cells from two different donors can be placed in the same chamber so that no direct contact between the cell populations occurs.

The outcome of the various combinations of cell preparations cultured either separately or together, is shown in Fig. 5. In each case, a shaded area means that the cell type was obtained from a sensitized individual and a non-shaded area indicates the reverse. The antigen used was Brucella bacteria. At the top the

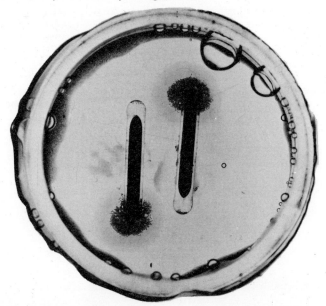

Fig. 4. Illustrating use of a single chamber in examining migration of cells from two different donors.

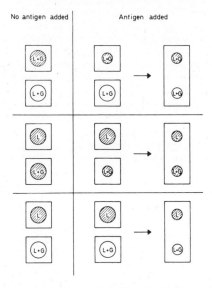

Fig. 5. Diagrammatic representation of studies of migration with different cell preparations.

results using a mixed cell preparation are shown. As expected, when the sensitized and non-sensitized cells are incubated separately in the presence of antigen, the migration of the sensitized cells is inhibited and that of the non-sensitized is not. When these mixed cell preparations are cultured in the same chamber the migration of both sensitized and non-sensitized cells is inhibited. This is a practical demonstration that inhibition is mediated by a soluble substance derived from the sensitized cells.

The middle part of the figure illustrates the outcome of exposing pure sensitized lymphocytes to specific antigen. No inhibition can be observed. However, if these lymphocytes are cultured in the same chamber as a mixed cell preparation from a sensitized donor, then inhibition of the migration of the pure lymphocytes is induced. This implies that inhibition of lymphocyte migration does not depend on mechanical hindrance due to clumped granulocytes. On the other hand, it is clear that the granulocytes must be present in order for a soluble factor, able to inhibit cell migration, to be produced.

The lower part of the figure, shows that when sensitized lymphocytes are incubated in the same chamber as a non-sensitized mixed cell preparation, the migration of both is inhibited. When incubated separately, no inhibition is seen.

On this evidence it seems that the sensitized lymphocyte is the immunologically specific cell, but the granulocytes, which must be present for inhibition to occur, do not need to be sensitized. Recently Falk *et al.,* (1970) from Uppsala have published some experiments in which the migration of an almost pure population of human peripheral lymphocytes was inhibited by antigen in a specific manner. So, although lymphocytes can be inhibited without participation of clumping granulocytes, the latter act as a kind of amplifier in the system.

IMPORTANCE OF AGGLUTINATION IN MECHANISM OF INHIBITION

I will now go on to another important question: Why do the cells, on contact with the antigen, cease to migrate? One explanation could be that the inhibition was an expression of agglutination of the migrating cells. This does not seem likely for the following reasons: Agglutination due to circulating agglutinating antibodies cannot be a factor because antibodies have never been demonstrated after the cells have been washed four times, which is done routinely before the cells are allowed to migrate. Furthermore, the migration of non-sensitized granulocytes can be inhibited by the addition of MIF, which does not contain conventional antibodies. MIF alone might, however, have agglutinating activity, and this hypothesis cannot be excluded. MIF has been shown in animal experiments to have an aggregating effect on peritoneal macrophages, which are usually used as indicator cells. It is quite likely that some degree of cell agglutination is instrumental in the production of inhibition. The agglutinating effect, however, might just as well be the expression of an increased stickiness of the cells which makes them adhere to the glass. Lastly, the idea that agglutination is important does not fit with the phenomenon of stimulation of migration which, as we shall see later, is closely related to inhibition.

Another theory to account for inhibition of migration is that decreased cell viability or even cell death is responsible. However, in animal studies, although a decrease in cell viability has been demonstrated in some experiments, in others no decrease, or even an increase in viability, has been found. Similarly, in the leucocyte migration test we have been unable to find any difference in viability after 24 hours incubation between cells in control chambers and those exposed to antigen.

OCCURRENCE OF STIMULATION OF MIGRATION UNDER CERTAIN CONDITIONS

Thus, damage of cells does not seem to be a necessary condition for inhibition to occur. This antigen-induced influence on the migration is also subject to variations which make it unlikely that cell damage is an important feature. During the first few hours after addition of antigen to the sensitized cells, a stimulation of migration can be seen which is later followed by the usual inhibition of migration. However, if low antigen concentrations are used, this stimulatory effect is not superseded by inhibition and at 24 hours a migration index of greater than 1·00 is found.

Figure 6 shows the mean values of the migration indices at different antigen concentrations, from cell donors with Brucella hypersensitivity. The highest antigen concentration in the test chambers is 50 million Brucella bacteria/ml. of

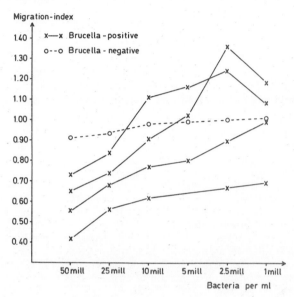

Fig. 6. Illustrating occurrence of stimulation and inhibition at different antigen concentrations in subjects with various degrees of brucellin hypersensitivity.

tissue culture medium and the lowest is 1 million/ml. Observations on the Brucella positive patients have been arbitrarily divided into four groups, according to the degree of sensitization, i.e., the migration indices at an antigen concentration of 50 million bacteria/ml. In the least sensitive group migration indices range from 0·71 to 0·76. In the next two groups values from 0·61 to 0·70 and 0·51 to 60, respectively are found: in the most sensitive group migration indices are below 0·50. This separation is justified by the finding that the migration indices at 50 million bacteria/ml., as I have previously mentioned, were closely correlated with the sensitivity of the cell donor, as shown by the delayed intracutaneous reaction. At the high antigen concentrations the migration indices from Brucella positive persons are all well below 1·00, whereas the migration indices of the Brucella negative controls at the various antigen concentrations are all centred around 1·00. Considering the least sensitive group first, with decreasing antigen concentrations the inhibition of migration is replaced by stimulation (Fig. 6). The migration in the most sensitive group, however, remains inhibited even at the lowest concentrations, although to a lesser degree.

Thus the curve seems to be biphasic, starting with low migration indices followed by an interval within the normal range, continuing with high indices and finally returning to the normal range. The diagram also shows that, at a fixed low antigen concentration, a wide distribution of indices can be observed, indicating that in some cases the migration has been stimulated, in some inhibited, and in some apparently uninfluenced by the antigen. In this situation the outcome depends upon the sensitivity of the cells, a highly sensitive culture being inhibited and a less sensitive culture stimulated or perhaps apparently uninfluenced. Conversely, with a fixed sensitivity, the outcome will depend upon the antigen concentration, i.e., the higher concentrations will induce inhibition and the lower concentrations a stimulation of migration.

So, inhibition and stimulation may both be considered expressions of cellular hypersensitivity *in vitro,* and moreover they appear to be closely interdependent. Whether stimulation or inhibition of cell migration results from antigenic action thus depends upon (1) the time after exposure to the antigen; (2) the concentration of the antigen, and (3) the sensitivity of the cells, or more correctly the sensitivity of the cell donor.

INHIBITION OF MIGRATION AND PHAGOCYTIC ACTIVITY

Finally, I would like to draw attention to a possible relationship between inhibition of migration and phagocytic activity. In 1959 Allgower and Bloch, and later others, demonstrated an inverse correlation *in vitro* between the motility of granulocytes and other cells, and the phagocytic activity of each cell type: in other words, the more the cell phagocytosed, the slower it moved. Barnet *et al.,* (1968) showed that the phagocytic activity of rabbit macrophages was stimulated by the presence of sensitized lymphocytes and the appropriate antigen. Dumonde *et al.,* (1969) have shown an increased phagocytic activity of guinea pig macrophages after addition of migration inhibitory factor. There might, therefore be an inverse relation between cell motility and phagocytic activity for an individual cell. If this was so, increased phagocytic activity by itself could be a contributory cause to the inhibition of migration. The latter might therefore be just another measure of the phenomenon of phagocytosis.

SUMMARY

In summary, I believe that the contact between sensitized lymphocytes and specific antigen results in the release of a soluble substance — MIF — which either alone or together with granulocytes produces inhibition of the migration of peripheral leucocytes. This inhibition is based on active cell processes and may perhaps be related to increased phagocytic activity of the migrating cells.

REFERENCES

Barnet, K., Pekarek, J., Johanovsky, J. (1968) Experientia 24, 9.
Clausen (1970) Acta Med. Scand. 188, 59.
David, J. R., Al-Askari, H. S., Lawrence, H. S., Thomas, L. (1964) J. Immunol. 93, 514.
Dumonde, D. C., Wolstencroft, R. A., Panayi, G. S., Matthew, M., Maley, J., Howson, J. T. (1969) Nature (Lond.) 224, 38.
Falk, R. E., Thorsby, E., Moller, E., Moller, G. (1970) Clin. Exp. Immunol. 6, 445.
George, M., Vaughan, J. H. (1962) Proc. Soc. Exp. Biol. (N.Y.) 111, 514.
Nerup, J., Bendixen, G. (1969) J. Clin. Exp. Imm. 5, 358.
Rich, A. R., Lewis, M. R. (1932) Bull. Johns. Hopk. Hosp. 50, 115.
Søborg, M. (1967) Acta Med. Scand. 182, 167.
Søborg, M. (1969) Acta Med. Scand. 185, 229.
Søborg, M., and Bendixen, G. (1967) Acta Med. Scand. 181, 247.
Thor, D. E., Jureziz, R. E., Veach, S. R., Miller, E., Dray, S. (1968) Nature (Lond.) 219, 755.

DISCUSSION
Chairman: Dr. D. C. Dumonde

SODOMANN

It might be of some interest that Rorsman has described a different method of using peripheral leucocytes in the migration inhibition test. After producing migration areas in the usual way he inverted the slides for about six hours and then measured the area remaining on the glass, which consisted mostly of monocytes. The majority of the other cells had sedimented away from the glass into the culture chamber. We have used a similar technique to isolate human peripheral monocytes by their ability to stick to glass and have obtained a cell population of approximately 80 per cent monocytes, 10 per cent polymorphs and 10 per cent lymphocytes. Our results were comparable to those of Rorsman: in tuberculin hypersensitivity the correlation between migration inhibition and the skin reactivity was very good. Have you shown a correlation in this situation with your method?

SØBORG

Yes, we have. Using PPD as antigen we have found a good correlation between the degree of migration inhibition and the delayed intracutaneous reaction. It is very interesting that you have been able to isolate so many monocytes, because I find great difficulty in getting a pure monocyte preparation.

CHAIRMAN

Have you found any differences when using soluble or insoluble antigens in your chamber?

SØBORG

No.

CHAIRMAN

Does this affect the sensitivity of the test? Does it affect the extent to which migration inhibition can be detected? Does it affect any correlation with clinical 48 hour skin reactions?

SØBORG

I do not think so, but I must admit that with Brucella bacteria, the test seemed a little more sensitive than with PPD. But we have not tried to use the whole tubercle bacillus.

CHAIRMAN

Have you compared the effects of Brucella whole bacteria and Brucellin?

SØBORG

Only in a very few experiments and there was no difference.

CHAIRMAN

One of the great problems about the application of this test to clinical medicine is the fact that in some situations one appears to get stimulation of cell migration. People have criticized the test because it is not clear what you should be looking for. Do you have any comments on that?

SØBORG

At the transition from stimulation to inhibition it is difficult to evaluate the degree of sensitivity in the cell donor. You should always try to work in the range in which inhibition is produced. One way of doing this is by increasing the antigen concentration in the system; to do this it may be necessary to purify the antigen to avoid non-specific toxic depression of the migration. By such means, inhibition only will be produced if the cells are sensitized, as can be shown in animal experiments.

CHAIRMAN

This paper is obviously of positive help to those utilizing the test for clinical purposes. Are you saying that you must employ dose-response-relationships in the test, and that it is no good doing the test under one or perhaps even two antigen concentrations?

SØBORG

If you are in the transitional range then you must use different antigen concentrations to titrate out the sensitivity of the donor.

CHAIRMAN

But if you do not know the degree of sensitivity of the donor, you might have to employ quite a wide range of antigen concentrations in the putatively hypersensitive or diseased subjects?

SØBORG

That is right, yes.

FEDERLIN

To what extent do you think contamination with erythrocytes will influence the migration? You said that only a few erythrocytes are allowable and yet I could see some in the slide.

SØBORG

Contaminating erythrocytes, provided that there are not too many, will remain in the centre of the migration areas. The outer area consists purely of granulocytes and lymphocytes.

FEDERLIN

Did you try any techniques to lyse the red cells?

SØBORG

This is really quite easy to do and we have used lysis to remove erythrocytes. However, we do not do it routinely as simple sedimentation is quite satisfactory.

FEDERLIN

Do techniques used for lysing red cells influence the ability of the leucocytes to migrate?

SØBORG

Not in our hands, but dextran sedimentation, where you may get a very high degree of contamination with erythrocytes, could do so. We feel that this may be one of the explanations for the poor results obtained elsewhere.

BENDIXEN

It has been shown experimentally in the cow and the pig that insufficient simple sedimentation occurs in 1 hour at 37°C for the leucocyte migration test to be carried out. However, it is possible to partially purify the leucocytes by centrifugation and then to remove the last remaining erythrocytes by osmotic shock. This technique does not damage the leucocytes, and allows the tests to be done in these animals. In this way cellular hypersensitivity to paratubercular bacteria in cattle can be detected. This method might also be useful in patients with a very low erythrocyte sedimentation rate.

LEUCOCYTE MIGRATION IN ACTIVE CHRONIC HEPATITIS AND PRIMARY BILIARY CIRRHOSIS

M. G. M. Smith, A. L. W. F. Eddleston and Roger Williams

In recent years, most of the interest in the immunology of liver disease has centred on circulating antibody. The persistently high titres of auto-antibodies found in active chronic hepatitis and primary biliary cirrhosis have been cited as convincing evidence of an auto-immune process occurring in these diseases (Doniach, 1970). However, an inherent weakness in the hypothesis has been the non-specific nature of most of these antibodies and, at the moment, no primary pathogenic role has been demonstrated for circulating antibody in the production or the perpetuation of human liver disease.

Cell mediated immunity has been little studied in liver disease. We now know from transplantation studies that sensitized cells can attack and destroy the liver, and the histological similarities between acute rejection and active chronic hepatitis (Paronetto and Popper, 1969) may therefore be highly significant. Consequently we were greatly interested when Dr. Søborg described the leucocyte migration test (Søborg and Bendixen, 1967) as this seemed to be a simple method of measuring delayed hypersensitivity responses to liver antigens *in vitro*. Since his original description, opinion has been divided as to the validity and inter- pretation of this test — some reports have been in favour (Mookerjee *et al.*, 1969) and some against (Kaltreider *et al.*, 1969). Our experience with leucocyte migration supports Dr. Søborg's findings, and in this paper we present additional evidence as to the validity of the test and report the results of its use in liver disease.

LEUCOCYTE MIGRATION TECHNIQUE

The method that we employ (Smith *et al.*, 1969) is basically the same as Dr. Søborg has just described. A minor difference is that we have found it necessary to use high molecular weight Dextran to aid the sedimentation of red cells in the initial separation of mixed leucocytes from peripheral blood. We do not find that this leads to excessive erythrocyte contamination as others have suggested (Bendixen and Søborg, 1970). The leucocytes are washed in Hanks Balanced Salt solution and subsequently packed into capillary tubes and incubated in tissue culture medium for 20 hours. The cells migrate to form circular areas on the cover slip during this time (Fig. 1). A migration index is calculated by dividing the mean area of migration in the antigen-containing chambers by the mean area of control migration. A figure of less than 1·0 indicates inhibition of migration and of greater than 1·0 stimulation of migration.

EFFECT OF TEMPERATURE AND ENZYME INHIBITION ON MIGRATION

Towards the end of last year, Kaltreider *et al.*, (1969) suggested that leucocyte migration was not a biological process — they felt that the leucocytes did not migrate from the capillary tubes, but fell out due to gravity and the cell areas then expanded by Brownian diffusion. We designed two simple experiments to examine this possibility.

Figure 2 illustrates the effect of temperature on the migration areas of leucocytes from normal subjects incubated in control medium. There is an exponential increase in the areas at 37°C when compared to those at 4°C and

135

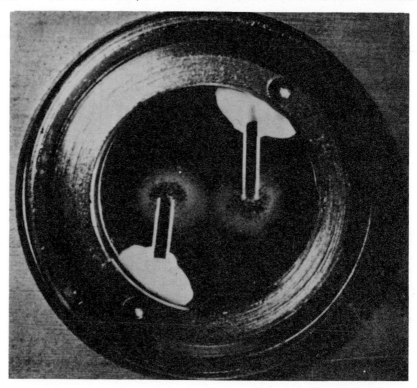

Fig. 1. Illustrating the migration areas of mixed leucocytes in control medium.

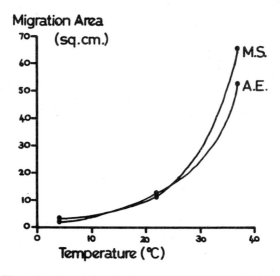

Fig. 2. Illustrating the relationship between temperature and migration area.

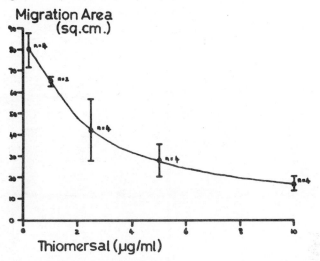

Fig. 3. Demonstrating the effect of an enzyme inhibitor on migration area.
(mean ± 1SD. n = numbers of observations).

22°C, as would be expected in a biologically active process. In Fig. 3 the effect
of an enzyme inhibitor on leucocyte migration areas is shown. Thiomersal was
added to the culture chambers in increasing amounts before incubation, and the
migration areas measured at 20 hours. The dose response curve shown on this
slide was the result; an appreciable reduction in migration area being found even
at concentrations as low as 1 μg. of inhibitor per ml. of tissue culture medium.
Again, this finding suggests that leucocyte migration is an active rather than a
passive process.

PREPARATION OF FOETAL LIVER ANTIGEN AND ITS EFFECT ON
NORMAL LEUCOCYTES

The antigen was prepared from freshly pooled human foetal liver. The liver
was homogenized in an equal volume of Hank's Balanced salt solution and the
suspension centrifuged at 1500 G — the supernatant was used as antigen in
concentrations of 40–400 μg. of protein per ml. of tissue culture medium. The
effect of this antigen on the leucocytes from normal subjects was then
investigated as illustrated in Fig. 4. The first three columns concern normal
subjects; each dot represents a measurement of the migration index at a certain
concentration of foetal liver antigen, shown here at 0, 200 and 400 μg. protein/ml.
In these normal subjects a narrow range of migration indices is found. The effect
of adding protein antigen to the test chambers is to produce slight, progressive
depression of the mean value from 1·0 without antigen, to 0·9 with a scatter
from 0·8 to 1·07 in the presence of 400 μg.

RELATIONSHIP BETWEEN STIMULATION AND
INHIBITION OF MIGRATION

When the migration of cells from patients with active chronic hepatitis and
primary biliary cirrhosis was examined, using 400 μg./ml. of liver antigen a very
different picture emerged. A wide range of values was found, from marked
inhibition to pronounced stimulation of migration (Fig. 4). However the value
for some patients still fell within the normal range. In an attempt to emphasize

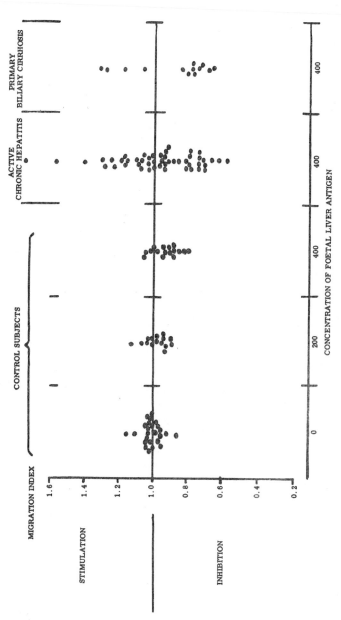

Fig. 4. Illustrating the effect of foetal liver homogenate on the migration of leucocytes from normal subjects and from patients with active chronic hepatitis and primary biliary cirrhosis.

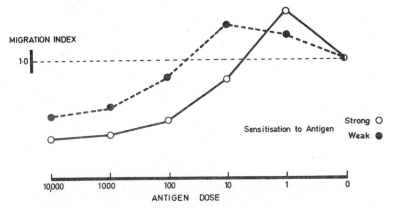

Fig. 5. Diagrammatic representation of studies on Brucellin hypersensitivity by courtesy of Dr. Søborg (1968).

this difference in behaviour from normal subjects, the relationship between stimulation and inhibition with particular reference to these apparently normal values was re-examined.

Dr. Søborg has kindly allowed me to show part of his data. Figure 5 shows diagrammatically some of the results of migration studies on patients with Brucellin +ve skin tests, using Brucella bacteria as antigen. The closed circles represent mean values for the migration index with increasing concentrations of antigen in a group of patients showing weakly +ve skin tests. The open circles represent a group of patients with strongly +ve skin tests. At high antigen concentrations inhibition of migration is found which is more marked in the strongly sensitized group. At low concentrations of antigen, stimulation of migration is found, occurring first in the group which is weakly sensitized. At a fixed antigen concentration, inhibition represents relatively strong *in vivo* sensitization as compared to stimulation.

If a single concentration of antigen is used in the test system, a migration index of 1·0 might represent a point at which there was truly no reaction, but could equally well be at the transition from inhibition to stimulation. This confusion can only be clarified by using more than one concentration of antigen: at a transitional point the use of a more dilute antigen will produce stimulation whereas at a truly normal point alteration of the antigen concentration will not change the result.

On the basis of Dr. Søborg's studies, we have plotted the scale on the ordinate so as to represent increasing sensitization (Fig. 6). All the subsequent data is expressed in this way. The result actually charted on each graph is the value of the migration index obtained using 400 μg. protein antigen; the position of the result on the graph depending on simultaneous consideration of the migration index measured at 200 μg. ml. and sometimes 50 μg. ml.

RESULTS IN LIVER DISEASE

The diagnosis in the 29 patients with active chronic hepatitis, was made after consideration of the clinical history, the physical examination, and the results of biochemical and serological studies. The liver histology of each of these patients was that of chronic aggressive hepatitis with or without cirrhosis. 12 patients with primary biliary cirrhosis were also studied and a small number of patients with other liver diseases (Table 1).

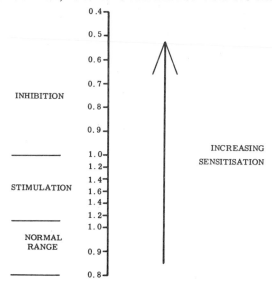

Fig. 6. Scale representing increasing sensitization. (From Eddleston *et al.*, 1970).

A comparison of the migration indices in the various groups is shown in Fig. 7. The normal range was established by measurement of the migration index at

TABLE 1

	No. Of Patients
Active Chronic Hepatitis	29
Primary Biliary Cirrhosis	12
Obstructive Jaundice	8
Inactive Cirrhosis	13
Acute Hepatitis	16

various antigen concentrations in 21 normal individuals. It is clear that readings on patients with primary biliary cirrhosis and active chronic hepatitis stand out from the others in the degree of abnormality of the migration index. In only one other patient was there inhibition of migration; this was a case of acute hepatitis in a young girl of 17 who gave a history suggestive of viral hepatitis, a short prodromal illness leading to acute epigastric pain and jaundice. She had associated with known cases of serum hepatitis some weeks before and it is possible that she herself took drugs. Physical examination was unremarkable, and both the liver function tests and the liver biopsy were compatible with hepatitis. The serum aspartate aminotransferase and bilirubin levels are shown in Fig. 8. The striking feature of this case was that not only was inhibition of migration found on 3 occasions, but also low titres of mitochondrial antibodies were present in the serum. These antibodies were found to be stable on storage, and are therefore of the type found in primary biliary cirrhosis as Dr. Walker reported yesterday. As you can see however, her liver function improved rapidly and now the auto-antibodies have vanished and the migration index is normal.

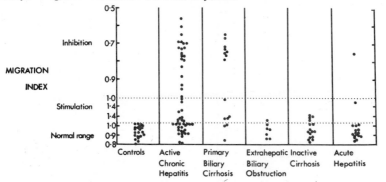

Fig. 7. Overall results of the leucocyte migration test in liver disease. (From Smith *et al.*, 1971).

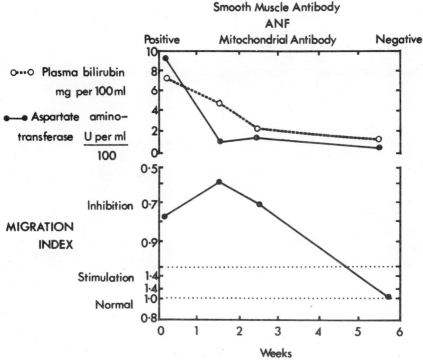

Fig. 8. Serial measurements of liver function, migration index and serum auto-antibodies in a young girl with acute hepatitis. (From Smith *et al.*, 1971).

RELATION OF MIGRATION INDEX TO TREATMENT AND LIVER FUNCTION

A more detailed analysis of the results obtained in the cases of active chronic hepatitis with reference to change in liver function is shown in Fig. 9. On the basis of the results of liver function tests, the patients were grouped into those with normal liver function, those with mild derangement of liver function (bilirubin < 5·0 mg./100 ml. and serum aspartate aminotransferase < 100 u/ml.)

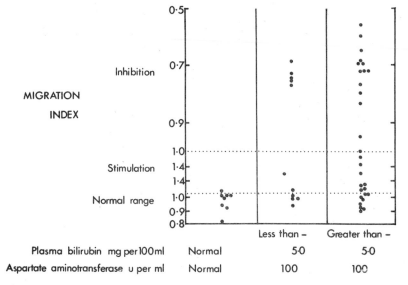

Fig. 9. Illustrating the relation between liver function and migration index in patients with active chronic hepatitis. (From Smith *et al.*, 1971).

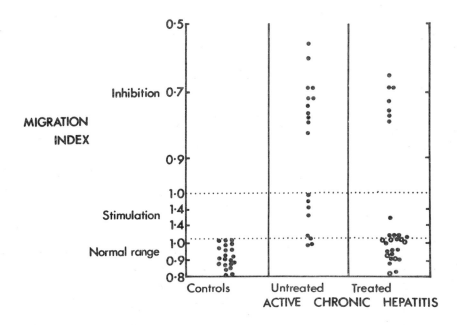

Fig. 10. Illustrating the relation between migration index and immunosuppressive therapy in patients with active chronic hepatitis. The open circles represent patients with normal liver function tests. (From Smith *et al.*, 1971).

and those with severe dysfunction (bilirubin > 5·0 mg./100 ml. or aspartate aminotransferase > 100 u/ml.). It can be seen that those patients with normal liver function had normal or nearly normal migration indices. However, there was no difference in the degree of abnormality between the two groups of patients with disordered liver function.

Most of these patients with active chronic hepatitis are participating in a double blind controlled therapeutic trial of prednisone against azathioprine. A comparison of the migration indices of the treated patients with the untreated is shown in Fig. 10. No attempt was made to take into account the amount or the duration of therapy. Despite these inherent disadvantages, it is still clear that more patients in the treated group have normal migration indices than in the untreated group. The difference between the two is statistically significant using Wilcoxson's rank test (p = <0·01). The patients in the treated group with normal migration indices are also those with normal liver function tests.

CONCLUSIONS AND MODEL OF AUTO-IMMUNE LIVER DISEASE

These present studies show without doubt that there are disordered delayed hypersensitivity responses to foetal liver antigens in patients with "auto-immune" liver disease. Our results in patients with active chronic hepatitis also suggest that the intensity of this delayed hypersensitivity response may correlate with the activity of the disease as assessed by results of liver function tests. Moreover, it would appear that in the patients receiving therapy with immunosuppressive drugs, changes in the migration index and liver function were running in parallel. However, to substantiate these observations the studies must be expanded into sequential investigations on individual patients. Purification of the antigens used in the test is also necessary to allow the sensitivity of the method to be increased and the difficulties of stimulation to be avoided.

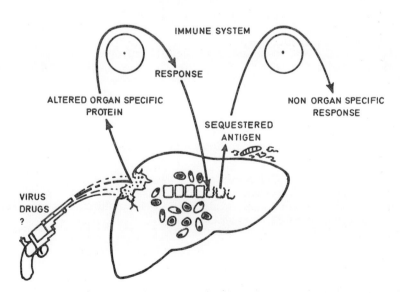

Fig. 11. Illustrating a hypothetical concept of auto-immune liver disease.

Finally I would like to show our current concept of the role of delayed hypersensitivity responses in "auto-immune" liver disease, (Fig. 11). We envisage an exogenous stimulus of some kind, perhaps a virus or a drug, damaging the liver and releasing or altering a liver specific protein. It is likely that this protein would be a surface antigen. This process stimulates a genetically predisposed immune system into attacking the liver. We think that the damage produced is mediated by lymphocytes sensitized to the liver specific antigen. The disrupted liver cells release sequestered antigens, such as nuclear fragments or mitochondria, which secondarily stimulate the immune system into producing excess amounts of various auto-antibodies which have already been recognized as markers of an underlying auto-immune process.

REFERENCES

Bendixen, G., Søborg, M. (1970) J. Immunol. 104, 1551.
Doniach, D. (1970) Proc. Roy. Soc. Med. 63, 528.
Kaltreider, H. B., Soghor, D., Taylor, J. B., Decker, J. L. (1969) J. Immunol., 103. 179.
Mookerjee, B., Ackman, C. F. D., Dossetor, J. B. (1969) Transplantation 8, 745.
Paronetto, F., and Popper, H. (1969) Hetero-iso- and Auto-immune phenomena in the liver.
    In: Textbook of Immunopathology, Ed. Miescher. P. A. and Muller—Eberhard, H. J.
    Publ. Grune and Stratton. New York and London, II, 562.
Smith, M. G. M., Eddleston, A. L. W. F., Dominguez, J. A., Evans, D. B., Bewick, M., and
    Williams, R. (1969) Brit. Med. J. 4, 275.
Smith, M. G. M., Eddleston A. L. W. F., and Williams, R. (1971) In Preparation.
Søborg, M. (1968) Acta. Med. Scand. 184, 135.
Søborg, M., Bendixen, G. (1967) Acta. Scand. 181, 247.

DISCUSSION
Chairman: Dr. D. C. Dumonde

BENDIXEN

Have you tried other tissue antigens in control experiments besides the foetal liver extract?

SMITH

We have tried foetal kidney and various other antigens, including glutein and the leucocyte extracts used in our transplantation studies.

BENDIXEN

And have you only found a reaction with foetal liver extract?

SMITH

In a limited number of observations on some patients with active chronic hepatitis or primary biliary cirrhosis, we have found some cross-reaction with foetal kidney. We shall have to try and isolate organ-specific antigens for use in this system to make the results more meaningful.

BENDIXEN

Of 15 patients with glomerulonephritis that I studied, there were actually 2 who cross-reacted with liver extract, so there might be some cross-reactivity.

Did you find any correlation between positive reactivity in the leucocyte migration and the clinical condition of the patients? Did you also examine other comparably ill patients, to see if it might have been a non-specific response?

SMITH

I did try to show you some relationship with liver function in the patients with active chronic hepatitis. Although I could not directly relate the amount of tissue damage to the degree of positivity, those with normal liver function had normal migration indices.

As to your second point concerning comparably sick patients, I must point out that the patients with acute hepatic necrosis who were in deep coma had normal migration indices.

BENDIXEN

You do not think if a patient is feverish then perhaps there might be some non-specific leucocyte reaction?

SMITH

I can only reply by saying that such states tend to depress immune responses rather than to excite them.

HAVEMANN

Have you used autologous liver antigens in your studies?

SMITH

No. But I believe Dr. Finlayson in New York has used autologous liver in about 15 studies on patients with liver disease, and observed inhibition of migration in some cases.

HAVEMANN

We have studied autologous liver antigen in lymphocyte cultures from patients with active chronic hepatitis, but we have not been able to show any reaction to the antigen in different concentrations. We did not find any increase of RNA or DNA synthesis with autologous antigen, nor were we able to show skin reactivity with it.

SMITH

That may well be so, but other workers have described positive results; both Pipitone from Italy, and Schaffner from the States.

HAVEMANN

This may depend on the technique.

SCHAFFNER

We have reported positive results; it is important to use foetal calf serum in the system and not autologous plasma.

HAVEMANN

We do not use autologous plasma, but normal human AB serum.

SCHAFFNER

Neither does that work as well as foetal calf serum.

SODOMANN

Did you use different concentrations of your antigenically effective substance in the cases with primary biliary cirrhosis or active chronic hepatitis? You did so in the control patients, I noticed.

SMITH

All the values shown on the patients with active chronic hepatitis were obtained by doing the test at several antigen concentrations. The ones actually charted on the graph were the results obtained using 400 μg protein.

SODOMANN

Can you give any figures about the variation between serial readings on any one patient?

SMITH

We have not done many sequential studies yet on individual patients. In most we have retested, we have found reasonable agreement. For instance on the young girl with acute hepatitis, there were three figures for inhibition of migration — 0·75, 0·67, and 0·6, all obtained within ten days.

McINTYRE

What happens if you use adult liver?

SMITH

I do not know; we use foetal liver because it is sterile and it happened to be readily available.

THE ANERGIC STATE AND OTHER IMMUNOLOGICAL CHANGES IN PRIMARY BILIARY CIRRHOSIS

R. A. Fox, F. J. Dudley and Sheila Sherlock

The possibility that primary biliary cirrhosis is an auto-immune disease has already been discussed. In this talk I wish to concentrate on other aspects of this disease. The earliest detectable lesion in primary biliary cirrhosis appears to be damage to intermediate sized bile ducts with surrounding chronic inflammatory infiltration. In some places this inflammatory infiltrate takes on the form of granulomas. It would appear that the granulomas occur early in the disease and this was the conclusion reached by Rubin, Schaffner and Popper in 1965. We have studied 105 sections of liver obtained at autopsy or biopsy and each section has been staged histologically. The histological staging is that already described by Dr. Scheuer and it was found that 81 per cent of Stage I patients had granulomas present in the liver compared with 27 per cent of Stage II, 12 per cent of Stage III and in Stage IV — when macronodular cirrhosis was present — no granulomas were found. The overall incidence of granulomas in the patients reported here is 42 per cent (Table 1). Most of these granulomas are found within the portal zones but in one patient studied there were a large number of granulomas and they were found in both central and portal zones. Other tissues have been available for examination in 12 patients and of these granulomas were found in 5; 3 in hepatic hilar lymph nodes, 1 in the omentum and in one patient in both lung and mesenteric nodes (Table 1). These findings are taken as evidence of a widespread granulomatous response in this disease.

Generalized lymphadenopathy is a well recognized feature of primary biliary cirrhosis and in the classical paper of Ahrens *et al.,* in 1950, 8 out of their 17 patients with primary biliary cirrhosis had generalized lymphadenopathy. Histological examination of these lymph nodes reveals germinal centre hyperplasia, sinus histiocytosis and occasional granulomas. The finding of lymphadenopathy and generalized granulomas has some similarity to the findings

Table 1

Incidence of Granulomas in Primary Biliary Cirrhosis

Total Number Examined		69
Intrahepatic Granulomas		29 (42%)
Portal Zones		27
Central and Portal Zones		1
Unclassified		1
Extrahepatic Granulomas		5
Hepatic Hilar Nodes	3	
Omentum	1	
Lung and Mesentric Nodes	1	

147

Table 2

Tuberculin Status

GROUP	TOTAL	POSITIVE		NEGATIVE	
		No.	%	No.	%
Control	45	32	71	13	29
Cirrhosis	71	42	59	29	41
Cholestasis	32	19	59	13	41
Primary Biliary Cirrhosis	51	21	41	30	59

in sarcoidosis. In some patients it is extremely difficult to differentiate these two conditions. However, we have performed Kveim skin tests on 16 patients with primary biliary cirrhosis and granulomas, and the Kveim test has been consistently negative. These tests were carried out with known potent Kveim antigen, the skin tests were read at one month but no biopsies of the test site were carried out. It was these similarities with sarcoidosis that led us to investigate primary biliary cirrhosis to see if the normal mechanisms of delayed hypersensitivity which are known to be affected in a significant proportion of patients with sarcoidosis, were similarly affected in primary biliary cirrhosis.

SKIN TESTING WITH TUBERCULIN OR DNCB

Tuberculin skin testing provides a means of testing for the expression of delayed hypersensitivity to an antigen that has been met at some time in the past. Four groups of patients were studied, all matched for age and sex (Table 2):

1. Control hospital ward in-patients without evidence of liver or auto-immune disease.

2. Patients with cirrhosis, cryptogenic or alcoholic.

3. Patients with cholestasis from some cause other than primary biliary cirrhosis, such as calculus, stricture, neoplasm or drugs.

4. Patients with primary biliary cirrhosis.

71 per cent of the control subjects were positive to tuberculin and 29 per cent were negative when the test was repeated with 10 and, if necessary, 100 tuberculin units. In contrast, 59 per cent of patients with primary biliary cirrhosis were consistently tuberculin negative, a difference that is statistically significant. 41 per cent of patients with other forms of cirrhosis and 41 per cent of patients with cholestasis were consistently tuberculin negative. This incidence did not differ statistically from the control subjects. There appears to be a difference between the patients with cholestasis and cirrhosis and primary biliary cirrhosis but again this difference is not statistically significant.

2, 4-dinitro 1-chlorobenzene (DNCB) is a chemical contact sensitizing agent which is used to investigate both the induction and expression of delayed hypersensitivity. The regimen used to sensitize these patients has been described (Fox *et al.,* 1969) and 21 out of 22 control subjects could be sensitized with DNCB. Only 1 control subject failed to be sensitized, an incidence of 4 per cent. 16 patients out of 30 with primary biliary cirrhosis tested, could be sensitized. In 14 there was failure of sensitization, an incidence of 47 per cent. These groups were matched for age and sex and the difference is statistically significant.

LYMPHOCYTE TRANSFORMATION TO PHYTOHAEMAGGLUTININ

In vitro lymphocyte transformation in response to a non-specific mitogen phytohaemagglutinin (pHA) has been a third method of assessing immunological competence. The results from normal control subjects and patients with primary biliary cirrhosis can be seen in Fig. 1. Lymphocyte transformation was assessed by measuring the rate of incorporation of tritiated thymidine by means of

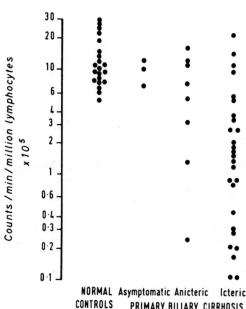

Fig. 1.

a liquid scintillation counting technique. The results were expressed as counts per minute/per million lymphocytes x 10^5 and expressed on a logarithmic scale. There is quite a wide range seen in control subjects. The patients with primary biliary cirrhosis were sub-divided into three groups:

1. Asymptomatic — these were three healthy middle aged females who were detected incidentally by the finding of a positive mitochondrial antibody test and subsequently shown to have the histological and biochemical features of primary biliary cirrhosis. One of these individuals has subsequently become symptomatic. All three had normal lymphocyte transformation.

2. Anicteric primary biliary cirrhosis — patients whose main symptom was pruritus but who had not yet become jaundiced.

3. Icteric — patients with symptomatic primary biliary cirrhosis who had the features of both jaundice and generalized pruritus.

A proportion of patients in groups 2 and 3 show impairment of lymphocyte transformation and a proportion of patients in both groups have obviously normal lymphocyte transformation. It would appear from these findings that impairment of lymphocyte transformation is not related to the serum bilirubin concentration. There is no good correlation between lymphocyte transformation and serum bilirubin, albumin, globulin, or IgM levels or the serum mitochondrial antibody titre.

It would appear unlikely that the depression of lymphocyte transformation in this disease is related to an inhibitory serum factor. Several experiments have been carried out in which the lymphocytes from control subjects, either normal individuals or patients with other forms of liver disease, have been used. In this situation plasma from a patient with primary biliary cirrhosis who has been shown to be anergic has no effect on the lymphocyte transformation. These experiments have been performed using isolated washed lymphocytes which were separated by preferential sedimentation in methylcellulose after the phagocytosis of particulate iron. Anergic primary biliary cirrhotic serum has no consistent effect on lymphocyte transformation. Lymphocytes from primary biliary cirrhotic patients have also been isolated and re-suspended in normal or calf serum and again there has been no significant elevation of lymphocyte transformation. On no occasion has the lymphocyte transformation returned to the normal range. It is concluded that the impaired lymphocyte transformation appears to be a true cellular defect and is not related to an inhibitory factor in the serum.

RELATION OF ANERGY TO CLINICAL AND PATHOLOGICAL GRADE

There is no good correlation between impairment of lymphocyte transformation and the duration of symptoms (Fig. 2). However, all patients with symptoms for more than 6 years show impairment of lymphocyte transformation. Duration of symptoms is a poor index of duration of disease and this conclusion is confirmed by the finding of asymptomatic or pre-symptomatic individuals. One never knows how long the disease has been

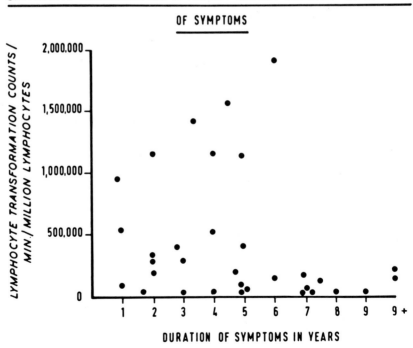

Fig. 2.

present before the symptoms develop. Probably the best method of assessing severity of disease is by the histological staging. All stage I patients show normal lymphocyte transformation and all the patients with stage IV disease show impairment of lymphocyte transformation. The results of stages II and III are varied. It would appear that anergy develops with the disease. Another feature of interest is that anergy is a feature when the granulomas have disappeared and when the granulomas are most prominent, in the early stages of the disease, lymphocyte transformation is normal. This finding militates against the hypothesis that anergy occurs as the result of antigenic competition.

RELATION BETWEEN LYMPHOCYTE TRANSFORMATION, TUBERCULIN AND DNCB TESTING

Lymphocyte transformation does not correlate with tuberculin status, neither does tuberculin status correlate with DNCB status, a finding which has been reported by many other workers in other diseased states. There is reasonable correlation between lymphocyte transformation and DNCB status (Table 3).

Table 3

In Vitro Lymphocyte Transformation and DNCB Skin Sensitization

Lymphocyte Transformation		+		−		+		−
DNCB		+		−		−		+
Control	21	18	86	1	5	0	0	2	10
Primary Biliary Cirrhosis	28	9	32	14	50	3	11	2	7
	Total	No.	%	No.	%	No.	%	No.	%

2 patients who were DNCB positive showed impaired lymphocyte transformation and 3 patients who were DNCB negative had normal lymphocyte transformation. 83 per cent of the patients with primary biliary cirrhosis and 91 per cent of the control subjects had either positive DNCB sensitization and normal lymphocyte transformation or failed to be sensitized with DNCB and had impaired lymphocyte transformation.

STUDIES WITH HAEMOCYANIN

The results reported so far demonstrate that there is a degree of anergy in a proportion of patients with primary biliary cirrhosis. The abnormality appears to be in the delayed hypersensitivity mechanisms related to thymic derived lymphocytes. We are currently investigating the response of these patients to a primary antigenic stimulus. The antigen that is used is haemocyanin, prepared from the haemolymph of Californian Keyhole limpets (megathura crenulata). This is a high molecular weight antigen which can be obtained very pure. The regimen that we have followed is to inject 5 mg. of haemocyanin subcutaneously on day one. Blood is removed at this time for baseline studies of antibodies, lymphocyte transformation and leucocyte migration inhibition to haemocyanin. On days 5–7, 100 mg. of haemocyanin are injected intradermally and at 48 hours the skin test is read. The preliminary results with haemocyanin skin test indicate that 100 per cent of control subjects react to haemocyanin and to date 21 controls have been tested. 6 of the 15 patients with primary biliary cirrhosis produced a positive skin test. 60 per cent failed to be sensitized. This finding correlates closely with the incidence of DNCB sensitization. In patients with cholestasis or cirrhosis, the majority — 90 per cent and 89 per cent respectively — have reacted by producing a positive skin test. The *in vitro* tests of delayed hypersensitivity that have so far been investigated are leucocyte migration inhibition and lymphocyte transformation. In the control subjects all patients showed inhibition of leucocyte migration after immunization with haemocyanin. In primary biliary cirrhosis a significant proportion of the patients failed to show inhibition of leucocyte migration after immunization and the results correlated closely with the results of the skin test, though it would appear that the skin test is slightly more sensitive. The results for lymphocyte transformation and also the haemocyanin haemagglutinating antibodies are too preliminary to be reported at this stage.

CONCLUSIONS

We have demonstrated that granulomas are found within the liver and in extrahepatic sites in primary biliary cirrhosis. A significant proportion of patients are anergic as demonstrated by negative tuberculin skin tests, failure to be sensitized with DNCB and impaired lymphocyte transformation to phytohaemagglutinin. It is concluded that there is impairment of normal mechanisms of delayed hypersensitivity which appears to occur as a result of the disease and is probably not aetiologically related.

REFERENCES

Ahrens, E. H. Jr., Payne, M. A., Kunkel, M. G., Eisenmenger, W. J., Blondheim, S. H. (1950) Medicine, Baltimore, 29, 299.
Fox, R. A., James, D. G., Scheuer, P. J., Sharma, O., Sheila Sherlock (1969) Lancet, i, 959.
Rubin, E., Schaffner, F., Popper, H. (1965) Amer. J. Path., 46, 387.

DISCUSSION
Chairman: Dr. D. C. Dumonde

CHAIRMAN
You suggested in a provocative way that you have not exhaustively excluded the participation of a serum factor in depressing antigen-specific cell mediated immunity — would you like to enlarge on that?

FOX
In our initial studies we could not be sure that all serum had been removed from the lymphocytes. In the later studies we have washed them very thoroughly and separated them. However, I have found that with too much washing one destroys the lymphocytes.

CHAIRMAN
Have you looked to see whether plasma or serum from an anergic patient will depress the tuberculin-stimulated lymphocyte transformation of a normal tuberculin-sensitive individual?

FOX
  I have not done that.

MacLAURIN
  In the phytohaemagglutinin study, I wondered whether you had assessed the responses of both age-matched controls and of patients with a comparable degree of illness but with normal livers? I ask this because in a large control series that I have been doing, there are quite a number of patients of 60 or 70 years who come well below the lower limit of your normal range.

FOX
  Yes, but that depends on how much tritiated thymidine you add.

MacLAURIN
  That is true, but nonetheless, some elderly normal subjects and certainly some elderly ill subjects can show very low levels of thymidine incorporation; so have you made any attempt to either study age-matched controls or to assess comparably debilitated patients?

FOX
  Most of these subjects were out-patients with very few complaints apart from pruritus. In fact, of all the patients, only 2 or 3 were in hospital, one with fractures and the other two for assessment. So really, the majority were not debilitated.
  We now do lymphocyte transformation with phytohaemagglutinin in parallel with the haemocyanin study and we use matched controls at the same time. In the future we shall express the results as a percentage of the matched control value on each occasion, following Levene's example.

WILLIAMS
  Is it fair to call a Kveim test negative without doing a biopsy?

FOX
  There is divided opinion on this. Dr. James at the Royal Northern Hospital does not feel that it is necessary if there is no macroscopic reaction. On the other hand, I know that Dr. Willoughby, who has worked on Crohn's disease, and others feel that a biopsy is mandatory.

WILLIAMS
  In the literature there are a number of papers on the concurrence of primary biliary cirrhosis with sarcoidosis, and we have seen one patient in whom the Kveim test was positive. Would you clarify for me the relationship between the anergic state as shown by impaired lymphocyte transformation and the stage of the primary biliary cirrhosis?

FOX
  The anergic state appears late in the disease. One of the possible mechanisms for the anergy is antigenic competition; i.e., the lymphocytes are so taken up with forming granulomas in the liver that they do not have time to transform with PHA. Our finding militates against that particular hypothesis as the granulomas tend to occur early.

EDDLESTON
  I wonder, Dr. Fox, if the difference between the tuberculin results and the DNCB results might suggest that it was the sensitization phase of the immune system which was abnormal? Secondly, if there really is a circulating inhibitory factor, Dr. Dumonde, do you think it could have been produced by the lymphocytes?

FOX

Your explanation for the discrepancies between the DNCB and the tuberculin results may well be right — there could be a great difference between eliciting a secondary response to an antigen acquired in childhood or at least some years previously, and giving them an antigenic stimulus to which they have not been exposed before. In sarcoidosis, Hodgkins disease and in most of the other diseases that have been studied there is poor agreement between DNCB and the tuberculin status.

CHAIRMAN

To answer your second question, we and others have some evidence that antigen-stimulated lymphocytes can release an inhibitor of thymidine incorporation. This, of course, does not necessarily relate to primary biliary cirrhosis.

INDUCTION AND TRANSFER OF AUTO-IMMUNE PERIDUCTULAR FIBROSIS IN INBRED RAT STRAINS – WITH EVIDENCE FOR PREDOMINANTLY CELL-MEDIATED PATHOGENESIS

B. P. MacLaurin

As discussed yesterday and again to-day, there are a great variety of auto-antibodies present in the serum of patients with liver disease. Most of these antibodies do not seem to be directed against the right things, for example they react with intracellular constituents, such as mitochondria, rather than cell surface components. Moreover, the majority of them, with the possible exception of antiductular antibodies, also react with cells in other tissues in the body.

In auto-immune thyroiditis, there is evidence that patients' lymphocytes are cytotoxic for thyroid cells in tissue culture. A similar finding has been reported by Perlmann and Broberger (1963) in ulcerative colitis. Lymphocytes from patients with ulcerative colitis are toxic to tissue cultures of foetal colon cells. Perlmann has further shown that when target cell monolayers (Chang liver cells) are coated with a specific antibody they remain intact in the absence of complement. If you then add normal (non-sensitized) lymphocytes to that monolayer, the Chang cells are promptly destroyed (Perlmann and Holm, 1968). I have recently shown somewhat similar findings using a tissue culture line of Burkitt lymphoma cells as the target tissue. These cell lines carry EB virus and also EB virus-determined antigens on their surface. They appear to be identical to similar lines produced from the lymphocytes of patients with infectious mononucleosis. If the Burkitt lymphoma cells are coated with antibody from the serum of a patient with infectious mononucleosis, nothing happens even if complement is present. However, if normal lymphocytes are then added, the Burkitt cells are promptly lysed within a six-hour period. So I wonder if these models give us an indication of what might be happening in liver disease in which there are numerous serum antibodies present and also, as was shown this morning, immune lymphocytes directed against the liver. The question is: can these two immune components combine to produce the lesions seen in liver disease?

DEVELOPMENT OF ANIMAL MODEL

In order to determine the relative significance of cell-mediated versus antibody-mediated immune damage, it seemed desirable to develop an animal model (MacLaurin and Humm, 1968 and 1969). In this paper I shall describe a periductular fibrotic liver lesion in rats, produced by prolonged immunization with isologous liver homogenate in complete Freund's adjuvant. This lesion is partially transferrable by spleen cell injections to isologous animals and is associated with some degree of delayed skin hypersensitivity to a supernatant fraction of liver. It is also associated with auto-antibody formation.

The animals used were two pure-line strains. The AS2 strain was the recipient animal in all tests, and was either immunized with isologous liver or with hybrid liver or with a strongly incompatible liver. The latter was obtained from pure strain BS black rats, there being a histocompatibility difference at the AgB[3] locus between these strains. As shown in Table 1, four groups of animals were immunized with liver homogenate in Freund's adjuvant. There were two sets of

155

Table 1
Experimental Groups of AS_2

RECIPIENT RATS

Animal Group Direct Liver Immunization	Number of animals
A	6
B	6
C	4
D	4
Controls	
E(untreated)	5
F(with adjuvant)	6
Spleen Cell Transfer	
G(Immunized cells)	11
H(sonicated cells)	6
K(normal cells)	5

Table 2
Liver Immunization Schedule

Animal Group Direct Liver Immunization	Source Strain	Inj. No.	+/− C.F.A.*
A	AS_2 BS	16	+
B	AS_2 BS	13	+
C	AS_2	10	+
D	BS	10	+
Controls			
E(untreated)	—	—	—
F(with adjuvant)	—	12	+

*C.F.A. = Complete Freund's Adjuvant.

control animals, one untreated and one treated with adjuvant alone. Two sets of animals received repeated intravenous injections either of intact or sonicated spleen cells, obtained from animals immunized with liver homogenate. Lastly a group of animals were immunized with spleen cells from normal animals.

The immunization schedule is shown in Table 2. The animals immunized with liver homogenate received a total of 10–16 injections at twice-weekly intervals, consisting of 0·5 ml. of homogenate in a water and oil suspension in Freund's complete adjuvant. The controls with adjuvant received the same amount of this agent.

HISTOLOGICAL APPEARANCES OF LIVER LESIONS

The appearance in unimmunized animals after van Giesen staining is shown in Fig. 1. The portal tracts are almost normal with very little cellular infiltration or

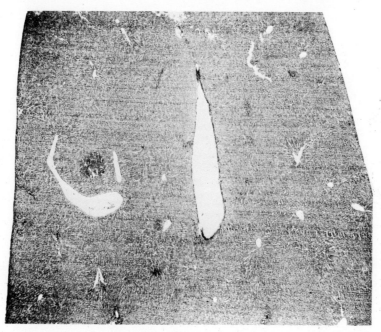

Fig. 1. Normal rat liver stained by the van Giesen method. There is negligible staining of fibrous tissue in the portal tracts. (Magnification x22).

fibrosis and the area around central veins is normal. In contrast, the appearances in immunized animals (Fig. 2) show red staining fibrous tissue around areas in which there are small and medium sized bile ducts, although the central veins are again normal. Under the high power, the changes are seen to be almost confined to the areas in the region of bile ducts and do not seem to involve the vessels to any significant extent. The fibrosis is patchy, involving some bile ducts and not others, and bile duct reduplication is common. Around the ducts a cuff of lymphoid cells was frequently seen (Fig. 3). No polymorph infiltrate was found and neither was there any particular increase of plasma cells on Unna Pappenheim staining.

Animals sacrificed shortly after the end of the immunization programme, showed a well-marked cellular infiltrate in the portal tracts in addition to the

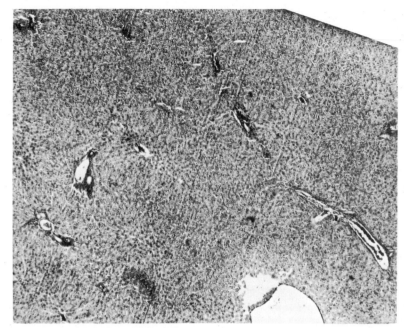

Fig. 2. Liver, following immunization with isologous liver and Freund's adjuvant (Group C), similarly stained, showing fibrous tissue densely stained, in relation to bile ducts in the portal tracts. (Magnification x44).

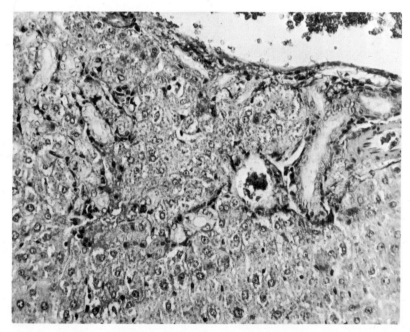

Fig. 3. Reduplication and distortion of small bile ducts following direct liver immunization. Note the cuff of lymphocytes surrounding each duct. (Magnification x240).

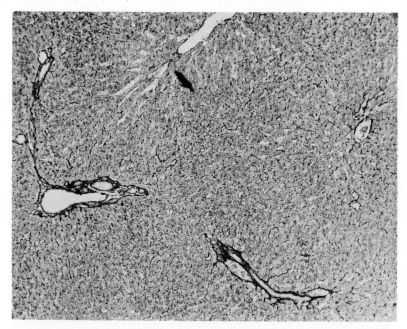

Fig. 4. Rat liver following direct immunization showing tendency for bridging between adjacent portal tracts, demonstrated by a reticulin stain. (Magnification x88).

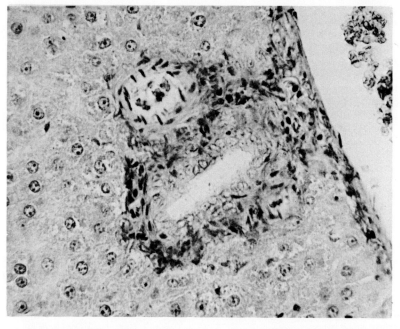

Fig. 5. Liver lesion produced by transfer of liver immunized spleen cells (Group G), showing distorted and thickened bile duct epithelium, with a surrounding dense fibrotic reaction. (Magnification x380).

fibrotic reaction. Later on the fibrotic reaction became the dominant feature and the cellular infiltrate had largely subsided. Reticulin stains in the more severely affected animals showed that there was a tendency for aggregation of adjacent portal areas (Fig. 4).

Antibody studies were carried out by Mr. Ken Couchman of the Palmerston North Medical Research Foundation in New Zealand. Using fluorescein isothiocyanate labelled antisera to rat globulin raised in rabbits on cryostat sections of liver from these immunized rats, he found specific fluorescence confined to the areas of the fibrotic reaction. The fluorescence did not appear to involve the liver cells to any significant extent, but seemed to outline some of the small bile ducts and bile duct canaliculi.

FINDINGS IN ANIMALS IMMUNIZED BY TRANSFER OF SPLEEN CELLS

These were normal animals which had received injections of spleen cells from the immunized group. Three successive intravenous injections of cells were given at monthly intervals — a total of 75×10^6 cells. Histological sections of the liver showed distorted bile ducts with some reduplication of the mucosa. Surrounding the bile ducts was a fibrotic reaction with a moderate cellular infiltrate. The neighbouring liver cells were unaffected except in the more severely involved areas where there was much cellular infiltrate. In such areas, minor degrees of liver cell damage were seen. Overall, the histological changes were comparable to, but not as severe as in the directly immunized group (Fig. 5).

QUANTITATION OF HISTOLOGICAL CHANGES

In an attempt to quantitate these findings, the slides were coded and, by "blind" assessment, an attempt was made to score the degree of change (Table 3). This is rather a crude method but I am reasonably confident that there were significant differences in the means for the group immunized with homogenate and the spleen cell transfer group as compared with the control animals. Thus, considering the fibrotic reaction, two of the groups of animals immunized with liver homogenate certainly showed a difference and one possibly; the fourth group showed very little change. The animals in this fourth group had been immunized from birth, whereas the others were immunized at three months of age; it may be that three weeks after birth is too early, although at that age this strain normally has full immunological competence.

The bile duct changes were largely confined to animals showing periductular fibrosis, and accordingly the bile duct changes in the group immunised with homogenate were quite well marked. Only minor bile duct changes were seen in animals who had received injections of sonicated cells even though there was quite marked periductular fibrosis in these animals. The finding of a histological lesion in the latter group raises the question of whether antibody or antibody-producing cells are transferred when the spleen cells are given, in addition to cellular-immune reactivity.

One other lesion was demonstrated in these animals. This was a change in the peribronchial region in the lungs. Animals immunized with liver homogenate and those immunized by spleen cell transfer, showed very striking lymphoid infiltration in the peribronchial region throughout the lung fields (Fig. 6). Germinal centres were frequently seen along the bronchi. This lesion was not seen either in control animals (Fig. 7), or in animals receiving normal spleen cells by injection. It was found only to a minor extent in animals receiving sonicated spleen cells from the immunized group.

Table 3

Mean Scores for Liver Histology

Animal Group	Liver Histology	
Direct	Periductular	Bile Duct
Liver	Fibrosis	Damage
Immunization		
A	2·5	1·5
B	1·3	0·2
C	4	1
D	1	0
Controls		
E	1	0
F	1	0·5
Spleen Cell Transfer		
G(Immunized cells)	1·8	1·1
H(Sonicated cells)	1·7	0·3
K(Normal cells)	0·5	0·4

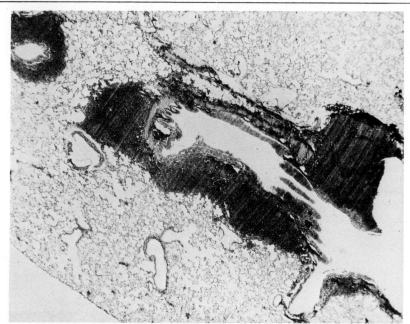

Fig. 6. Dense peribronchial lymphocytic infiltration with germinal centres and with some disruption of the bronchial epithelium as seen in the direct liver immunized animals (Group D). (Magnification x22).

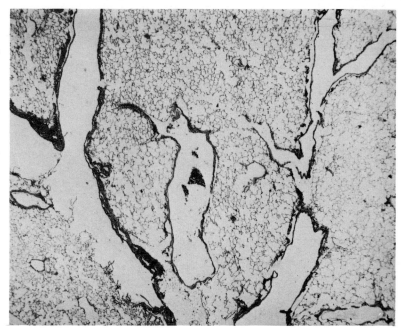

Fig. 7. Minimal peribronchial lymphocytic accumulation seen in non-immunized animals (Magnification x22).

CHANGES IN SKIN REACTIVITY

The next stage was to assess whether immunization had produced any alteration in skin reactivity to liver antigens. The liver homogenate was centrifuged at 15,000 G for 15 minutes and the resulting supernatant was used as the antigen. This was injected intradermally on one side of the back, and normal saline in similar amounts on the other side. Two of the groups of animals immunized with liver homogenate showed a definite reaction when compared with the control side. Comparison of skin thickness measured by calipers is shown shown in Table 4. This reaction developed at 24 hours and was maximal by 48 hours but regrettably no biopsy was taken of the lesion. In the spleen cell transfer group only a minor increase in skin thickness was found, of doubtful significance.

In order to assess this further, I also studied the behaviour of macrophages from the peritoneal cavity of the immunized animals, compared with macrophages from control animals. I did not feel justified in looking for inhibition of macrophage migration by antigen because I could not completely exclude particulate matter from the liver supernatant. However, I simply made an assessment of macrophage monolayers in the presence of the liver homogenate or in the presence of normal saline. Initially the cells were evenly dispersed but within two hours there was a definite aggregation of macrophages in the immunized group which was more marked by 12 hours (Fig. 8). This was not seen to any significant extent in the controls. This provides some further confirmation of cellular immune change.

Table 4

Skin Tests with Supernatant of Liver Homogenate

Animal Group	Mean Skin Thickness in mms at 48 Hrs.	
Direct	Test side	Control side
Liver		
Immunization		
A	3·3	2·0
B	3·0	1·9
C	2·4	2·0
D	2·0	1·7
Controls		
E	2·3	2·0
F	2·2	2·0

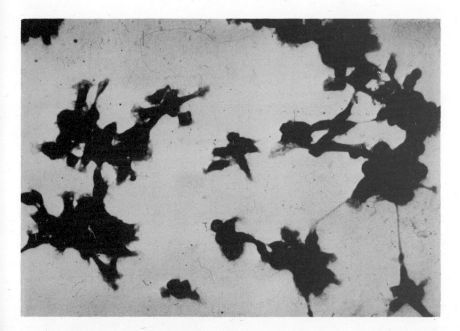

Fig. 8. Aggregation reaction in macrophage monolayer (previously evenly dispersed) 12 hours after the addition of the supernatant fraction of liver homogenate used for skin testing. (×230).

LYMPHOCYTES

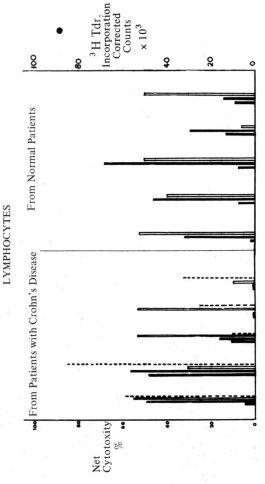

Fig. 9. Illustrating various responses of lymphocytes taken either from normal patients or from patients with Crohn's Disease. The solid black columns represent the cytotoxic activity of the cells on chromium-labelled Birkett lymphoma cells either with or without preincubation in the presence of irradiated tumour cells respectively. The open columns represent the proliferative response of the lymphocytes induced by Birkett lymphoma cells, and the dotted column the response of Crohn's lymphocytes to phytohaemagglutinin.

RELATIVE ROLES OF CELLULAR VERSUS ANTIBODY AUTO-IMMUNITY

The lesion I have demonstrated bears some resemblance to the liver lesion seen in ulcerative colitis and in Crohn's disease, and perhaps to the findings described in primary biliary cirrhosis. It is most marked after prolonged immunization. It was more marked in the animals receiving 16 injections than in the animals receiving 12, and it was more marked in the animals where immunization was commenced after three months of age. The changes were more evident in the group receiving isologous liver homogenate, as compared with homologous or hybrid liver homogenate, so I think it fair to describe the lesion as an auto-immune periductular fibrosis. In contrast to the findings of Scheiffarth *et al.*, (1967) who produced a temporary liver lesion in mice by a similar method, this lesion was persistent; at least, the fibrosis was persistent, the cellular infiltrate tending to diminish with time. It seems reasonable to suggest that the appearances result from a combined cellular and antibody-mediated immune response, possibly directed against bile duct constituents. The fact that this lesion is seen to a lesser degree in animals receiving a transfer of sonicated spleen cells from immunized animals would suggest that the production of damage was not solely a cellular immune process. Equally one can argue that it is not solely an antibody-mediated process.

The pulmonary lesion may also be "auto-immune" and could represent a cross-reaction with tissue of similar embryological origin. It is of interest that in the immunized animals, antibody against gastric parietal cells was demonstrated although no mitochondrial antibody was found.

CYTOTOXICITY OF LYMPHOCYTES

The evidence of anergy in primary biliary cirrhosis, might be considered to contradict the importance of cellular immunity in human liver disease. There is clearly a conflict between the findings of Dr. Smith and Dr. Fox. though admittedly these were with very different antigens. However it must be emphasized that only some parameters of cellular immunity have so far been studied in this disease and the crucial question of whether lymphocyte-cytotoxicity is impaired or not, remains unanswered. To me, the latter is the most important unanswered question still remaining in the study of "auto-immune" liver disease. Failure to demonstrate lymphokine factors may or may not be synonymous with absence of lymphocyte cytotoxic capacity on an antibody labelled target tissue.

To support this contention, I would like to describe some findings relating to the cytotoxic capacity of lymphocytes from patients with Crohn's disease and from normal subjects against Birkett lymphoma cells (Fig. 9). If one adds normal lymphocytes to tumour cells there is some cytotoxic response. If the lymphocytes are pre-incubated with irradiated tumour cells for 5 days beforehand, and then added to chromium-labelled lymphoma cells, there is a considerable increase in cytotoxicity. The important point is that some normal subjects showed a good cytotoxic response but a poor proliferative response measured by uptake of tritiated thymidine, against the surface antigens of the tumour cell. Other subjects showed rather poor cytotoxicity but a good proliferative response. Similarly, when one examined lymphocytes from the Crohn's patients, in some there was no cytotoxicity at all and yet one of them had a perfectly normal proliferative response and a reasonable phytohaemagglutinin response. Again, in other patients there was almost complete absence of cytotoxicity against the tumour cells but quite a reasonable phytohaemagglutinin response and a rather poor proliferative response. So there can be a separation between the cytotoxic capacity of lymphocytes and their proliferative capacity in the presence of the same antigen *in vitro* and perhaps between the ability to produce lymphokines and a cytotoxic reaction *in vivo*. In my view the cytotoxic reaction is paramount in immune reactions affecting the liver.

REFERENCES

MacLaurin, B. P. and Humm, J. A. (1968), 46, 3, 75–77.
MacLaurin, B. P. and Humm, J. A. (1969) Proceedings of the 3rd Asian-Pacific Congress of
    Gastroenterology, (Melbourne), Pages 46–54.
Perlman, P., Holm. G. (1968). In Mechanism of inflammation induced by Immune reactions.
    Eds. Miescher P. A. and Grabar P. (Schwabe, Basil). P. 325.
Perlman, P., Broberger, O., (1963) J. Exp. Med. 117, 717.
Scheiffarth, F., Warnatz, H., Mayer, K., (1967) J. Immunol. 98, 396.

DISCUSSION
Chairman: Dr. D. C. Dumonde

FOX

Yesterday, you mentioned that you had produced granulomas in some of your inbred rats. Was this another experiment?

MacLAURIN

Yes, that was a type of graft versus host reaction in which I endeavoured to accentuate the liver changes by injecting the spleen cells from an immunized animal into a F1 hybrid. By these means a very much more striking lesion was produced, but the appearance was different and no longer bore any resemblance to the human disease. In a typical graft versus host reaction there is a predominantly centrilobular lesion. There is also a portal reaction. I have some slides which demonstrate these changes but regrettably none which actually show a giant cell, although they were seen in some of these lesions. By direct injection into the liver a short lasting granuloma is produced resembling the Elkins lesion in the kidney. Here is a fairly large bile duct which is showing considerable change in the bile duct surface and the beginnings of invasion by lymphoid cells (Fig. 1). A higher power view is shown in Fig. 2. An enormous proliferation of lymphoid cells develops with a granuloma-type appearance with involvement of bile ducts in the periphery.

SMITH

In the present study, did you find any lesions in the kidneys or in the salivary glands of these rats?

MacLAURIN

There were no lesions in the kidneys. Neither was there any obvious abnormality in the salivary glands or thyroid.

EDDLESTON

Can you really say that if you fail to abolish the response by using sonicated cells, you have ruled out cell-mediated transfer; presumably you are likely to liberate transfer factors and possibly RNA.

MacLAURIN

The thesis I am putting forward is that there is a combined cellular and antibody-mediated response here. If this is solely a cell mediated response then the transfer of sonicated cells should not produce a lesion unless, as you suggest, transfer factors are involved. Indeed this may be so because the amount of antibody going across must be very small. I was very impressed by the relative absence of plasma cells in the liver itself.

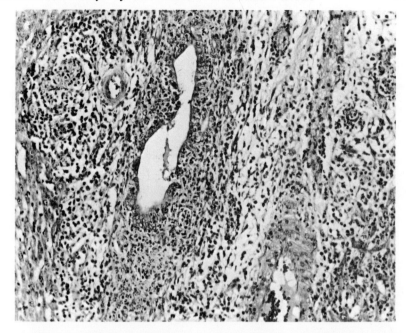

Fig. 1. Lesion produced by direct intrahepatic injection of liver immunized spleen cells into an F$_1$ hybrid rat. A local graft versus host reaction ensues, with production of some degree of piecemeal necrosis of liver cells and a rather granulomatous reaction about the bile ducts with some disruption of the mucosa.

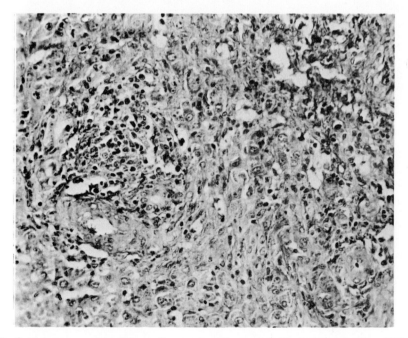

Fig. 2. Higher power view of the graft versus host liver seen in Fig. 8. (Magnification x240).

SMITH

Have you tried the effect of injecting kidney homogenate and then looking at the liver to see what lesions are produced, if any?

MacLAURIN

I have not. Scheiffarth *et al.,* did this experiment and did show minor changes. I believe that these changes could well have been produced by the Freund's adjuvant: after administration of adjuvant alone it has been reported that there may be an impressive increase in spleen weight and a tremendous increase in the number of macrophages and histiocytes in the liver.

CHARACTERIZATION AND ISOLATION OF LIVER SPECIFIC PROTEINS IN DIFFERENT SPECIES: THEIR IMPORTANCE FOR EXPERIMENTAL MODELS AND IN DIAGNOSIS OF CHRONIC HEPATITIS

K. H. Meyer zum Büschenfelde and F. K. Kössling

In 1963 as a result of clinical observations in active chronic hepatitis with hyper-gamma globulinaemia, we became interested in whether the liver possesses an immunological specificity. Our interest was further stimulated by the studies of Dumonde (1966), and by the reports of immune reactions after hepatic transplantation from Starzl *et al.* (1961), McBride *et al.* (1962) and Paronetto *et al.* (1965).

OCCURRENCE OF LIVER SPECIFIC AUTO-ANTIBODY

At the beginning of our studies we wanted to know whether or not liver specific auto-antibodies could be found in the serum of patients with active chronic hepatitis, antibodies which could not be absorbed with subcellular fractions of other organs of man and other species. From 1964 to 1968 we found such antibodies in the sera of 16 patients out of a group of 85 cases with active chronic hepatitis. On liver biopsy these 16 patients all showed the morphological changes of chronic agressive hepatitis at different stages, and hyper-gamma globulinaemia in their serum. The antibody was an IgG type of immunoglobulin and was not absorbed by soluble proteins of other organs. Complete species specificity could not be ascertained as hetero-immune sera against human liver specific protein showed lines of identity with the antibody found in these human sera. Complete absorption of the auto-antibody is only possible with the liver specific protein. The incidence of this antibody together with that of antinuclear factor, anti-mitochondrial antibody and anti-gamma globulin factors in 3 different groups of liver disease and a group of blood donors is shown in Table 1.

	Humoral Immunreactions in			
	acute Hepatitis	chronic active Hepatitis	Livercirrhosis (postnecrotic and alcoholic)	Blood donors
n	87/100 %	85/100 %	62/100 %	68/100 %
ANF	15/29 %	34/40 %	14/21 %	0 %
AMA	29/33 %	37/43 %	7/12 %	0 %
AGF	6/7 %	26/30 %	11/18 %	0 %
LSpA	> 1:8 0 %	> 1:8 16/19 %	> 1:8 0 %	0 %

Table 1. Spectrum of antinuclear factors (ANF), anti-mitochondrial antibodies (AMA), antigammaglobulin factors (GF) and liver specific antibodies (LSpA) in 3 groups of different liver diseases and a group of blood donors.

ISOLATION OF CORRESPONDING ANTIGEN

The antigens against which the liver specific auto-antibody is directed were found:

1. In the supernatant of a liver homogenate free of nuclei after ultra centrifugation at 150,000 G.

2. In the first peak of an eluate from Sephadex G. 100 column-chromatography after application of the 150,000 G. supernatant.

3. After purification accomplished by re-chromatography of the first peak mentioned above on Sephadex G 200.

Figure 1 demonstrates a typical chromatogram on Sephadex G 200 of an eluate from Sephadex G 100 (first peak) compared with normal human serum. Localized

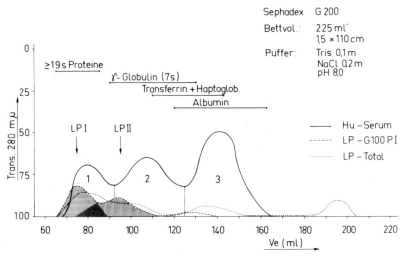

Fig. 1. Chromatogram on Sephadex G 200 of an eluate from Sephadex G 100 (first peak) compared with a normal human serum. LP 1 demonstrates the position of a lipoprotein, LP 2 of a liver specific cytoplasmic protein.

between the 19s and 7s globulins of normal human serum, a cytoplasmic protein with a molecular weight of approximately 190,000, could be eluted from the Sephadex G 200 column. The molecular weight was calculated from sucrose density gradient centrifugation. The position of this protein in immune electrophoretic and polyacrylamide electrophoretic studies can be seen in Fig. 2 and 3. Antibodies reacting with this protein could not be absorbed by corpuscular subcellular fractions of liver tissue. Chordi *et al.* (1969) have now confirmed our findings. The protein can be detected by hetero-immune sera in the blood of patients with severe necrotic episodes (Fig. 4).

In the first peak of the Sephadex G 200 eluate, occurring in the region where 19s globulins are localized, we found a lipoprotein which was different from serum-lipoprotein. The electrophoretic behaviour of this lipoprotein was studied in starch gel, agarose, cellulose acetate (Fig. 5a), and on Whatman 2' paper (Fig. 5b). Antibodies to this lipoprotein were localized to membranes of hepatocytes by the indirect Coon's technique of immuno-fluorescence (Fig. 6). However confirmation of this finding by electronmicroscopy is necessary.

We then set out to examine the biological significance of these proteins in experimental models.

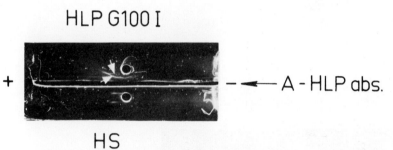

Fig. 2. Position of LP 1 and LP 2 in immuno-electrophoresis. The absorbed antihuman
LP serum (AHLP abs) from rabbits gives no reaction with human serum (HS),
with HLP G-200 II (LP 2) only 1 precipitate near the start, with HLP G-200 I
there are two precipitation lines.

INDUCTION OF TOLERANCE USING HUMAN LIVER PROTEIN

In the first place we tried to induce specific immunological tolerance to
soluble human liver protein in adult rabbits. The experiments published by
Mitchison (1964), Billingham (1961), and Moller (1967) as well as by
Thorbecke and Benaceraff (1967), showed the importance of using a very
small primary dose of antigen in initiating the induction. Furthermore it was
essential to use stable protein solutions, because aggregated proteins had proved
to be unsuitable. We used freshly eluted protein solutions for this reason, and
began the immunization procedure with repeated doses of 5 mg. of protein per
injection up to the 100th day. An antibody response could not be elicited
during this period and, even when the antigen dose was increased thereafter
to 275 mg and given in Freunds adjuvant, no antibody response could be
detected (Fig. 7).

We then attempted to break the established immunological tolerance by
using antigen conjugated with sulfanilic acid according to the method of
Baker *et al.* (1956). This was successful after the second immunization. The

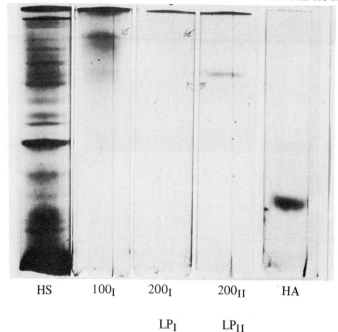

HS   100$_I$ 200$_I$ 200$_{II}$ HA

LP$_I$ LP$_{II}$

Fig. 3. The result of polyacrylamide-electrophoresis using LP 1 and LP 2 from
Sephadex G 200, the first peak of an eluate from Sephadex G 100, normal human
serum (HS) and human albumin (HA). Behringwerke, Marburg).

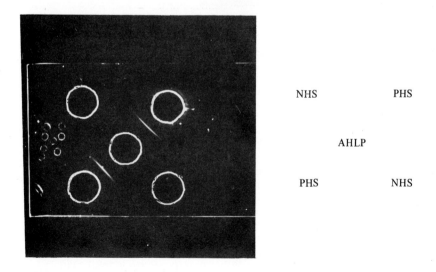

NHS   PHS

AHLP

PHS   NHS

Fig. 4. Demonstration of LP 2 in a serum of a patient with a severe necrotic using
hetero-immune sera from rabbits (central position). A normal human serum
shows no reaction.

    AHLP = antihuman LP-Serum
    NHS = normal human Serum
    PHS = pathologic human Serum

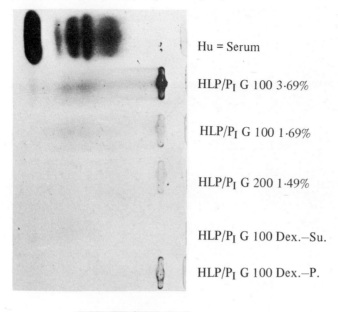

Hu = Serum

HLP/P$_I$ G 100 3·69%

HLP/P$_I$ G 100 1·69%

HLP/P$_I$ G 200 1·49%

HLP/P$_I$ G 100 Dex.—Su.

HLP/P$_I$ G 100 Dex.—P.

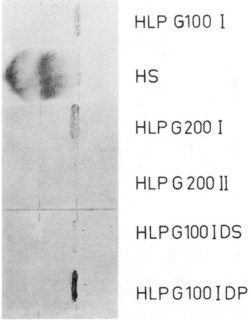

HLP G100 I

HS

HLP G 200 I

HLP G 200 II

HLP G100 I DS

HLP G100 I DP

Fig. 5. (a) Microzone electrophoresis on cellulose acetate. In the first peak (P$_I$) of eluates from Sephadex G 100 and G 200 as well as in the precipitate by dextran-Sulfate and calcium chloride (Burstein-Technik), there is a protein which stays at the point of application. This corresponds to the separation on (b) Whatman 2 paper. The coloration on Whatman 2 paper demonstrates a lipoprotein which migrates differently from serum lipoproteins.
DS = Dex.-Sup. = supernatant after precipitation with Dextran-Sulfat
PP = Dex.-Sup = precipitate by Dextran-Sulfat
HLP = human liver protein

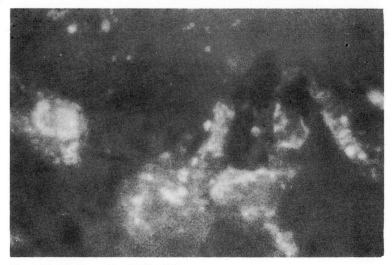

Fig. 6. Localization of antibodies against LP 1 by the indirect Coon's technique of immunofluorescence.

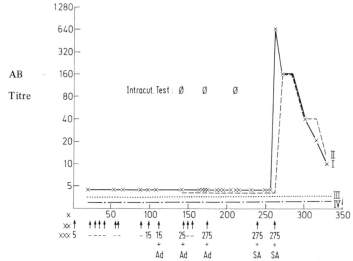

Fig. 7. Induction of immunotolerance towards organ specific soluble human liver protein by low dosage protein injections (5 mg./week/ 2000–3000 g. rabbit). After the 100th day it was not possible to break tolerance by higher doses of the native protein administered with complete Freund's adjuvant (Ad). Tolerance was broken after two injections of sulfanilic acid conjugated liver specific protein (SA). Following this, circulating antibodies both to the altered human liver protein and the native protein were found*.
　　* Days on which blood was taken.
　 ** Days on which protein was injected.
　*** Protein dosage in mg.

Curve 1: native human liver specific protein as antigen,

Curve 2: sulfanilic acid altered human liver protein as antigen,

Curve 3: native soluble human kidney protein as antigen,

Curve 4: native soluble rabbit liver protein as antigen for passive haemagglutination.

antibody response obtained was not only directed towards the altered, but also towards the native soluble liver protein. This finding seemed of basic importance with regard to the suspected role of auto-immune reactions involved in the self-perpetuation of active chronic hepatitis.

PRODUCTION OF ACTIVE CHRONIC HEPATITIS BY IMMUNIZATION PROCEDURES

The next step in our examination of the biological significance of the liver specific soluble protein was concerned with the induction of active chronic hepatitis by immunization with homologous and heterologous antigens. Our experiments were dependent on the finding that antibodies against homologous liver specific protein were not completely species specific. Dumonde (1966) and Hraba (1968) have reported that auto-immune reactions may be induced not only by homologous or autologous organ-bound antigens in Freund's adjuvant, but also by heterologous antigens, probably with less difficulty. They were able to show that immunization with heterologous organ protein produced a higher antibody titre to the corresponding homologous protein than did initial immunization with the homologous tissue. It is not yet clear whether tissue damage is produced more easily by immunization with heterologous rather than homologous antigens.

In our attempt to induce active chronic hepatitis in the rabbit, several different immunisation schedules were used. I want to confine my discussion to the following three:—

1. Immunization with heterologous (human) liver protein with and without adjuvant, for a long period of time.

2. Immunization with homologous (rabbit) protein and Freund's adjuvant.

3. Immunization with homologous (rabbit) protein conjugated with sulfanilic acid and administered in Freund's adjuvant.

Control animals were immunized for equivalent periods with nuclei of liver cells, human serum albumin, human Cohn's fraction II, adjuvant alone, and immune complexes.

Morphological changes similar to those seen in active chronic hepatitis were found in animals immunized with heterologous proteins. The addition of adjuvant had a marked accelerating effect — the typical lesions of piecemeal necrosis were detectable after an immunization period of 6 to 7 months (Fig. 8). Antibodies reacting with the homologous liver protein were demonstrable at this time by passive haemagglutination (Table 2).

With fluorescein isothiocyanate (FITC)-labelled rabbit liver protein and FITC-labelled antirabbit gamma globulin from the goat, specifically sensitized cells were detectable in the periportal field (Figs. 9 and 10). To-date the inflammatory liver disease has shown self-perpetuation for three to five months after the last immunization.

Contrary to the positive results with heterologous proteins, the histological lesions of active chronic hepatitis could not be produced in the rabbit by immunization with the homologous (rabbit) liver specific protein. However, after 6–7 months immunization with homologous liver proteins conjugated with sulfanilic acid, early histological changes were obtained. The control animals showed no evidence of an active chronic liver disease but did show non-specific sensitization reactions (Table 3).

	AHLP/ARLP from Rabbit after absorption with	
PH with	HLP	RLP
HLP	–	+
RLP	+/–	–

Table. 2. Summary of inhibition tests (pH = Passive haemagglutination). Anti-sera containing antibodies to human and rabbit LP's from rabbits with morphological changes similar to active chronic hepatitis tested after absorption with human LP and rabbit LP. It is uncertain why antibodies reacting with rabbit liver protein cannot be demonstrated in all cases.

Group	Rabbit n	Antigen for Immunization	Duration of Immunization (days)	Morphology chronic active hepatitis +	Morphology chronic active hepatitis –	Immunreactions Antibody RLP	Immunreactions Antibody HLP	Immunreactions Skintest RLP
1	7	HLP + FA[+]	400	7	O	4	7	7
2	16	HLP + FA	180–240	6	10	10	16	16
3	14	KLP + FA	180–300	O	14	O	O	O
4	20	KLP (altered) + FA	180	O	20	10	O	12
5	24	different controls	180–300	O	24	O	O	O

Table 3. Morphological changes and immune reactions in different groups of white New Zealand rabbits after immunization with different liver antigens and Freund's adjuvant.

        HLP = human liver protein
        KLP = Rabbit – liver protein
        FA = Freund's adjuvant

DEMONSTRATION OF SPECIFICALLY SENSITIZED CELLS IN HUMAN ACTIVE CHRONIC HEPATITIS

The demonstration of specifically sensitized cells using FITC-labelled homologous liver protein in active chronic hepatitis induced in rabbits led to similar studies in the human disease. We have now completed investigations in two series of cases with different liver diseases. The outstanding finding was that cells specifically sensitized to the liver protein were demonstrated

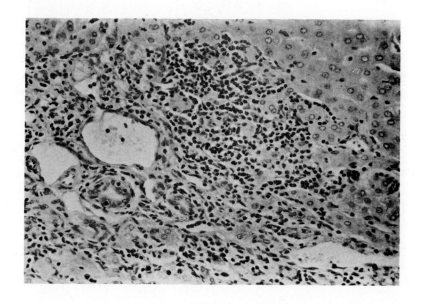

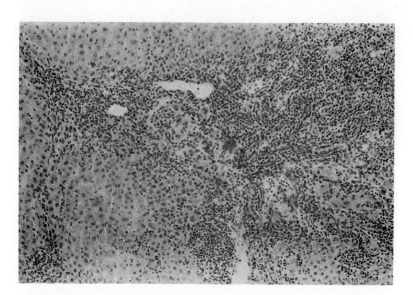

Fig. 8. Active chronic hepatitis induced in a rabbit by heterologous (human) liver protein and Freund's adjuvant. 5 months after the last immunization. (H and E ×400 and ×80).

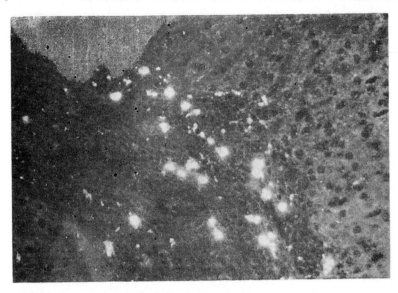

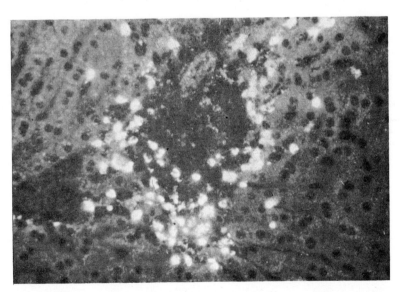

Fig. 9. Specifically sensitized cells demonstrated by direct immunofluorescence with FITC-marked rabbit liver protein in active chronic hepatitis in rabbits induced by human LPG 100 I. (5 months after the last immunization).

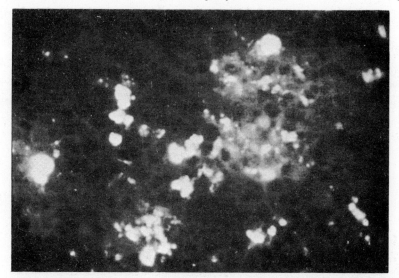

Fig. 10. Gamma globulin producing cells demonstrated by indirect immunofluorescence technique with FITC-marked antirabbit gamma globulin from the goat. Chronic active hepatitis in rabbits induced by human LPG 100 I. (5 months after the last immunization).

(Fig. 11), in more than 85% of patients with active chronic hepatitis. The detection of these cells in liver biopsy specimens by immuno-fluorescence has become an important criterion for selecting patients for immunosuppressive therapy.

In our most recent series of patients, gamma globulin producing cells demonstrated by using FITC labelled anti-human gamma globulin, were found in more than 90% of cases of active chronic hepatitis. However, as these cells could be detected frequently in other inflammatory liver disorders their presence is not specific for active chronic hepatitis. Moreover the frequency of positive results with this technique appears to be dependent on the quality and quantity of the labelled antisera used.

STUDIES WITH PERFUSED RAT LIVER

I should now like to describe some experiments performed in collaboration with Dr. Jeunet and Dr. Miescher in Geneva. Our aim was to discover why specific sensitized cells are so constantly detectable in the liver biopsies from patients with active chronic hepatitis, whereas circulating antibodies to liver specific proteins are found only inconstantly and in low titres. For this purpose we used the isolated, perfused rat liver shown in Fig. 12. The isolation and perfusion techniques have been reported elsewhere (Jeunet and Good, 1967, Jeunet and Good, in press). Antisera to rat liver specific protein were raised in rabbits and after absorption with rat kidney and rat plasma, those with significant titres to rat liver specific protein were used in the subsequent experiments.

The isolated rat liver was perfused at one hour intervals with small aliquots of the antiserum for a total time of five hours. The flow rate in the system was adjusted to 16 ml./minute and, for two minutes after each application of antiserum, samples were taken from the perfusate at 15 second intervals. Each sample was studied for the titre of antibody to liver specific protein, total

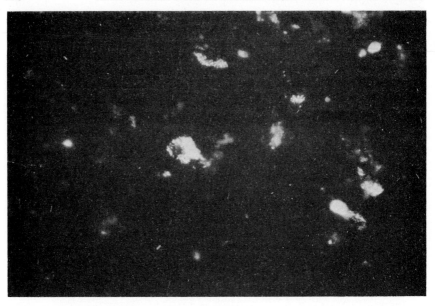

Fig. 11. Demonstration of specifically sensitized cells by FITC-labelled homologous
liver protein in active chronic hepatitis in man.

haemolytic complement levels and the aspartate and alanine aminotransferase
levels as well as for the pH. The flow rate in the system and the bile flow
served as an index of a correctly functioning perfusion.

Figure 13 illustrates the rate of antibody consumption. The longer the
duration of the perfusion the more the antibody against the cytoplasmic
protein (LP II) was used up. In contrast to the low consumption of the antibody
in the early stages, we observed a rapid decrease of total haemolytic complement
levels after the first antibody application (Fig. 14). This rather surprising
finding led us to repeat the experiment using antisera pretreated by differential
absorption. When an antiserum absorbed with the first peak of Sephadex
G 200 was used, there was no significant decrease of the total haemolytic
complement levels. However, perfusion with antiserum absorbed with the
second elution peak from Sephadex G 200, that is the cytoplasmic liver
specific protein, produced marked consumption of haemolytic complement.
This is shown in experiments numbers 27 and 28 respectively, in Fig. 14.
Control perfusion with Coombs sera and antihuman liver protein sera and
antirat mitochondrial sera showed little or no antibody consumption
(Fig. 15).

Immunofluorescent studies of the perfused liver showed localization of the
consumed antibodies to cytoplasmic and membrane structures of the hepatocytes (Fig. 16). To-date we have not used FITC-labelled anticomplement
in our studies. Further confirmation of these findings by electronmicroscopy
is necessary.

These results suggest that the liver specific auto-antibodies in human active
chronic hepatitis are also consumed. Membrane antibodies can probably fix
complement and be directly cytotoxic. The antibody directed against the
cytoplasmic protein can only produce damage by indirect means through
antigen antibody complex formation. Membrane lesions seem to be necessary

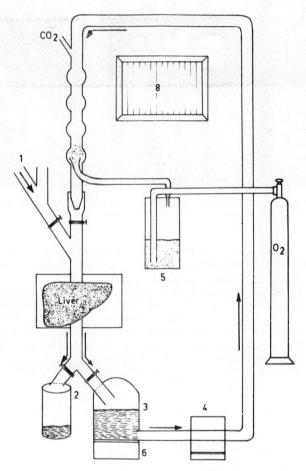

Fig. 12. Diagram of the experimental system of the perfused rat liver.

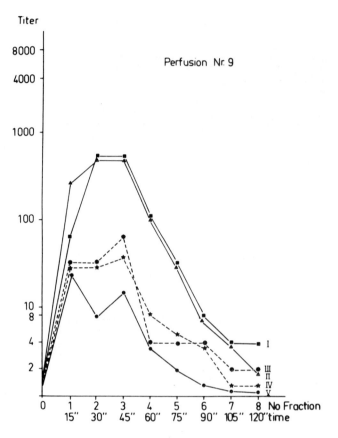

Fig. 13. Results of antibody consumption in the perfused rat liver after application of an hetero-immune-anti-rat liver serum raised in rabbits. The antibody was retained in progressively larger amounts the longer the duration of the perfusion.

I = application after 15 minutes
II = application after 1 hour
III = application after 2 hours
IV = application after 3 hours
V = application after 4 hours

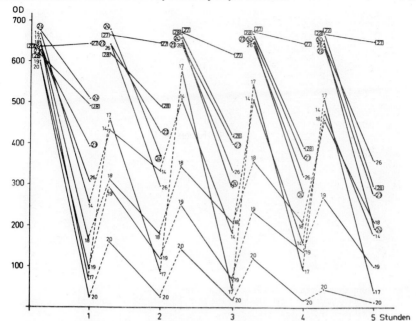

Fig. 14. In contrast to the slow antibody consumption, after the first antibody application a rapid decrease of the total complement OD = optical density.

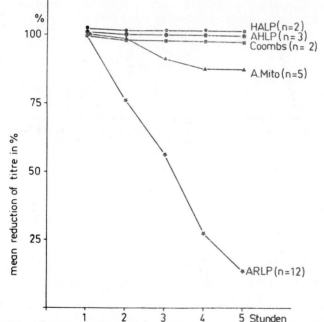

Fig. 15. Summary of results of antibody consumption. Mean reduction of titres in per cent.

HALP = human albumin protein.
AHLP = antihuman liver proteins serum raised in rabbits.
A.Mito = anti-rat mitochondrial antibodies.
Coombs = Coombs-serum from rabbits
ARLP = anti-rat liver protein raised in rabbits.

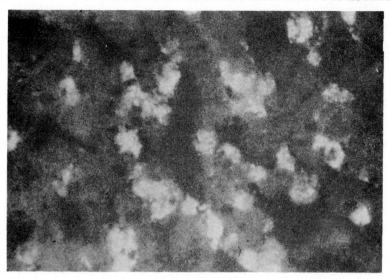

Fig. 16. Immunofluorescent studies of the perfused liver with FITC-marked anti-rabbit-gamma globulin raised in the goat. The consumed antibody is localized in cytoplasmic and membrane structures of hepatocytes.

for this antibody to gain access to the antigen. We believe that the delayed type of hypersensitivity reaction may not be the sole important immunological reaction in the self-perpetuation of active chronic hepatitis.

CONCLUSION

Our experimental models as well as immunological studies in different human liver diseases suggest that auto-immune reactions play an important role in the pathogenesis of active chronic hepatitis. In our studies the characterization and isolation of liver specific proteins was of basic importance. In future studies the isolated protein fractions (LP I and LP II) should be used for the induction of active chronic hepatitis. Furthermore the biochemical relationship of antigenic determinants characteristic of the group or species, and of the tissue or organ should be investigated.

Much of this work is reported in greater detail in:

Kössling, F. K. and Meyer zum Büschenfelde, K. H. (1968) Virchows Arch. Abt. A. path. Anat. 345, 365–376.
Kössling, F. K. and Meyer zum Büschenfelde, K. H. (1970) Ztschr. ges. exp. Med. In Press.
Meyer zum Büschenfelde, K. H. (1968) Arch. Klin. Med., 215, 107–132.
Meyer zum Büschenfelde, K. H., Jeunet, F. and Miescher, P. A.: In preparation.
Meyer zum Büschenfelde, K. H. (1968) Ztschr. ges. exp. Med. 148, 131–163.
Meyer zum Büschenfelde, K. H. (1969) Verh. dtsch. Ges. inn. med. 75, 72.

The remaining bibliography is to be found in:

Baker, M. C., Campbell, D. H., Epstein, S. I. and Singer, S. J. (1956) J. Am. Chem. Soc. 78, 312.
Billingham, R. E., Brown, J. B., Defendi, V., Silvers, W. K. and Steinmuller, D. (1961) Anns. N.Y. Acad. Sci. 87, 457.
Chordi, A., Lledias, T., Santamaria, P., Alvarez-Moreno, C. and Ortiz de Landazuri, E. (1969) Path. europ., vol. 4, No. 3, 209.

Dumonde, D. C. (1966) Advances of Immunology, 5, 245–412.
Hraba, T. (1968) Mechanism and Role of Immunological Tolerance. Monographs in
    Allergy 3, S. Karger–Basel–New York.
Jeunet, F. S. and Good, R. A. (1967) J. Reticuloendothelial. Soc. 4. 351–369.
Jeunet, F. S. and Good, R. A., J. Reticuloendothelial. Soc. In Press.
McBride, R. A., Wheeler, H. B., Smith, L. L., Moore, F. D. and Lamnin, G. J. (1962)
    Amer. J. Path. 41, 501–519.
Mitchison, N. A. (1964) Proc. Roy. Soc. B. 161, 275.
Moller, G., Gabl., F., Reithmuller, G., Schumacker, F. and Zeiss, I. (1967) Z. Immun.
    Forsch. 133, 413.
Paronetto, F., Horowitz, R. E., Sicular, A., Burrows, L., Karl, A. E. and Popper, H.
    (1965) Transplantation, 3, 303.
Starzl, T. E., Kaupp, H. A., Brock, D. A. and Linman, J. W. (1961) Surg. Gynaec.
    Obstr. 112, 135–144.
Thorbecke, G. J. and Benacerraf, B. (1967) B. Immunology, 13, 141.

DISCUSSION

Chairman: Dr. L. E. Glynn

SMITH

Did you look for anti-mitochondrial antibodies, or anti-smooth muscle antibodies in the rabbits with chronic aggressive hepatitis?

Meyer zum BÜSCHENFELDE

No, we did not.

EDDLESTON

Which of your two organ specific proteins did you use to produce the experimental disease?

Meyer zum BÜSCHENFELDE

We used both. To separate these proteins, we have to use Sephadex G 200 – and in our animal experiments we did not do this. Instead we took the first protein peak from the elution on Sephadex G 100 which consists of approximately 70% of liver specific protein. The contaminants are probably albumin and other plasma proteins, present in such low concentration that they do not provoke an immune response. We have carried out control experiments with human albumin.

IMMUNOLOGIC OBSERVATIONS AND ELECTRON MICROSCOPY OF HALOTHANE -INDUCED HEPATIC INJURY

Fenton Schaffner and Fiorenzo Paronetto

Halothane-induced liver damage is beyond the confines of this conference in that it is not an auto-immune liver disease, but we would like to marshal the evidence that at least one drug-induced hepatic injury is an example of immune liver disease. The observations presented include the work of many people: the pathological observations were made by Dr. Popper, the clinical observations by the Liver Group at Mount Sinai Hospital, and finally our own electron microscopic and immunological observations (Klion *et al.,* 1969; Rodriguez and Paronetto, 1969; Paronetto and Popper, 1970).

CERTAIN HISTOLOGICAL FEATURES

The first patients in whom halothane-induced hepatitis was recognized all died of hepatic necrosis, which was indistinguishable from the hepatic necrosis of viral hepatitis. As we became aware of this possible cause of liver injury we began to biopsy the liver in patients with post-operative jaundice. Some were found to have evidence of massive necrosis, and in some there was a typical spotty necrosis with the development of acidophilic bodies. Furthermore, the portal tracts in these biopsies sometimes contained numerous eosinophils with both lymphocytes and plasma cells. Because of the similarity of these pathological findings to those that occur in iproniazid hepatitis of which we have seen many examples, we reviewed some of the clinical aspects of these cases.

TIMING OF ONSET

We found that the severity of the operations made little difference to the incidence of post-operative jaundice. The majority of the patients developed the condition after laparotomy but some became jaundiced even after minor procedures such as endoscopy, saphenous vein ligation and the simple setting of Colles' fractures. In an attempt to separate halothane-induced hepatitis from post-operative cholestasis or toxic jaundice (whatever that condition is) we examined the timing of the onset of jaundice with respect to the operation.

A difference in the rapidity with which jaundice appeared was noted between the first exposure to halothane and subsequent exposures. Jaundice developed two weeks after the first exposure in the majority of cases. After two or more exposures the jaundice developed earlier, towards the end of the first week. Some patients, jaundiced after exposure to halothane, had been re-explored under halothane anaesthesia to exclude an obstructive cause. These patients died after a few days with massive hepatic necrosis. It was usually possible to separate halothane-induced hepatitis from simple post-operative cholestasis because the latter appeared on the first or second day and usually did not get progressively worse. Many of the patients with halothane hepatitis became progressively more jaundiced as time went by.

SIGNIFICANCE OF POST-OPERATIVE FEVER

Fever is an important point in the differential diagnosis of post-operative jaundice. In halothane-induced hepatitis spikes of fever, up to 102°F or more, preceded the development of jaundice by 2, 3 or 4 days. If the patient became jaundiced on the 14th post-operative day the fever usually began on the 10th day — but if the jaundice appeared earlier, for example on the 8th day, then the fever began on the 6th or 7th post-operative day. In contrast to acute viral hepatitis, the fever of halothane hepatitis persisted into the period of jaundice. Very early post-operative fever, on the first day, had to be disregarded as it occurred in more than half of all the surgical patients. In these cases the fever rarely reached 102°F.

OCCURRENCE OF MITOCHONDRIAL ANTIBODIES

Mitochondrial antibodies were found in the serum of several patients with halothane-induced hepatitis, in relatively low titres. In the initial survey, of 9 patients with halothane jaundice, 7 had positive sera: of 7 patients with jaundice due to chlorpromazine, 4 had positive sera. However, mitochondrial antibodies were *not* found in the sera of normal people, nor in patients who had received halothane or chlorpromazine but had not developed jaundice, nor in patients with viral hepatitis. Neither did patients with jaundice due to other drugs including erythromycin estolate, alpha-methyldopa and some oral contraceptives, develop these antibodies. In our most recent series of 15 patients with halothane-induced hepatitis, 10 have had the mitochondrial antibody in the serum.

After we had found mitochondrial antibodies in the sera of patients with halothane jaundice but not in those with viral hepatitis, we wondered if a morphological difference could be found by electron microscopy which was not visible under the light microscope. About the same time it had been reported from Germany that repeated injections of halothane into laboratory animals produced abnormalities in the liver mitochondria (Schaude *et al.,* 1967).

ELECTRON MICROSCOPY CHANGES

Under the electron microscope hepatic necrosis is characterized by the engulfment of acidophilic bodies by macrophages, whether the necrosis is due to halothane hepatitis, viral hepatitis or any other cause. Cholestasis is recognized by the finding of dilated bile canaliculi with loss of canalicular microvilli, and the presence in the hepatocytes of liquid crystals and other debris with the appearance of retained bile.

In the livers of patients with halothane-induced hepatitis some of the damaged hepatocytes with large autophagic vacuoles contained diminished amounts of endoplasmic reticulum, particularly of the rough form. However, in the majority of the cells the rough endoplasmic reticulum was present, although in parts it was rather dilated. The ribosomes were seen to line the membranes of the endoplasmic reticulum in a normal fashion. The striking feature in all the 8 cases that we have examined, has been the peculiar appearance of the mitochondria. They were clumped together and there were membrane abnormalities not seen in viral hepatitis. At high magnification, the adjacent mitochondria have electron-lucent areas between them and part of the membrane of one mitochondrion was invaginated into the next one. Light and dark cells were seen but it was difficult to know whether this finding represented an early stage of the formation of acidophilic bodies or whether it was an artefact resulting from the fixation technique. The mitochondrial abnormalities were present in both types of cell but were more clearly seen in the darker cell, perhaps because of the contrast of the dark hyaloplasm and the lighter invaginations.

Very rarely the same appearance had been seen in severe alcoholic hepatitis and also in some animals with experimental liver injury produced by methyl butter yellow (3′ methylaminoazobenzene).In these animals, the activity of the mitochondrial enzymes succinic dehydrogenase and proline oxidase was diminished. We take this to indicate mitochondrial injury, which was absent in acute viral hepatitis. No correlation was found between the occurrence of mitochondrial antibodies and the abnormal appearance of the mitochondria in the patients with halothane-induced hepatitis.

Comparison with other drug jaundice

Liver histology was examined in patients with a comparable period of jaundice due to alpha methyldopa. Although cholestasis with dilatation of bile canaliculi and loss of microvilli was found, the endoplasmic reticulum was the main site of abnormality just as it is in viral hepatitis. There was loss of rough endoplasmic reticulum with dilatation, and an increase in the amount of smooth endoplasmic reticulum. The mitochondria were normal. We did not find mitochondrial abnormality in chlorpromazine jaundice either. However, mitochondrial abnormalities were found in one patient with anicteric hepatitis due to allopurinol. This patient did not become jaundiced although the serum aminotransferase and alkaline phosphatase levels were slightly elevated. The conventional liver histology showed a non-specific hepatitis, but under the electron microscope mitochondrial changes almost identical with those seen in halothane hepatitis were found.

LYMPHOCYTE TRANSFORMATION

At this point, the evidence that some immune reaction is responsible for halothane-induced hepatitis may be summarized as follows:— (1) Fever, (2) Circulating and tissue eosinophilia in half the cases, (3) The higher incidence of hepatitis after multiple exposures, (4) A shorter latent period after repeated exposure, (5) The two anaesthesiologists who were deliberately challenged with halothane and who developed typical halothane hepatitis (Klatskin and Kimberg, 1969), (6) The presence of mitochondrial antibodies.

In the search for additional and perhaps more direct evidence that immune reactions are fundamental to the development of jaundice after halothane exposure, we decided to investigate prospectively the effect of halothane in stimulating a proliferative response by the lymphocytes of patients, *in vitro.* Fifteen patients were studied, using lymphocyte cultures with uptake of tritiated thymidine as a measure of lymphocyte stimulation. Of the 15 patients, one had been exposed to methoxyflurane, a closely related drug, instead of to halothane. Three patients who had been exposed to halothane but did not develop any evidence of liver disease were also studied and finally, there were 9 patients with other liver diseases and 6 healthy controls.

Blood was collected in sterile tubes with pure heparin. In 6 instances blood collected elsewhere was kept at 5°C and sent to our laboratory within a day. The rest were collected at the Mount Sinai Hospital. Lymphocyte stimulation was measured following the method of Robbins *et al.,* (1969). Phytohaemagglutinin was used as a non-specific mitogenic stimulant to show that the lymphocytes were reactive. The antigens were prepared as follows: Halothane or methoxyflurane was diluted a hundredfold in Medium 199 containing 20 per cent autologous plasma, and this was sonicated at 5°C for 30 seconds. The suspension was then centrifuged at 200 G for 5 minutes in a refrigerated centrifuge. Most of the halothane or methoxyflurane remained in the precipitate. The supernatant was further diluted 10 times with the medium and 25, or 5 μl. of this solution was used as the stimulating antigen. Higher concentrations of halothane were toxic for the lymphocytes. To avoid the possibility that circulating inhibitory substances might prevent lymphocyte stimulation, a series of parallel cultures were set up using washed lymphocytes and tissue culture medium 199 containing 20% foetal calf serum rather than autologous plasma. All tests were carried out in duplicate.

Lymphocyte stimulation in the presence of halothane was not observed in the healthy controls nor in the 9 patients with various other liver diseases, which included primary biliary cirrhosis, active chronic hepatitis, acute viral hepatitis and alcoholic cirrhosis. An increase in tritiated thymidine uptake in the DNA of the lymphocytes incubated with halothane as compared with control values was seen in 9 of the 15 patients with jaundice after halothane exposure. 2 of the 6 negative patients had penicillin-hypersensitivity and, as penicillin was present in the tissue culture medium, uptake of tritiated thymidine also occurred in the control tubes. 2 showed lymphocyte stimulation when foetal calf serum was used instead of auologous plasma. Similarly lymphocytes from a patient with methoxyflurane hepatitis were stimulated by incubation with methoxyflurane in medium containing foetal calf serum, but not in medium containing autologous plasma. The lymphocytes of these three patients above exhibited grossly reduced stimulation after incubation with autologous plasma and phytohaemagglutinin; normal reactivity was restored by using foetal calf serum instead of autologous plasma.

In two patients the test was repeated after they had recovered from the jaundice. The increased lymphocyte stimulation that had previously been found had disappeared by the time the serum aminotransferase and bilirubin levels had returned to normal. Another interesting finding was that lymphocytes from two patients with halothane hepatitis reacted to methoxyflurane as well as to halothane, whereas the lymphocytes from cases of methoxyflurane induced hepatitis did not react to halothane. Finally lymphocyte stimulation was not observed in those patients exposed to halothane who did not develop any evidence of hepatic damage.

None of the patients with jaundice after halothane had Australia antigen positive sera. The presence of the latter was sought both by the gel diffusion method and by complement-fixation.

ROLE OF SENSITIZATION

These last investigations, we feel, have added an additional parameter in the differential diagnosis between halothane-induced and viral hepatitis. The enhanced incorporation of tritiated thymidine into the DNA of lymphocytes from patients with halothane-induced hepatitis incubated with halothane, indicates sensitization to the anaesthetic. This supports the hypothesis that sensitization may play a role in the pathogenesis of the disease and it also seems to hold true for methoxyflurane. That halothane does not stimulate the lymphocytes non-specifically, as phytohaemagglutinin does, has been demonstrated by the fact that in the control patients halothane had no effect. A simple exposure to halothane does not sensitize all patients since those who did not develop overt liver damage did not show lymphocyte stimulation. In the one or two instances that it was sought, sensitization to halothane was not detectable before the appearance of clinical liver disease. Some patients who had fever in whom we had collected lymphocytes serially, did not develop increased lymphocyte stimulation until the onset of clinically recognizable liver disease. The disappearance of increased lymphocyte stimulation with recovery indicates that this sensitization is very transient.

Whether the sensitizing agent is unmodified halothane or a metabolite, or a halothane protein complex, we do not know. Halothane and methoxyflurane are metabolically related, one being derived from the other. Whether this indicates that the culprit could be a metabolic product is not known. Failure to demonstrate Australia antigen in the serum of our patients following exposure to halothane, and electron microscopic differences constitute circumstantial evidence against the thought that halothane hepatitis might be due to activation of latent hepatitis virus. More important and offering much firmer support, is the finding that the mitochondrial antibodies are present in most of the patients, whereas they are not present in viral hepatitis. The demonstration of the sensitization of the lymphocytes to halothane is the strongest evidence for a pathogenic role of a cell-mediated hypersensitivity reaction. We think that the lymphocyte-transformation test is a safer method of demonstrating hypersensitivity to a drug than a direct challenge to the patient. The combined morphological and immunological evidence points to the fact that halothane-induced hepatitis is a distinct disease, separate from viral hepatitis and probably mediated in some way by hypersensitivity.

ACKNOWLEDGEMENT

This work was supported by U.S.P.H.S. Grant No. AM 03846 and U.S. Army Medical Research and Development Command, Contract No. DA-49-193-MD-2822.

REFERENCES

Klatskin, G. and Kimberg, D. V. (1969) New Eng. J. Med. 280, 515.
Klion, F. M., Schaffner, F. and Popper, H. (1969) Ann. Intern. Med. 71, 467–477.
Paronetto, F. and Popper, H. (1970) New Eng. J. Med. 283, 277–280.
Robbins, J. H., Burn, P. G. and Levis, W. R. (1969) Fed. Proc. 28, 363.
Rodriguez, M.,and Paronetto, F. (1969) JAMA 208, 148–150.
Schaude, G. von, Seiss, M., Vogell, W. and Niessing, J. (1967) Acta Histochem, 26, 185.

DISCUSSION
Chairman: Dr. L. E. Glynn

SØBORG

Was there any correlation between the occurrence of lymphocyte transformation and the finding of mitochondrial antibodies in the patients you investigated?

SCHAFFNER

I cannot give you the exact numbers. In most cases it occurred in the same patients. However, some patients without antibodies were penicillin-sensitive and in the technique used, this led to lymphocyte transformation. The patients who reacted to the foetal calf serum alone tended to have antimitochondrial antibodies.

SØBORG

Heterologous serum has been shown in other experiments to produce lymphocyte transformation — could that not explain the reaction to foetal calf serum?

SCHAFFNER

It did not in our material — in all the studies that Dr. Paronetto had done, the lymphocytes behaved quite well with heat-inactivated foetal calf serum. Although the extent of transformation was less than with autologous plasma or AB plasma, in his hands, it proved more reliable. However, there is certainly a need for standardization of this method.

SAUNDERS

Dr. Klatskin has told me of two patients; one working in a factory where halothane is manufactured, who had recurrent hepatitis until he was removed from exposure. The other, a Professor of Surgery at Stanford, is now working in a special operating theatre, where halothane is never used, after having had recurrent hepatitis for a year previously. Have other studies been done on lymphocyte transformation in viral hepatitis? In the data you gave, only 3 jaundiced patients with viral hepatitis had been studied. Without further information on such patients is it justifiable to conclude that your method gives a true idea as to whether people are sensitive to halothane, if it is only positive while they are jaundiced?

SCHAFFNER

Several studies have been done on viral hepatitis. The first came from New York, in which inhibition of phytohaemagglutinin induced transformation was demonstrated during the early stages of the illness and then later stimulation. Dr. Paronetto has since repeated these observations and, using foetal calf serum, does not find this inhibitory phase. He therefore feels that it may be due to a circulating factor.

HAVEMANN

We have studied lymphocyte transformation in acute and chronic hepatitis using purified lymphocytes. The RNA and DNA is then extracted and the specific activity per mg. of nucleic acid is calculated for each culture. In acute hepatitis, for 10 days during the acute phase, we found a depressed response to phytohaemagglutinin (PHA) in 10 patients (Fig. 1). Most then return to normal, but 2 of our patients have retained a depressed response over a period of more than 5 months — histologically they show a persistent hepatitis.

The next slide (Fig. 2) shows the reaction in chronic liver disease. The control values for percentage activity per mg. of RNA and DNA at 72 hours after

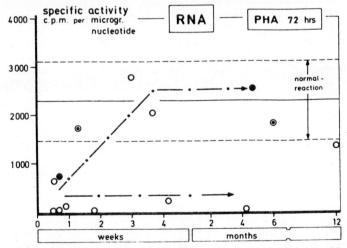

Fig. 1. PHA response of lymphocytes from patients with acute infectious hepatitis obtained at different times after the onset of jaundice.

——— · ——— different possibilities for the time-course of the lymphocytic PHA reaction (qualitatively drawn). (Reprinted from the New England Journal of Medicine, 283, 271–280, 1970, with permission).

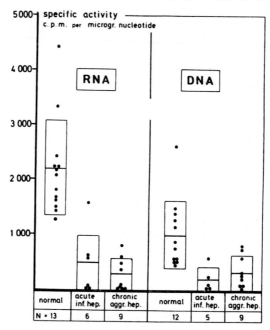

Fig. 2. RNA and DNA synthesis in lymphocytes stimulated by PHA *in vitro* normal = healthy persons, acute inf. hep. = acute infectious hepatitis during the first 10 days of jaundice, chronic aggr. hep. = chronic aggressive hepatitis. Mean and standard deviation. (Reprinted from the New England Journal of Medicine, 283, 271–280, 1970, with permission).

exposure to PHA are also shown. The lymphocytes from patients with chronic aggressive hepatitis have all shown a depressed response to PHA. We could not find this in patients with hepatitis due to alcohol or drugs. Our observations have been repeated on several occasions and have been confirmed by studies from elsewhere in Germany in which dose/response curves to PHA are described. This depressed response might imply persistence of virus infection within the cells, particularly as cells infected by rubeola virus lose their capacity for reacting to PHA.

FOX

Can you tell us how big the molecule of halothane is? Is it of the size likely to provoke an immune response? Has anybody attempted to immunize animals with halothane? Lymphocyte transformation by halothane does not necessarily imply a cell-mediated response, since transformation can be produced by an antigen which evokes a humoral rather than a cell-mediated response *in vivo*.

SCHAFFNER

The molecule looks like this.

$$\begin{array}{cc} F & H \\ | & | \\ F-C-C-Br \\ | & | \\ F & Cl \end{array}$$

What causes the response and what the sensitization means is difficult to say. The fact that it is not present either in halothane-exposed people without hepatitis, in normal individuals or in individuals who have other liver diseases must mean something.

DONIACH

Is it not rather extraordinary that you can get symptoms of sensitization within a day of the anaesthetic even after the first exposure?

SCHAFFNER

We do not think that happens. After the first exposure, the symptoms of the hepatitis do not occur earlier than the 8th day.

SAUNDERS

To refer to the question of the experimental animal. — If rats are repeatedly exposed to halothane, the activity of BSP-conjugating enzymes, measured in the isolated, perfused rat liver, can be inhibited. However, one should take care before interpreting this as sensitization, because as Himsworth showed a long time ago, a single dose of direct toxin in an experimental animal might produce no effect whereas repeated small doses can be toxic through a cumulative effect.

SCHAFFNER

I did not mean to imply that the animal work from Germany was an indication of sensitization. I think it is toxicity, because it occurs in all animals exposed and is dose-related.

CHAIRMAN

It is clear that halothane belongs to that group of drugs which very rarely produce massive necrosis of the liver, of which you will perhaps recall that TNT was an outstanding example in both the first and the second world wars. Its effect then was thought equally mysterious; it may well be, had we known how to test for lymphocyte transformation in 1939, we might have shown the same result.

STUDIES ON MULTI-SYSTEM INVOLVEMENT IN ACTIVE CHRONIC HEPATITIS AND PRIMARY BILIARY CIRRHOSIS

P. L. Golding, R. Bown and A. Stuart-Mason

In several series of patients with "auto-immune" liver disease, involvement of other organs has been noted (Read, *et al.,* 1963, Doniach, *et al.,* 1966). But to our knowledge no systematic study of the type or prevalence of organ; involvement has been reported. We are currently studying patients with liver disease for evidence of Sjögren's syndrome, renal tubular acidosis, fibrosing alveolitis, peripheral neuropathy and cardiomyopathy and in this paper I would like to report our findings to-date.

In all, 63 patients have been studied. These were classified into 4 groups on the basis of clinical, biochemical and histological criteria (Table 1). For the

Table 1

Numbers of Patients in the Four Groups Examined

Group	Total No. Of Patients	Male	Female	Diagnosis
1	24	2	22	Active chronic hepatitis
2	18	1	17	Primary biliary cirrhosis
3	13	10	3	Cryptogenic cirrhosis
4	8	7	1	Alcoholic cirrhosis

purposes of this paper, we have grouped the first three conditions together under the heading of auto-immune liver disease, although we fully realize this aetiology is by no means proven, particularly in the case of cryptogenic cirrhosis.

DEFINITION OF SJÖGREN'S SYNDROME

By general usage, Sjögren's syndrome comprises the triad keratoconjunctivitis sicca, xerostomia and rheumatoid arthritis. Every patient was investigated for each component. The diagnosis of keratoconjunctivitis sicca was made on the basis of Schirmer's Type I and II tests and also on corneal staining with Rose Bengal. Schirmer's test was considered positive if there was less than 10 mm. of moistening of a strip of filter paper held suspended from the unanesthertized conjunctival sac, first without lachrymal stimulation, then with stimulation. Figure 1 illustrates the small punctate staining of devitalized corneal epithelium seen with Rose Bengal in a patient with keratoconjunctivitis sicca.

Xerostomia was diagnosed if the total salivary flow whilst chewing paraffin wax or gum for a 10 minute period was less than 10 ml. In some cases sialograms and labial salivary gland biopsies were obtained.

The diagnosis of rheumatoid arthritis was made using the criteria of the American Rheumatism Association (Ropes *et al.,* 1958).

194

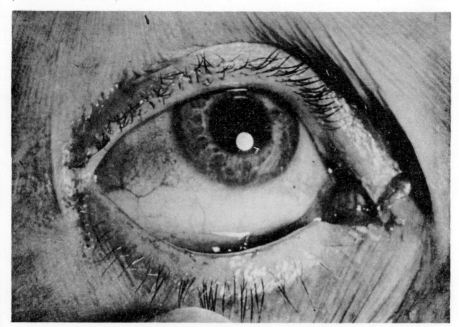

Fig. 1. Illustrating the appearances of the eye in Sjögren's syndrome with staining of cornea and conjuctiva by the Rose Bengal dye.

SJÖGREN'S SYNDROME IN AUTO-IMMUNE LIVER DISEASE

Of the 24 patients with active chronic hepatitis, 41 per cent had keratoconjunctivitis sicca, and 38 per cent also had xerostomia (Table 2). Rheumatoid arthritis was found in only 4 per cent. In the primary biliary cirrhosis group, 73 per cent had keratoconjunctivitis sicca, 61 per cent had xerostomia as well, and 6 per cent had rheumatoid arthritis. In the group with cryptogenic cirrhosis there were fewer patients with keratoconjunctivitis sicca and xerostomia. In the alcoholic cirrhosis group, we found no evidence of Sjögren's syndrome. Thus the sicca component of Sjögren's syndrome, keratoconjunctivitis sicca with or without xerostomia, was found in 51 per cent of patients with auto-immune liver disease (Table 2).

Table 2

*Incidence of Different Features of Sjögren's Syndrome in
Various Groups of Auto-immune Liver Disease*

	No. Of Patients	Incidence of		
		K.C.S. %	Xerostomia %	RH. Arthritis %
Active chronic hepatitis	24	41	38	4
Primary biliary cirrhosis	18	73	61	6
Cryptogenic cirrhosis	13	38	14	0
Total	55	51	40	4

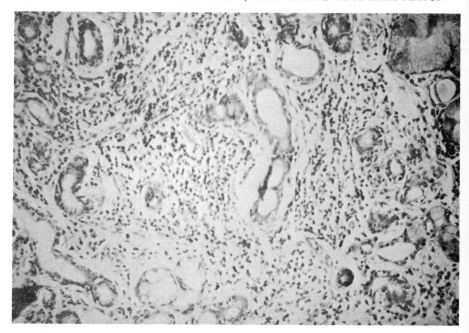

Fig. 2. Labial gland biopsy showing marked lymphocyte infiltration with acinar atrophy.

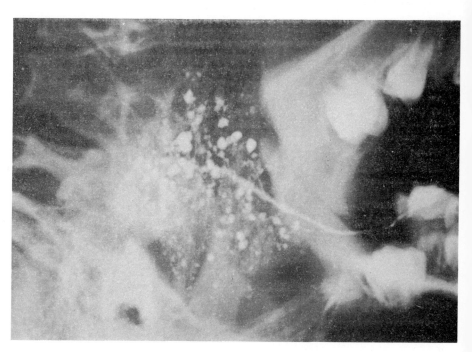

Fig. 3. Sialogram showing the characteristic changes of punctate sialectasis. (By courtesy of Prof. G. Seeward, Dental Department, London. Hospital).

All of the 8 labial biopsies showed marked lymphocytic infiltration and acinar atrophy (Fig. 2). Five patients had sialograms performed and all showed a characteristic punctate sialectasis (Fig. 3). Parotid enlargement was found in only 3 of the 55 cases with auto-immune liver disease and in 1 case of alcoholic cirrhosis.

Relation of Sicca Complex to Liver Function and Serum Antibodies

The presence of the sicca complex did not correlate with the degree of hepatocellular dysfunction. Patients with alcoholic cirrhosis in which the sicca complex did not occur often showed an equivalent degree of abnormality in liver function.

Table 3

The Incidence of Serum Auto-antibodies in Patients with Auto-immune Liver Disease Separated into those with and without Sicca Complex

| | Sicca Complex | | | |
| | Present | | Absent | |
	No.	%	No.	%
Total	28		27	
Rheumatoid factor	15	53	12	45
Anti-nuclear factor	12	43	9	33
Smooth muscle antibody	12	43	7	26
Mitochondrial antibody	17	61	8	30

Serum auto-antibodies were found in rather more patients with the sicca complex (Table 3). IgG, IgA and IgM levels were measured in each case and are expressed as a percentage of the mean value in the normal adult (Fig. 4). It can be seen that the presence of sicca is related neither to the level nor to the actual class of immunoglobin elevated.

RENAL TUBULAR ACIDOSIS

This may be defined as an inability of the renal tubule to acidify urine out of proportion to any reduction in glomerular filtration rate. Renal tubular acidosis may present clinically as an overt type in which the urine pH is greater than 6, despite a systemic metabolic acidosis with a serum bicarbonate of less than 20 mEq./litre. An "incomplete" variety also occurs in which case the defect is only detected when the patient is stressed with an acid load. To detect the latter we used an ammonium chloride load according to the method of Wrong and Davies (1959). In a normal response the patient should be able to acidify his urine to a pH of less than 5·2, and achieve a maximum titratable acidity in the urine of greater than 24 μEq./min. with a maximum ammonia excretion of 33 μEq./min. or more.

The incidence with which these two forms of renal tubular acidosis were found in the different varieties of "auto-immune" liver disease is shown in Table 4. Overall 38 per cent of patients had incomplete or overt renal tubular acidosis. The highest incidence, particularly of the overt form, was found in primary biliary cirrhosis. At the time of the testing only 3 patients, all with

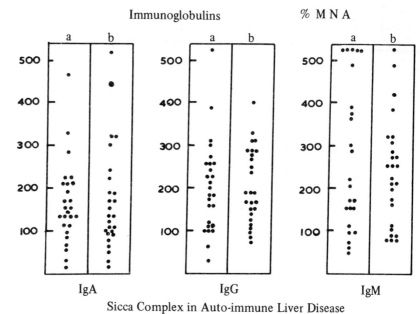

Sicca Complex in Auto-immune Liver Disease

Fig. 4. A comparison of the serum immunoglobulins in those with (a) and those with (b) the sicca complex, expressed as a percentage of the normal mean adult value. (% MNA) 2 patients with monomer "M" protein are not shown in this figure.

Table 4

The Incidence of Two Forms of Renal Tubular Acidosis in Auto-immune Liver Disease

| | No. Of Patients | Renal Tubular Acidosis | | | |
| | | Incomplete | | Overt | |
		No.	%	No.	%
Active chronic hepatitis	20	5	25	1	5
Primary biliary cirrhosis	15	5	33	4	26
Cryptogenic cirrhosis	7	1	14	0	0
Total	42	11	26	5	12

overt renal tubular acidosis were hypokalaemic, and none were on diuretics.

As in the case of the sicca complex, we could find no correlation between hepatic dysfunction and renal tubular acidosis. Neither was there any particular pattern of serum auto-antibody nor immunoglobulin level which was more frequently present in those with renal tubular acidosis.

Copper deposition in renal tubules as a result of a high serum copper levels has been suggested as a cause of renal tubular dysfunction in primary biliary cirrhosis (Leeson and Fourman, 1967). However, we could find no difference in serum copper levels between the patients with renal tubular acidosis and those without (Fig. 5). Another suggested cause for this condition has been peritubular vascular abnormalities resulting from high globulin levels (Morris *et al.*, 1964). Our evidence does not support this hypothesis as there was no significant correlation between the presence of renal tubular acidosis and the level of total serum globulin (Fig. 5).

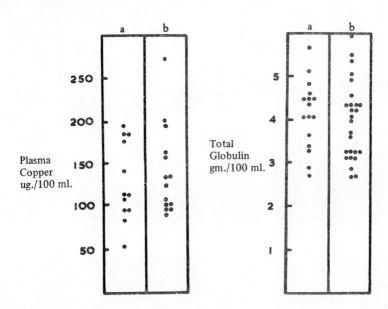

Fig. 5. Comparison of serum copper and globulin levels in patients with (a) and without (b) renal tubular acidosis.

There have been several reports of the concurrence of renal tubular acidosis and Sjögren's syndrome (Kaltreider and Talal, 1969; Shiopi, *et al.*, 1970) but there was no mention of hepatic abnormality in these cases. However, it is interesting to note that lymphocytic infiltration of both the kidney and salivary gland was found in such cases. In one of our patients we were also able to demonstrate marked lymphocytic infiltration of the salivary gland (Fig. 6a) and to a lesser extent, lymphocytic infiltration of the kidney, with tubular atrophy (Fig. 6b). At no time did we find any evidence of urinary tract infection in this patient, but the renal biopsy was not cultured.

In our series, a combination of renal tubular acidosis and sicca complex occurred in 20 per cent of cases of active chronic hepatitis, and 60 per cent of cases of primary biliary cirrhosis. No patients with cryptogenic cirrhosis showed both lesions. Thus the overall incidence in our patients with "auto-immune" liver disease was 31 per cent (Table 5).

OTHER SYSTEMIC MANIFESTATIONS

In conclusion, I would like to briefly mention other systemic manifestations found in the patients with "auto-immune" liver disease. Ulcerative colitis, peripheral neuropathy both sensory and motor, and auto-immune thyroid disease

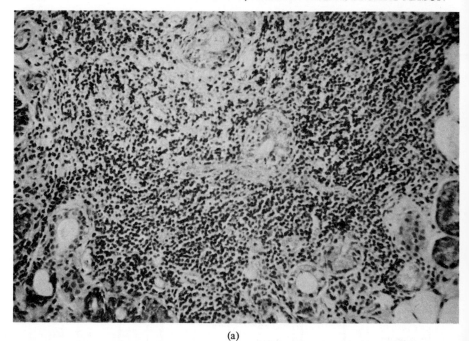

(a)

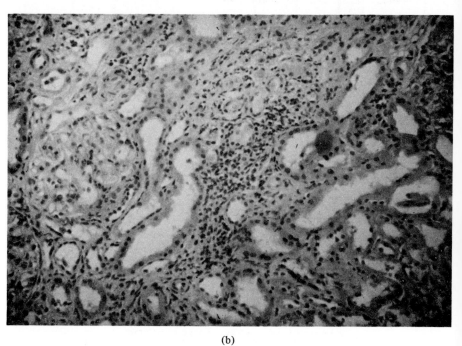

(b)

Fig. 6. (a) Labial gland biopsy showing marked lymphocytic infiltration. (b) Renal biopsy showing lymphocytic infiltration and tubular atrophy from patient with primary biliary cirrhosis.

Table 5

"Sicca Complex" and R.T.A. in Auto-immune Liver Disease

	No.	R.T.A. + Sicca %	R.T.A. %	Sicca %
Active chronic hepatitis	20	20	10	15
Primary biliary cirrhosis	15	60	0	13
Cryptogenic cirrhosis	7	0	14	59
Total	42	31	7	20

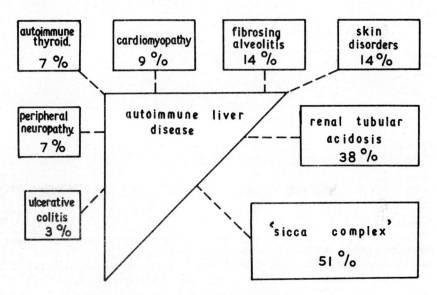

THE SPECTRUM OF AUTOIMMUNE LIVER
DISEASE

Fig. 7. Illustrating the incidence of the various systemic manifestations of auto-immune liver disease.

were found in various patients (Fig. 7), as has been observed in other series (Read *et al.*, (1963; Doniach *et al.*, 1966). A systemic manifestation not previously described was cardiomyopathy which we found in 5 patients, an incidence of 9 per cent. One of these had definite hypertrophic obstructive cardiomyopathy, and another had a constrictive cardiomyopathy. The diagnosis in the other 3 patients has not finally been decided.

Fibrosing alveolitis (Scadding, 1964), a syndrome of reduced vital capacity, grossly reduced transfer factor, normal forced expiratory volume, and an abnormal chest x-ray, was found in 8 patients (14 per cent). None of these had obvious portal hypertension or a low serum albumin, two conditions that may produce a reduction in transfer factor. Skin disorders, excluding acne, were found in a further 8 patients, 14 per cent of the series. The majority of these patients had allergic capillaritis as has been described by Sarkany (1966). Finally to this list should be added the high incidence of renal tubular acidosis and the sicca complex as described in this paper.

REFERENCES

Doniach, D., Roitt, I. M., Walker, J. G. and Sherlock, S. (1966) Clin. Exp. Immunol, 1, 237–262.
Kaltrieder, H. B. and Talal, N., (1969) Arthr. and Rheum. 12, 538–541.
Leeson, P. M. and Fourman, P. (1967) Amer. J. Med. 43, 620–634.
Morris, R. C., Johnson, L. and Fudenberg, M. A. (1964) J. Clin. Invest. 43, 1293.
Read, A. E., Sherlock, S. and Harrison, C. V. (1963) Gut 4, 378–393.
Ropes, M. W., Bennett, G. A., Cobb, S., Jacox, R. and Jesaar, R. A. (1958) Bull Rheum Dis. 9, 175.
Sarkany, I. (1966) Lancet 2, 666.
Scadding, J. G. (1964) Brit. Med. J. 2, 686.
Shioji, R., Furayama, T., Onodera, S., Saito, H., Ito, H. and Sasaki, Y. (1970) Amer. J. Med. 48, 456–463.
Wrong, O. and Davies, H. F. (1959) Q.J.M. 28, 259–313.

DISCUSSION
Chairman: Dr. L. E. Glynn

SØBORG
Did you look for salivary gland antibodies?

GOLDING
Only in a few patients. We found some but their significance is uncertain at the moment.

MacLAURIN
You may be aware that in the sicca syndrome many patients show a depressed response to DNCB. Williams, from Minnesota, has reported that of 20 patients with rheumatoid arthritis, some of whom had the sicca complex, about 75 per cent showed diminished reactivity in a one-way mixed lymphocyte reaction. So this would imply impairment of cellular immunity and perhaps similar to that described by Dr. Fox this morning.

GOLDING
We have not really studied this aspect but lymphocytes from a few of our patients showed a diminished response to phytohaemagglutinin. In particular the family of one of our patients is interesting in that most of the relatives show a diminished response.

MacLAURIN
I think that PHA reactivity may be a separate expression of cell mediated immunity. I have examined several rheumatoids now and find that some have quite high PHA responses and yet have grossly imparied mixed lymphocyte reactivities.

Meyer Zum BÜSCHENFELDE
Which method did you use to detect the rheumatoid factor? Did you use the Rose Waaler test, the sheep cell test, or the latex test; and did you inactivate the serum? I ask because we have found anti-gamma globulin factors different

from the rheumatoid factor in a high proportion of liver diseases. Bonomo was able to separate these anti-gamma globulin factors on anion columns; he eluted three different fractions, one at pH 6, another at pH 5 and the last at pH 7, whereas the rheumatoid factor is found at pH 6·5. Did you bear these possibilities in mind?

GOLDING

We did not look into the rheumatoid factor in great detail — the test was a simple latex slide agglutination.

Meyer Zum BÜSCHENFELDE

Did you work with native serum, which may contain a high proportion of anti-gamma globulin factors? If so — did you heat inactivate the serum? As the rheumatoid factor is stable at 65°C, this is a very simple way of separating these antibodies.

GOLDING

No, we did not.

McINTYRE

Surely you have found a remarkably high incidence of these abnormalities in your patients with liver disease. Could you tell us what possible selection there may have been? Clearly this report has come from a rheumatology group — to what extent do you think this might have affected the incidence? I am sure most of us would find lower figures if we looked.

GOLDING

There are several points here. First and foremost, we were also very surprised by the figures when we analysed our results. Nevertheless were you to specifically question your liver clinic patients, I think you would find many of them would admit to having dry and sore eyes and a dry mouth. It is interesting to note that Mackay in his initial description of the systemic manifestations of primary biliary cirrhosis, comments that, "the patient first complained of a dryness of the eyes". Mackay then goes on to describe lymphocytic infiltration in the kidneys and in the stomach. The next point is that the eyes of a patient with Sjögren's syndrome may look reasonably normal, they are not usually red but have a mucous film over them giving a shiny impression. So even if the patient does complain of dry gritty eyes — the cause may be overlooked.

Finally — these patients have not been specially selected in any way and they do not come from a rheumatology group. This study was started in Southampton, where every possible patient with liver disease was examined and was then continued at the London hospital. More recently, we have joined forces with Dr. Bown and Dr. Dawson at St. Bartholomew's Hospital and have examined every other patient from their Portal Hypertension Clinic.

DAWSON

The sicca syndrome can be very severe, 3 of these patients were taking artificial saliva. Another point is that renal tubular acidosis, can also be easily overlooked. Many of the incomplete cases are really only found by investigation although the overt ones may present with electrolyte disturbances which are quite difficult to manage. Would you not agree?

GOLDING

This is certainly a major problem. One might easily say that they are "acidotic", simply as a part of the cirrhosis rather than anything else, if the urine pH is not tested.

SOME ASPECTS OF HUMORAL AND DELAYED HYPERSENSITIVITY IN CHRONIC HEPATITIS

V. Pipitone and O. Albano

In this paper we describe studies which provide some support for the possible pathogenic role of the immune system in certain forms of liver disease with particular emphasis on delayed hypersensitivity. Others have emphasized that immunological phenomena may be responsible for the transition of acute to chronic hepatitis and its subsequent perpetuation (Paronetto and Popper, 1969).

We understand the term chronic hepatitis to imply chronic inflammation of the liver without the special characteristics of cirrhosis. On histological grounds this form of hepatitis has been divided into two types (De Groote et al., 1968). Chronic aggressive hepatitis is characterized by fibrosis and inflammation both in the portal zones and in the hepatic parenchyma with piecemeal necrosis. These histological appearances are associated with the clinical syndrome of active chronic hepatitis or lupoid hepatitis. In contrast chronic persistent hepatitis is characterized by an inflammatory infiltrate confined to the portal tracts without parenchymal involvement or portal fibrosis.

Certain histological features suggest that cell mediated immunity may be involved in these two sorts of hepatitis. Under the electron microscope large lymphoid cells with polysomes indicating protein synthesis may be seen in the portal zone. These cells do not show the prominent endoplasmic reticulum of the plasma cells in which there is also protein secretion (Klion and Schaffner, 1967).

LYMPHOCYTE TRANSFORMATION IN LIVER DISEASE

It is well known that sensitized lymphocytes when cultured for 72 hours or more, with the appropriate antigen will undergo blast transformation and proliferation *in vitro* (Hinz et al., 1970; Valentine and Lawrence, 1969; Marshall et al., 1969). Using the same antigen *in vivo* it is possible to obtain a delayed intracutaneous reaction. We therefore believe that lymphocyte proliferation after antigen stimulation may be positively correlated with the delayed hypersensitivity response, as others have suggested (Loewi et al., 1967; Oppenheim et al., 1967).

By applying this technique to patients with liver disease we have previously shown that delayed hypersensitivity responses to liver antigens are commonly found in patients with chronic hepatitis or post necrotic cirrhosis (Pipitone, 1967 and 1968) and also primary biliary cirrhosis (Pipitone et al., 1967). The antigens used were mitochondrial and ribosomal fractions of liver (Table 1). Our results indicated that lymphocyte transformation by these antigens was commonly found in chronic, but not in acute hepatitis. Similar results to these have been obtained by Tobias et al., (1967); Hoenig and Possnerova (1967) and Ortona et al., (1970).

One of the main objectives of the present study was to further investigate delayed hypersensitivity responses in these cases. Dumonde et al., (1969) have reported that after incubation with the appropriate antigen, thymus dependent sensitized lymphocytes produce at least five active substances, the so called lymphokines, that are non-antibody mediators of cellular immunity. The substances include a cytotoxic factor, a skin reactive factor, a transfer factor,

Table 1.

Blast Transformation of Lymphocytes in Various Liver Diseases
(From Pipitone, 1965 and 1966)

Diagnosis	Liver Antigen	
	Mitochondrial Fraction	Ribosomal Fraction
Acute hepatitis	3/34	4/34
Persistent chronic hepatitis	20/34	22/34
Postnecrotic cirrhosis	9/29	11/29
Primary biliary cirrhosis	3/3	3/3

a mitogenic factor and lastly a macrophage migration inhibitory factor (MIF) as shown in Fig. 1. We decided to study the production of the last of these factors, MIF, by the lymphocytes of patients with various liver diseases.

PATIENTS STUDIED AND TECHNIQUES

20 patients were examined, consisting of 3 cases of acute hepatitis, 4 with chronic persistent hepatitis, 1 with chronic aggressive hepatitis, 10 with post necrotic cirrhosis and lastly 2 with primary biliary cirrhosis.

Macrophage migration inhibition test (modified from Bloom and Bennett, 1969)

For each patient three "short term" lymphocyte cultures were prepared, a control culture, a culture containing a non-specific stimulant (such as PHA) and lastly, an antigen containing culture. The antigen used was the combined mito-chondrial and ribosomal liver cell fraction. After 72 hours incubation, the cultures were centrifuged for 10 minutes at 250 g. The pellet was transferred onto slides and stained with May Grunwald Giemsa. The supernatant was added to Mackaness culture chambers containing capillary tubes in which there were guinea pig macrophages. The latter were obtained by the intraperitoneal inoculation of 10 ml. 2% sodium caseinate solution into guinea pigs with subsequent drainage (Bartfield *et al.,* 1969). The culture chambers were incubated for 18 to 24 hours and then the area of macrophage migration was measured. The area of the control culture is considered equal to 100% migration: if the migration area in the test chamber is less than 60%, it means that migration has been inhibited.

In all patients the following were also investigated.
(1) The serum immunoglobulin levels.
(2) Antiliver antibodies, detected both by haemagglutination and by complement fixation.
(3) Antigammaglobulin factors using both the RA test and the Rose Waaler test.

RESULTS

Immunoglobulin levels

Raised levels of IgG and IgM were found in both chronic persistent and chronic aggressive hepatitis (Table 2). High IgA levels were found to be characteristic of cirrhosis of any cause. These findings are similar to those of Pirotte *et al.,* (1970) and Walker and Doniach (1968).

DELAYED AND HUMORAL IMMUNITY

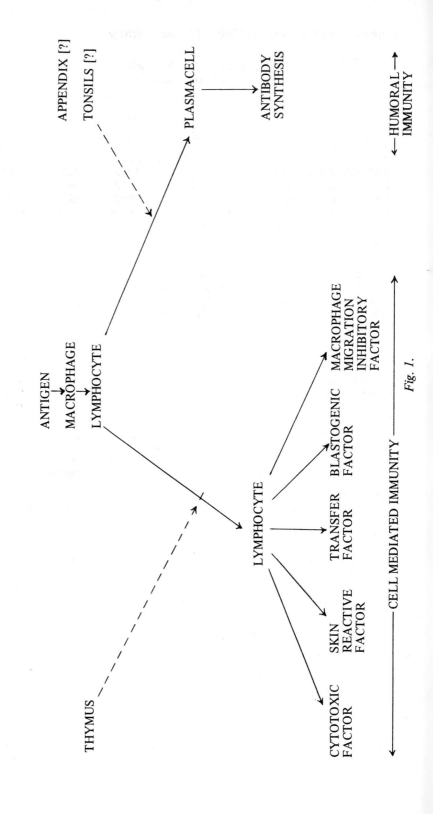

Fig. 1.

Table 2.
Immunoglobulin (mg%)
(Mean of values)

Diagnosis	Number of cases	1gG	1gA	1gM
Acute hepatitis	3	1080	295	180
Persistent chronic hepatitis	4	2040	320	195
Aggressive chronic hepatitis	1	1900	125	270
Postnecrotic cirrhosis	10	1460	540	380
Primary biliary cirrhosis	2	1900	600	265

Normal Value: 1gG = 1300 ± 200
                  1gA = 288 ± 121
                  1gM = 80 ± 29

Table 3.
Antiliver Antibodies
Boyden's haemagglutination technique and auto-immune complement fixation (AICF) test

Diagnosis	Subjects tested	Boyden technique*	AICF*
Acute hepatitis	3	0/3	1/3
Persistent chronic hepatitis	4	4/4	4/4
Aggressive chronic hepatitis	1	1/1	1/1
Postnecrotic cirrhosis	10	4/10	5/10
Primary biliary cirrhosis	2	2/2	2/2

* — Serum-positive cases out of total
  — Boyden's technique = serum-positive at titre 1/16 or more
  — AICF test = serum-positive at titre 1/16 or more (50% haemolytic units)

Antiliver antibodies

These were common in chronic hepatitis and in primary biliary cirrhosis (Table 3). A rather lower incidence in post necrotic cirrhosis was found. 1 of the 3 cases of acute hepatitis showed antibodies on complement fixation but not on haemagglutination.

Antigammaglobulin factors

As in our previous experiments (Carozzo *et al.*, 1968) rheumatoid factors (RF) have been distinguished from antigammaglobulin factors (AGF). The former are almost confined to rheumatoid arthritis, whereas the latter are present in numerous diseases and especially in chronic liver disease. We have reported an incidence of AGF of 52·9% in acute liver disease, 78·1% in chronic disease and of 81% in evolutive forms of liver disease (Pipitone, 1968). In the present studies the highest titres of AGF occurred in the chronic and progressive forms (Table 4).

Macrophage migration inhibition test

Table 5 summarizes the findings related to MIF production and to blast transformation in these patients. A relationship between the two phenomena can be seen. We feel that although the transformation test is more sensitive, the biological assay of MIF as a measure of delayed hypersensitivity is more specific. We found that the highest incidence of MIF production was in the evolutive forms of liver disease (chronic persistent or chronic aggressive

Table 4.

Antigammaglobulin Factors — Anti-human: RA test
Anti-rabbit: Waaler Rose
(Mean of titres)

Diagnosis	Number of cases	RA test	Waaler Rose
Acute hepatitis	3	1/40	1/32
Persistent chronic hepatitis	4	1/40	1/128
Aggressive chronic hepatitis	1	1/80	1/64
Postnecrotic cirrhosis	10	1/80	1/64
Primary biliary cirrhosis	2	1/40	1/32

Waaler Rose (Heller): Normal Value = ≤ 1/32

Table 5.
Delayed Hypersensitivity Phenomena
(a) Blast Transformation of Lymphocytes (b) Migration Inhibitory Factor
Production

Diagnosis	Subjects tested	Blast transformation incidence*	M.I.F. production incidence*
Acute hepatitis	3	0/3	0/3
Persistent chronic hepatitis	4	3/4	3/4
Aggressive chronic hepatitis	1	1/1	1/1
Postnecrotic cirrhosis	10	4/10	2/10
Primary biliary cirrhosis	2	1/2	1/2

*   Blast transformation and MIF production positive cases out of total examined
Blast transformation positive if higher than 10%.
M.I.F. production in lymphocyte supernates positive if macrophage migration
area is smaller than 60%.

Table 6.
Delayed Hypersensitivity Phenomena in Rheumatoid Arthritis
(from Pipitone, 1968 and 1969)

Blast transformation of stimulated lymphocytes*

Diagnosis	Blast incidence
Rheumatoid arthritis	18/37
Other diseases	4/23

Migration inhibitory factor production in supernates of stimulated
lymphocyte cultures*

Diagnosis	M.I.F. production
Rheumatoid arthritis	13/33
Osteoarthritis	0/19

*Lymphocytes are stimulated by synovial membrane antigen

hepatitis), and the lowest in chronic forms (post necrotic cirrhosis). Lympho-cytes from cases of acute hepatitis did not produce MIF in these circumstances.

These findings are in agreement with our previous studies on patients with rheumatoid arthritis (Pipitone *et al.*, 1969). The latter are illustrated in Table 6 in which it can be seen that when synovial membrane was used as antigen, MIF production was specific for rheumatoid arthritis lymphocytes. Furthermore there was a close correlation between MIF production and the severity of the disease.

CONCLUSIONS

Although our patients had the high incidence of antiliver antibodies that others have reported, the significance of these antibodies is not known. In some instances they may be of great diagnostic importance and some have suggested that under some circumstances they may even be protective (Waller *et al.*, 1969). Our experiments also show that MIF production by circulating lymphocytes is a suitable tool for investigation of delayed hypersensitivity reactions in liver disease particularly when liver antigens are used in the system. This is in keeping with the idea that delayed hypersensitivity is of importance in the pathogenesis of these diseases.

REFERENCES

Bartfield, H., Atoynatan, T. and Kelly, R. (1969) 7, 242.
Bloom, B. and Bennett, B. (1970) Rev. Europ. Etudes clin. biol. 15, 460.
Carrozzo, M., Arbore, S., Numo, R., La Torre, F. and Pipitone, V. (1968) Gazz. int. Med. Chir. 73, 3224.
De Groote, J., Desmet, V. J., Gedik, P., Korb, G., Popper, H., Poulsen, H., Scheuer, P. J., Schmid, M., Thaler, H. and Vehlinger, E. (1968) Lancet 2, 626.
Dumonde, D. C., Wolstencroft, R. A., Panayi, G. S., Matthew, M., Morley, J. and Howson, W. T. (1969) Nature 224, 38.
Hinz, C. F., Daniel, T. M. and Baum, G. L. (1970) Int. Arch. Allergy, 38, 119.
Hoenig, V. and Possnerova, V. (1967) Zeit. Imm. Allergie Klin. Immunol. 133, 199.
Klion, F. M. and Schaffner, F. (1967) Exp. molec. Path. 6, 361.
Loewi, G., Temple, A. and Vischer, T. L. (1968) Immunology 14, 257.
Marshall, W. H., Valentine, F. T. and Lawrence, H. S. (1969) J. Exp. Med. 130, 327.
Oppenheim, J. J., Walstencraft, R. A. and Gell, P. G. H. (1967) Immunology 12, 89.
Ortona, L., Ciarla, O., Pozzigallo, E. and Laghi, G. (1970) Min. medica. 61, 2611.
Paronetto, F. and Popper, H. (1969) Bayer Symposium – Ed. Springer Verlag – 213.
Pipitone, V. (1967) Lancet 1, 849.
Pipitone, V. (1968) Carlo Erba Foundation. International Symposium on "Gammopathies, Infections, Cancer and Immunity".
Pipitone, V., Carrozzo, M. and Albano, O. (1967) Arch it. Mal. App. Dig. 34, 418.
Pipitone, V., Chériè Ligniére, G., Caruso, I., Numo, R. and Arbore, S. (1969) Report at International Congress of Rheumatology – Praha.
Pirotte, J., Royters, L. and Salmon, J. (1970) Acta Gastro-enterol. belgica. 33, 9.
Tobias, H., Safran, A. F. and Schaffner, F. (1967) Lancet 1, 193.
Valentine, F. T. and Lawrence, H. S. (1969) Science, 165, 1014.
Waller, M. V., Richard, A. J. and Mallory, J. (1969) Immunochemistry 6, 207.
Walker, G. and Doniach, D. (1968) Gut. 9, 266.

ROUND TABLE DISCUSSION ON CELL MEDIATED RESPONSES AND MANIFESTATIONS OF IMMUNOLOGICAL DAMAGE
Chairman: Dr. L. E. Glynn

POPPER

Yesterday I asked a question but did not quite get an answer and I would like to ask it today again. But first, would it be permissible to see again that very elegant slide that Dr. Smith showed? Fig. 11 page 144.

We are all puzzled by a series of questions: firstly, are we observing an immune reaction or a true auto-immune reaction? Secondly, the terrible question, why should auto-immune disease develop in one patient and not in another who may have the same type of history? And why should it stop in some, and not continue despite the same factors, both cell-mediated and humoral being present? Perhaps I may be permitted to divide it into four separate questions:—

(1) We have here a beautiful slide showing a gun shooting various question marks at the liver! But Dr. Smith has told us about a case of acute viral hepatitis in which apparently, manifestations of auto-immune disease were present — antibody markers and abnormalities of cell-mediated immunity. We know that in primary biliary cirrhosis if a drug is given, jaundice may appear which was not present before, and many of us think that although drugs cannot produce primary biliary cirrhosis, they may unmask it. So can viral hepatitis unmask — be a second gun? Dr. Smith has mentioned the possibility of a "double-barrelled gun" being involved.

(2) We see here, and I am in full agreement with what is drawn, that in genetically prepared people a cell-mediated response occurs. This then leads to release of normally sequestered antigens. Is that damaging, or may it not even be protecting? There are some people in our own Department who claim that circulating antibody protects against immune damage.

(3) Could the antigen/antibody complexes, which are obviously formed as a result of the release of sequestered antigen, be responsible for the whole beautiful gamut of diseases which Dr. Golding has just described? Because at least in the skin and in the kidney, immune complexes can be demonstrated, although not in the liver, except in the case of primary biliary cirrhosis. I would like to hear whether these diseases could be related to circulating immune complexes from which the liver is protected by its Kupffer cells.

(4) What is the relation of fibrosis to this? This is the most difficult because I still believe that cirrhosis is not produced by the immune reaction directly but is produced by another mesenchymal response, namely, fibrosis.

GOLDING

It is difficult to believe that renal tubular acidosis is produced by antigen/antibody complexes. Damage from such complexes in the kidney is classically glomerular. Admittedly, we have not got biopsies from all of these patients but in case reports of liver disease with Sjögren's and renal tubular acidosis, glomerular lesions are not described. What has been postulated is a distal tubular lesion. This is interesting in view of the mitochondrial fluorescence Dr. Doniach showed yesterday which was concentrated at the distal tubules, and was also very marked in the salivary glands. Furthermore, if you give patients malleic acid you can induce renal tubular acidosis because of its action on succinic dehydrogenase, which also happens to be mitochondrial marker. So I wonder whether these ancillary diseases are more closely related to anti-mitochondrial antibody rather than to immune complexes.

SMITH

Dr. Popper, did you not show in the experimental Auer hepatitis that with a previously damaged liver, antigen/antibody complexes introduced into the portal vein or into the systemic circulation, may overcome the Kupffer cells? In such cases antigen/antibody complexes are found in the hepatic parenchyma, where they do produce damage. It is perfectly possible that such mechanisms are involved in active chronic hepatitis and primary biliary cirrhosis, perhaps in the perpetuation of the disease processes. Of course, it is rather difficult that one does not find immune complexes in the liver in active chronic hepatitis.

MacLAURIN

If, in the Perlmann system, an IgG antibody is put on to a monolayer, the latter is destroyed. On the other hand, if an IgM antibody is used nothing happens. If the Birkett lymphoma system is used the same results are obtained. So there may be a critical balance between the two types of antibody.

In relation to the fluctuation of auto-immune disease, one can draw a parallel here to the local graft-versus-host disease produced in the liver of an F_1 hybrid by the direct intrahepatic injection of parental lymphocytes. Now, the extraordinary thing about this lesion is that it increases to a certain size and then suddenly disappears. Elkins has described the same in the kidney. When insufficient parental cells are introduced into an F_1 hybrid kidney, although a mild graft-versus-host reaction develops to begin with, it then disappears by six months. The recipient animal may produce a circulating inhibitor which acts on the parental cells. A similar phenomenon might explain the fluctuation in human liver disease.

SMITH

Most of us feel that the immune system in these patients is abnormal, and I believe Dr. Golding has evidence that this is genetically determined.

GOLDING

The propositus (A) in one of our families presented with overt renal tubular acidosis; in addition she was found to have Sjögren's syndrome, Hashimoto's disease, a peripheral neuropathy and fibrosing alveolitis (Fig. 1). Her twin sister (B) had a high titre of both smooth muscle antibody and mitochondrial antibody, and a liver biopsy showed chronic aggressive hepatitis. A brother (C) had high titres of auto-antibodies without any other evidence of disease, and another sister (D) had Sjögren's syndrome, hepatomegaly, abnormal liver function tests but a normal liver biopsy. The daughter of the woman with chronic aggressive hepatitis had schizophrenia — even this has been suggested as being auto-immune! — and also had abnormal gamma globulins. Finally, another brother (E) with a +ve antinuclear factor had two daughters with abnormal globulins and antibody titres diagnostic of Hashimoto's thyroiditis! (Fig. 1). So there certainly seemed to be a genetic predisposition to auto-immune disease in that family.

We are now studying the family of a patient with primary biliary cirrhosis, whose sister appears to have active chronic hepatitis — she certainly has abnormal liver function tests and smooth muscle antibodies. Furthermore, both sets of children have also got smooth muscle antibodies and high IgM levels.

SCHAFFNER

There is no doubt that all of us accept that there is immunological abnormality in these patients. What is difficult to understand is the step from an

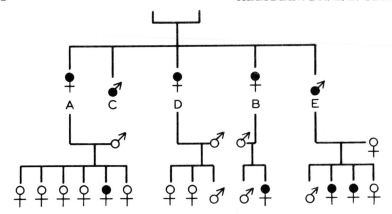

Fig. 1. Showing the family tree of a patient (A) with multiple "auto-immune" disorders. The patients A–E are referred to in the text. Closed circles represent members of family known to be affected.

immunological abnormality to a fibrous septum in cirrhosis or a destroyed bile duct in primary biliary cirrhosis. There is a gap. Dr. Popper was attempting to provoke somebody to answer the question, and I still feel that it has not been answered.

SMITH

May I ask Dr. Schaffner what view he takes of the experiments that Dr. Meyer Zum Büschenfelde has shown us?

SCHAFFNER

I think that the demonstration of cell injury to the point of death where it is replaced by a fibrous scar and can no longer regenerate, still has not been shown; that antigen/antibody complexes injure cells, that there may be all types of interference with membrane exchange for one reason or another – this I can accept. But why the cell dies and is replaced by a collagen scar, I do not know.

SMITH

Dr. Schaffner, do you think that Dr. Meyer Zum Büschenfelde has produced a model of active chronic hepatitis?

SCHAFFNER

He has produced a disease in his animals – I do not think that this is the same disease that we are seeing in our patients.

MacLAURIN

I was very impressed with Dr. Meyer Zum Büschenfelde's paper because, in the lesions demonstrated, there seemed more similarity to active chronic hepatitis than to primary biliary cirrhosis. In the rat lesions that I discussed the emphasis was on the bile duct and on fibrosis. In our study the liver homogenate with adjuvant was injected alternately intramuscularly and intraperitoneally, and from the peritoneal surface lymphocytes could be seen migrating in through the liver capsule. Where they had travelled there was a line of fibrous tissue following along behind. Thus, wherever the lymphocytes localized they stimulated a fibrotic reaction.

DUMONDE

As many people must obviously realize, the mechanism which provides the stimulus for fibrosis is not fully known. Under certain circumstances, in delayed hypersensitivity reactions one can demonstrate it. Exudation of fibrinogen can be shown for quite a lengthy period of time after the initiation of a tuberculin skin reaction. Thus, extravascular accumulation of fibrinogen might be one initiating mechanism for fibrosis. It could be argued that the lymphocyte-induced reaction of cell-mediated immunity in the liver might also induce a fibrinogen exudate. Maybe this also occurs in the Arthus reaction. It is clear that further fundamental studies on the nature of the stimulus producing fibrosis are needed.

SCHAFFNER

One human situation which was interesting to us was the fibrosis of chronic passive congestion, for this occurs in the absence of significant lymphocytic infiltration. I had wondered from my own electron microscopic observations whether the macrophage and not the lymphocyte was the mediator in this transfer of information to the fibroblasts.

DUMONDE

The only model systems which have been set up for fibroblast/lymphoid cell interaction are the cytotoxic ones. In these, monolayers of fibroblasts have been taken and to them activated lymphoid cells have been added together with soluble or insoluble antigen. Under these circumstances, the fibroblast monolayers become destroyed. Stimulation of the fibroblasts does not seem to occur under these highly artificial circumstances, protein synthesis and other functions are impaired. It would require a very curious sort of model to demonstrate whether a cell-mediated immune reaction can result in the stimulation of fibroblasts. Recently, a factor has been recognized which activates macrophage metabolism and lymphocyte DNA synthesis, resulting from interaction of lymphocytes with antigen. It would be interesting to investigate this in relation to the activation of fibroblasts.

EDDLESTON

Some of us who were at the Liver Club the other day, heard Dr. MacLean give the other side of this picture. If you implant a piece of fibrous tissue into a cirrhotic liver it is not removed, whereas it is in a normal liver.

PART IV
Results of Immunosuppressive Therapy

PROBLEMS OF MULTI-CENTRE TRIALS, ILLUSTRATED BY THE COPENHAGEN TRIAL OF STEROID THERAPY IN CIRRHOSIS

Niels Tygstrup

I understand that the main purpose of this afternoon is to discuss controlled trials in general, and perhaps multi-centre trials in particular. I have the honour to present some of the experience gained by the Copenhagen Study Group for Liver Disease in doing such a trial. In view of our purpose I think it best to start with the results and then go backwards to methods and end with the planning.

THE RESULTS

After 5 years the group had collected 334 patients with cirrhosis, half of whom were treated with prednisone. The results are shown in Fig. 1. The shaded

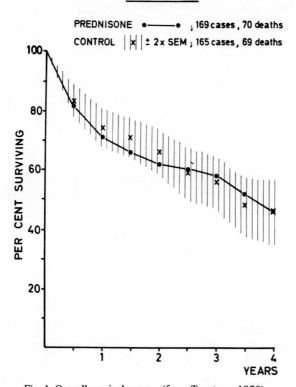

ALL CASES

PREDNISONE ●———● ; 169 cases, 70 deaths
CONTROL | |x| | ± 2x SEM ; 165 cases, 69 deaths

Fig. 1. Overall survival curves, (from Tygstrup, 1970).

area represents the percentage survival of control patients ± double the standard error. It is seen that the survival curve of the prednisone treated patients remains within this area. Thus, if survival was the only parameter studied, the conclusion

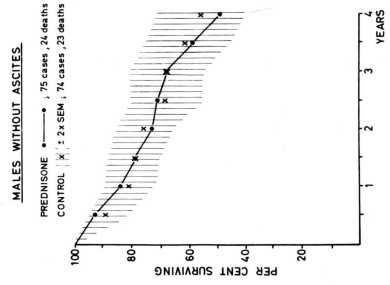

MALES WITHOUT ASCITES

PREDNISONE ●———● ; 75 cases , 24 deaths

CONTROL |x| ± 2 x SEM ; 74 cases ,23 deaths

PER CENT SURVIVING

Fig. 3. Survival curves in all male patients without ascites, (from Tygstrup, 1970).

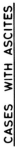
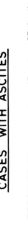
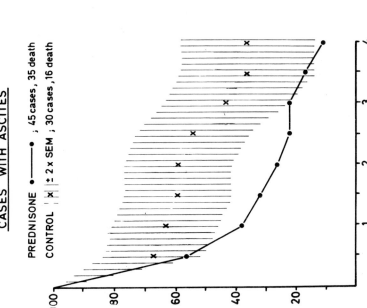

CASES WITH ASCITES

PREDNISONE ●———● ; 45 cases, 35 death

CONTROL |x| ± 2 x SEM ; 30 cases ,16 death

Fig. 2. Survival curves in all patients with ascites, (from Tygstrup, 1970).

would be that prednisone, as used in this study, does neither harm nor good. However, there are two other possibilities:

(1) it is due to a beneficial effect in one category of patient, balanced by a detrimental effect in another group.

(2) a beneficial effect of prednisone on the cirrhosis is counteracted by the side effects of prednisone therapy, or in other words, some of the treated patients die from complications of steroid therapy.

Both possibilities have been examined and more or less confirmed. We do find a group in which prednisone decreases the survival significantly, namely in patients with ascites as shown in Fig. 2. Correspondingly, in patients without ascites, the survival is increased. It appears, however, that this group is not homogeneous. When divided according to sex, male patients show no difference (Fig. 3) whereas a clear difference is noted in female patients (Fig. 4).

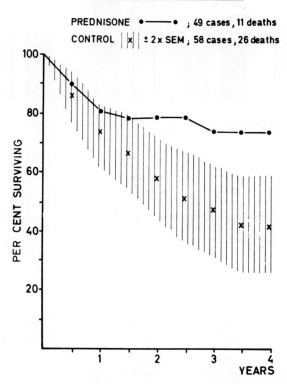

Fig. 4. Survival curves in female patients without ascites, (from Tygstrup, 1970).

We have tried to isolate a group with a greater difference between prednisone treated and controls, by using clinical, laboratory and histological criteria of "activity" and "auto-immunity", but so far in vain. One difficulty is that the groups become too small when combined criteria are applied.

The second question, namely death from cirrhosis versus death from side

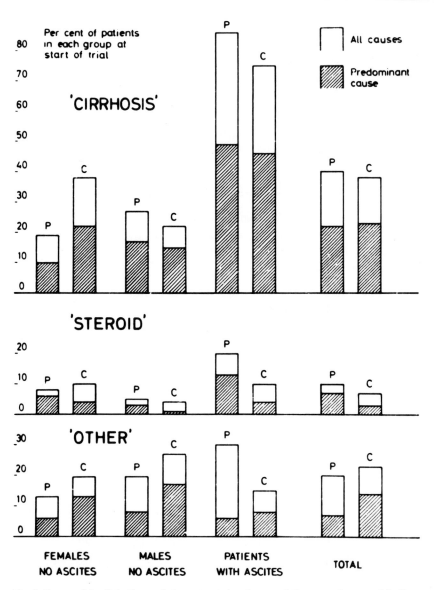

Fig. 5. Causes of death in the prednisone treated patients and the control groups (c), (from Sloth *et al.*, 1970).

effects to treatment, is examined in Fig. 5. The causes of death are divided into 3 groups:

(1) "cirrhosis-induced", e.g., liver failure, haemorrhage from varices and hepatoma.
(2) "prednisone-induced", e.g., bleeding peptic ulcer, perforated ulcer and sepsis, and
(3) other causes, such as arteriosclerosis and extrahepatic malignant tumours.

If we concentrate on the predominant cause of death it is seen that in the total material, death from cirrhosis is equally frequent in both prednisone treated and control groups. However, in females without ascites, death from cirrhosis is significantly reduced in the treated group. Steroid-induced causes are relatively infrequent, but in the total material they are significantly more frequent in the prednisone group. Finally, and unexpectedly, other causes are less frequent in prednisone treated patients without ascites, male and females considered together.

This gives us some practical guidelines in the use of prednisone therapy but many questions remain open. We hope to be able to answer some of them, because of the rather elaborate system of registration, and this brings us to the discussion of the methods used.

REGISTRATION AND PROCESSING SYSTEM

If a liver biopsy from a patient in one of the 7 participating departments shows cirrhosis, according to established criteria, the detailed histological findings are recorded on a data sheet, together with the clinical and laboratory findings (Fig. 6). The sheets are collected and registered at a central office and transferred to punched cards. A working group plans and elaborates programmes for processing, and the output is discussed by the whole study group at regular intervals, controlled by the central office.

Figure 7 shows the programme system which permits any classification of the material from the input data and comparison of the categories with respect to all registered data. As an example Fig. 8 shows the distribution of prothrombin values at initial registration in the prednisone group and a test of the distribution function. It is automatically compared statistically with similar data of the control group. Figure 9 shows a comparison of clinical oedema in male and female patients. The difference is not significant. Figure 10 shows the survival curves as obtained by the BMD programme, which some of you probably know.

I think that this type of registration and processing is essential for multi-centre trials for several reasons.

(1) The amount of data will inevitably be great. We must learn to swim in data without drowning. Electronic data processing is no guarantee, but probably the only lifebuoy.
(2) Each centre can easily isolate its own data and use them alone or in combination with those from other centres or the whole group.
(3) It is easily controlled if the material from different centres is comparable, and if the planned schedule is followed.
(4) Electronic data processing cannot be started without careful definition of the questions, planning, and standardization. I consider this to be an advantage, because without these preparations the results will be useless.

CONCLUSIONS

From the technical point of view multi-centre trials are possible. However, it is a great mistake to believe that these technical facilities make trials easy, and it

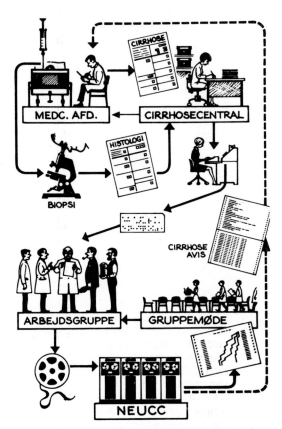

Fig. 6. Illustrating the registration system.

is not difficult to see why few multi-centre trials exist despite the fact that most of us agree that the therapy of liver diseases largely rests on very fragile ground.

(1) Such trials are very time consuming and require continuous and long lasting surveillance.

(2) The number of co-workers is inevitably high, and each will get a rather small amount of credit for his work. He may even fear that other members will take his share of this volatile, though essential substance!

(3) Such trials do not at the moment have a very high scientific esteem. They are considered less meritorious than experimental laboratory work.

Therefore, only clinicians who believe in this approach and who are ready to pay the costs, should embark on such a project. Personally I believe that it is one of the most important methods for making clinical medicine more scientific than it is today.

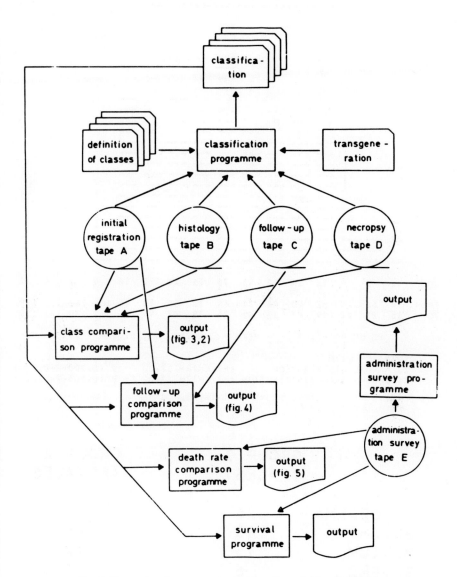

Fig. 7. Illustrating the programme system, (from Juhl *et al.*, 1970).

VARIABLE A 119 - PROTHROMBIN
****

```
                                    ---                    GROUP 1
                                    ---                (PREDNISONE TREATED)
                                    ---
                                    ---
                   L                ---
                         L   -N-  N
            L            N   ---
                            -L-       -N-          ---
                            ---                    ---
         ---   N            ---   L   ---          ---
         ---         --- --- --- --- ---    N      ---
 -L-  --- --- --- --- --- --- ---                  ---
 ---  -N- --- --- --- --- --- ---    -L-           ---
 ---  --- --- --- --- --- --- --- ---    --- ---   ---
 ---  --- --- --- --- --- --- --- ---   -L- -N-
 -N-  --- --- --- --- --- --- --- --- ---               L
 ---  --- --- --- --- --- --- --- ---   -L-
    L --- --- --- --- --- --- --- --- ---      N
    N --- --- --- --- --- --- --- --- ---      L
      --- --- --- --- --- --- --- --- --- --- N   ---
 N -N- --- --- --- --- --- --- --- --- --- --- L  -L-
 ---  --- --- --- --- --- --- --- --- --- ---     -N- -N-
 --- -L- --- --- --- --- --- --- --- --- --- --- --- ---
```

NO	1	3	4	12	14	12	13	23	13	16	10	16	4	1	4	2
FROM	8	16	24	32	40	48	56	64	72	80	88	96	104	112	120	128
TO	15	23	31	39	47	55	63	71	79	87	95	103	111	119	127	135

NO OF PT - 148   MEAN -   69.34   S.D. -   25.58

COMPARISON WITH
  1. NORMAL DISTRIBUTION   (N) CHI2- 12.20 F- 9 (0.300-P-0.200)
  2. LOG.-NORMAL DISTRIBUTION (L) CHI2- 27.00 F- 9 (0.005-P-0.001)

Fig. 8. Distribution of prothrombin values at initial registration in one of the patient groups, (from Juhl *et al.*, 1970).

	GROUP 1 (MALES)	GROUP 2 (FEMALES
NO OEDEMA	226	91
SLIGHT	41	26
MEDIUM	15	12
SEVERE	6	3
UNKNOWN	0	0
TOTAL	288	133

COMPARISON BETWEEN GROUP 1 AND 2
CHI2-   4.35 F- 2 (0.100-P-0.200)

Fig. 9. Clinical oedema in male and female patients, (from Juhl *et al.*, 1970).

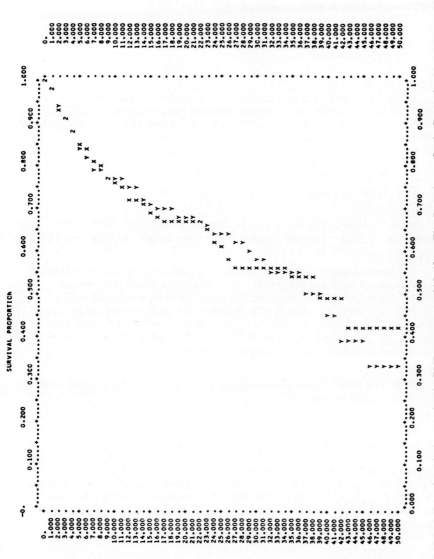

Fig. 10. Calculation of survival curves by the BMD programme 01S, (from The Copenhagen Study Group for Liver Disease, 1969).

REFERENCES

Juhl, E., Winkel, P., Frank, H., Tygstrup, N. and the Copenhagen Study Group for Liver
    Diseases (1970) Scand. J. Gastroent. Suppl. 7, 195–201.
Sloth, K., Juhl, E., Tygstrup, N. and The Copenhagen Study Group for Liver Diseases
    (1970) Scand. J. Gastroent. Suppl. 7, 189–193.
The Copenhagen Study Group for Liver Diseases (1969) Lancet 1, 119–121.
Tygstrup, N. (1970) Progress in Liver Disease III, 319–335.

DISCUSSION
Chairman: Dr. S. J. Saunders

CHAIRMAN
We are, of course, in a very fortunate position now, because we all understand very clearly, after the discussion of the last day and a half, what active chronic hepatitis is, what cryptogenic cirrhosis is and what primary biliary cirrhosis is; we know exactly how to distinguish between them pathologically and what the role of the immune mechanism is . . .! So really all we have to do now is to see whether we can help these patients with immunosuppressive therapy.   (LAUGHTER).

Prof. Tygstrup's paper is now open for discussion.

WILLIAMS
Is the Copenhagen study now to be changed in any way? Are more new cases going into it and are you still keeping it restricted to prednisolone versus placebo?

TYGSTRUP
It is being changed at the moment. The only new patients we now take are males without ascites as this was the one category in which there was no difference between the treated and untreated patients. We should like to continue to accept all patients with cirrhosis, but this raises ethical problems because, now knowing that we would prolong the survival of females without ascites, we felt obliged to give prednisolone to this group. On the other hand, we could not defensibly continue to give it to patients with ascites.

DAWSON
When one says "cirrhosis", what is the breakdown in terms of what we have heard in the last two days?

TYGSTRUP
We thought the only clear definition in this field was provided by the histological criteria of cirrhosis. Therefore, all cases that fulfilled these criteria were included. As I told you, the females without ascites consisted to a large extent of what we now refer to as active chronic hepatitis. However, as I illustrated in the distribution curve for prothrombin time, there was a smooth transition from one end of the distribution curve to the other and this also applied to the remaining liver function tests. So although we can clinically recognize typical cases of active chronic hepatitis, we cannot make a cut and say, "Above this, it is so, and below this, it is not".

De GROOTE
When patients had ascites, did you continue to treat them only with prednisolone?

TYGSTRUP
No. They then receive conventional treatment with diuretics, etc., and patients with hepatic coma also had conventional anti-coma treatment, both in the control and prednisolone groups.

PREDNISOLONE THERAPY IN ACTIVE CHRONIC HEPATITIS

G. C. Cook, Rosemary Mulligan and Sheila Sherlock

It is well known that corticosteroids improve the sense of well being in patients with active chronic hepatitis. They also favourably influence some of the biochemical indices of that disease. Whether they affect life expectancy is however unknown, and for this reason a controlled therapeutic trial of corticosteroid therapy in active chronic hepatitis has been carried out at the Royal Free Hospital, London, during a 6-year period, July 1963 to July 1969, (Cook *et al.*, 1970). Only patients who had not previously received immuno-suppressive agents were included in the study. The follow-up of individual patients varied between two and six years. The patients were randomly divided into treated and control groups by a method using sealed envelopes.

The criteria for inclusion were based on two or more of the following features: a clinical picture of active chronic hepatitis; the classical biochemistry of active chronic hepatitis, i.e. a raised serum bilirubin, transaminase and total globulin; and consistent liver histology. All except two of the patients ultimately accepted for the study had liver-biopsy histology examined. This showed features of chronic aggressive hepatitis, piecemeal necrosis usually with rosette formation, plasma cell infiltration, and fibrosis (Scheuer, 1968) in all the patients. In two-thirds of the patients cirrhosis was also considered to be present.

PATIENTS STUDIED AND BASE-LINE BIOCHEMICAL DATA

Initially 54 patients were included in the study but 5 were excluded at the final assessment in July 1969 because there was doubt about the diagnosis and the collective data were thought to favour another diagnosis. These 5 patients were ultimately considered to have persistent hepatitis (2), active alcoholic cirrhosis (1), partial biliary atresia (1), and Wilson's disease (1). A total of 49 patients was left of whom 22 were treated with corticosteroids (prednisolone, 15 mg. daily in the adults and a correspondingly lower dose on a weight basis in the children), and 27 acted as controls.

Figure 1 shows the ages and sex of the patients in the two groups. In the corticosteroid and control groups, the mean ages were 35 and 42 years respectively. The mean ± 1 standard deviation is shown in each case. The ultimate outcome in the individual patients is also shown. Figure 2 shows the length of the total history of disease at inclusion to the study — 21 and 16 months respectively, and Fig. 3 the length of jaundice — 10 and 9 months respectively. There was generalized systemic involvement in many of the patients in both groups: Arthropathy (4), colitis (4) and Hashimoto's thyroiditis (2) in the corticosteroid group; arthropathy (3), pleurisy (2) and aortic valve disease (2) in the control group. There were also a number of other associated features as one would expect in a group of patients with active chronic hepatitis.

Figure 4 shows the initial serum bilirubin concentrations in the two groups; the means were 2·9 and 3·8 mg./100 ml. respectively. Figure 5 gives the aspartate aminotransferase concentrations; the means were 157 and 118 i.u./1 respectively in the two groups. Figure 6 shows the total globulin concentrations in the two groups; the means were 5·7 and 4·7 g./100 ml. respectively. This difference between the means is significant ($p < 0.02$). Figure 7 gives the albumin concentrations in the groups; the means were 2·8 and 3·0 g./100 ml. respectively.

227

AGE AND SEX DISTRIBUTION AT INCLUSION
TO THE TRIAL

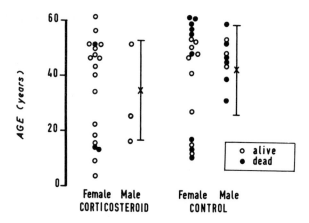

Fig. 1. Age and sex distribution of the patients studied. The mean ± 1 S.D. is shown for each group. O, alive at time of final assessment; ●, dead at time of assessment.

LENGTH OF TOTAL HISTORY AT INCLUSION TO THE TRIAL

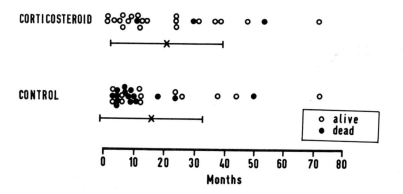

Fig. 2. Length of total history at inclusion to the study in the 2 groups. The mean ± 1 S.D. is shown for each group. O, alive at time of final assessment; ●, dead at time of assessment.

LENGTH OF JAUNDICE AT INCLUSION TO THE TRIAL

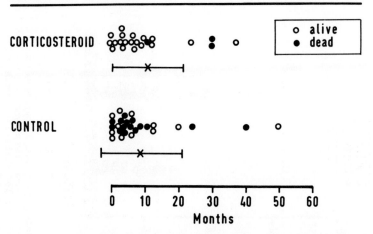

Fig. 3. Length of time since onset of jaundice at inclusion to the investigation in the 2 groups. The mean ± 1 S.D. is shown for each group. O, alive at time of final assessment; ●, dead at time of assessment.

TRANSAMINASE AT INCLUSION TO THE TRIAL

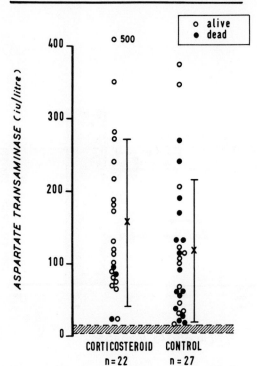

Fig. 4. Serum bilirubin in the 2 groups of patients at inclusion to the study. The mean ± 1 S.D. is shown for each group. O, alive at time of final assessment. ●, dead at time of assessment. The shaded area represents the normal range (0·3−1·0 mg./100 ml.).

TOTAL GLOBULIN AT INCLUSION TO THE TRIAL
o alive
● dead
GLOBULIN (g/100 ml)
10·0
8·0
6·0
4·0
2·0
0
CORTICOSTEROID
n=22
CONTROL
n=27

Fig. 5. Serum aspartate transaminase in the 2 groups of patients at inclusion to the study. The mean ± 1 S.D. is shown for each group. O, alive at time of final assessment; ●, dead at time of assessment. The shaded area represents the normal range (5–17 i.u./1).

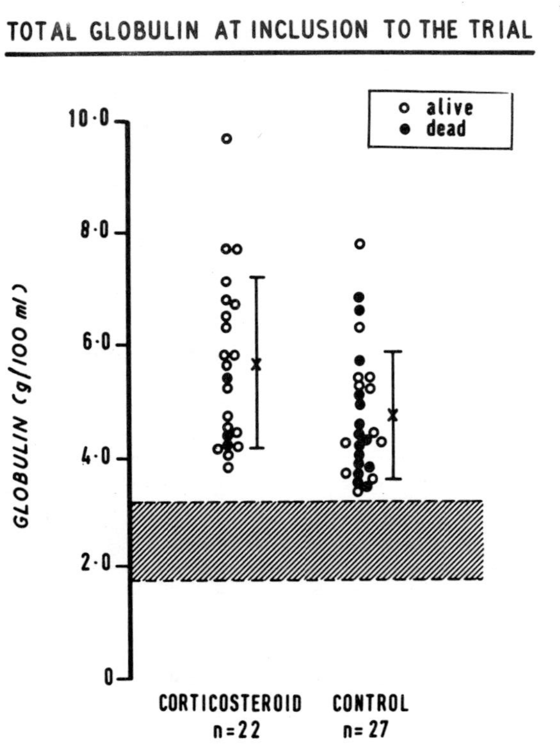

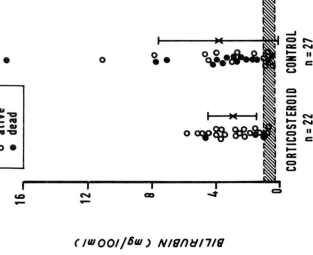

BILIRUBIN AT INCLUSION TO THE TRIAL
o alive
● dead
BILIRUBIN (mg/100ml)
16
12
8
4
0
CORTICOSTEROID
n = 22
CONTROL
n = 27

Fig. 6. Serum total globulin in the 2 groups of patients at inclusion to the study. The mean ± 1 S.D. is shown for each group. The difference between the means is significant ($p < 0{\cdot}02$). O, alive at time of final assessment; ●, dead at time of assessment. The shaded area represents the normal range (1·8–3·2 g/100 ml.).

ALBUMIN AT INCLUSION TO THE TRIAL

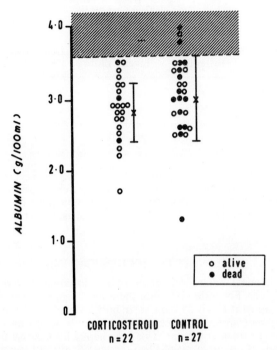

Fig. 7. Serum albumin in the 2 groups of patients at inclusion to the study. The mean ± 1 S.D. is shown for each group. O, alive at time of final assessment; ●, dead at time of assessment. The shaded area represents the lower part of the normal range (3·6−5·2 g./100 ml.).

CLINICAL COURSE AND MORTALITY

Table 1 summarizes the mortality in the two groups. In the treated group 3 of the 22 patients died during the study. In 8 of the surviving patients corticosteroid therapy was stopped during the trial, in 4 because the biochemical indices had completely returned to normal, and in 4 due to complications probably secondary to corticosteroid therapy. The 3 patients in this group who died, did so as a result of liver-cell failure. In the control group 15 of 27 patients died during the study. Thirteen of these died of liver-cell failure. The difference in mortality from liver-cell failure between the groups is significant (p < 0·05). The two other deaths in the control group were due to diseases not associated with liver-cell failure, an astrocytic glioma in one and carcinoma of the body of the uterus in another. However, both of these patients had severe liver-cell failure and it seems exceedingly unlikely that they would have been alive by the end of the study. If those deaths are also taken into account in the analysis of mortality, then the difference between the groups is significant at the 1·0 per cent level.

Complications probably associated with corticosteroid therapy were experienced during the study. The most severe were osteoporosis and vertebral collapse (2), perforated duodenal ulcer (1), steroid psychosis (1) and terminal bronchopneumonia (1). There were also a number of mild complications which were probably a result of corticosteroid therapy.

Table 1

Significance Between the Difference in Mortality Between the Two Groups

Group	Total No. Of Patients	Death Due To Liver Failure	Death Due To Other Causes	Total Deaths
Corticosteroid	22	3	0	3
Control	27	13	2	15
Significance		$p < 0.05$		$p < 0.01$

The status of the survivors in July 1969 was good or excellent in 13 and 4 patients in the treated and control groups respectively. Working capacity was normal in 15 and 7 respectively. The mean serum biochemical indices were very similar in the survivors of both groups at the final assessment.

CHANGES IN BIOCHEMICAL INDICES

The biochemical indices were observed at approximately 6-monthly intervals during the study. For serum bilirubin there was a significant trend to normal in the treated group at 6 and 24 months; in both cases at the 1·0 per cent level. Aspartate aminotransferase concentrations were not significantly different between the groups at any point. This is perhaps a little surprising since a previous study (Cook *et al.*, 1968) had shown a significant trend to normal in serum aspartate aminotransferase during the first few weeks of treatment with corticosteroids. Although there was a significant difference initially in the total globulin concentrations between the 2 groups ($p < 0.02$), this difference was reversed during the follow-up period and the level was significantly lower in the treated group at 12 months ($p < 0.02$) and at 24 months ($p < 0.01$). The most striking difference between the two groups was in the serum albumin concentrations — the treated patients showed a rise in the mean serum albumin and the difference between the groups was significant at 6 months ($p < 0.02$ and at 12, 18 and 24 months ($p < 0.01$).

Summary

The results of a controlled prospective trial of corticosteroids (using low dosage prednisolone, 15 mg./day) in active chronic hepatitis have been reported. There was a significant decrease in the mortality in the treated group. There was a significant trend to normal of serum bilirubin, total globulin and albumin in that group. It is concluded that corticosteroids in low dosage should be used in the early active phase of active chronic hepatitis.

REFERENCES

Cook, G. C., Mulligan, R. and Sherlock, S. (1970) Quart. J. Med. In Press.
Cook, G. C., Valasco, M. and Sherlock S. (1968) Gut 9, 270.
Scheuer, P. J. (1968) Liver Biopsy Interpretation. London, pp. 48–54.

DISCUSSION
Chairman: Dr. S. J. Saunders

CHAIRMAN

Do you think that your patients on steroids were eating better and that this might be why their serum albumins were higher than the controls.

COOK

This could be a factor, particularly as there was a greater weight increase which was not due to fluid retention as far as we could tell.

WILLIAMS

Perhaps the effect on the albumin levels is due to the stimulation of protein synthesis by steroids.

COOK

I think this is a much more likely explanation than Dr. Saunders'!

DAWSON

That cannot be the whole answer as I believe that there is an equal stimulation of protein degradation. The half-life of albumin is certainly decreased on steroids.

SODOMANN

Have you re-biopsied any of your patients treated with prednisolone and if so, have you seen any histological improvement?

COOK

We have got serial biopsies on a number of patients. They are at present being assessed.

DAWSON

The male/female ratio in the two groups is slightly different. If you deal with males and females separately, do you still get significant results?

COOK

Neither sex nor age were statistically important.

GEALL

If the trial is randomized could you explain why there was a significant difference in globulin levels between the two groups at the start.

COOK

This occurred purely by chance.

GEALL

The incidence of cirrhosis on first liver biopsy in patients with high gamma globulin levels and L.E. cells is only 35 per cent whereas it is 60 per cent when patients without L.E. cells and with lower gamma globulin level are considered. This might explain some of the differences in the responses of your two groups.

NEALE

Have you measured bromsulphthalein retention on these patients? You have shown very little change in liver function tests and perhaps BSP retention would be a more sensitive index.

COOK

A significant improvement in the storage capacity of BSP occurs early on but no improvement in transport maximum is found.

A LONG-TERM STUDY OF IMMUNOSUPPRESSIVE THERAPY IN ACTIVE CHRONIC HEPATITIS

J. Knolle, K. H. Meyer Zum Büschenfelde and H. Schonborn

As has been reported previously, therapy with corticosteroids gives controversial results in patients with active chronic hepatitis (Mackay *et al.,* 1963; Read *et al.,* 1963). In search of more effective means of influencing the underlying auto-immune process, the therapeutic effects of 6-mercaptopurine and azathioprine have been investigated. However, the numerous reports on this subject which have appeared in the past seven years, have not definitely established when and how these substances may be of benefit in the treatment of active chronic hepatitis (Page *et al.,* 1964; Weinreich, J., 1967; Mackay *et al.,* 1968; Farhlander *et al.,* 1968; Editorial, 1968). Assessment of the reported therapeutic value in these studies is difficult for two main reasons:—

(1) Frequently, information as to the stage of the disease process with respect to fibrotic change is lacking.

(2) The therapeutic procedure varies widely in the different studies with regard to drug combinations and duration of treatment.

In 1965 at our hospital, we started to treat 5 cases of active chronic hepatitis with azathioprine only. After six months, the serum aminotransferases were not completely normal, the values for gammaglobulin concentrations were almost unchanged and the patients still complained of fatigue. We then started them on a combination of 5 mg. prednisone and 2—3 mg./kg. body weight of azathioprine per day and since 1966, we have used this combination initially in all our patients. We now have 35 cases which have received this treatment for at least six months. The mean observation period to date is 22 months and some patients have received treatment for as long as 42 months.

SELECTION OF PATIENTS

All our patients were selected according to the following criteria:

(1) a pre-treatment observation period of about six months either in the hospital or on an out-patient basis, with examinations at 2—4 weekly intervals.

(2) a history of chronic hepatitis with or without jaundice, lasting for months or years without evidence of acute hepatitis in half the cases.

(3) hepatomegaly and splenomegaly.

(4) a continuous elevation of serum aminotransferase levels, hypergammaglobulinaemia, and hypoalbuminaemia. The erythrocyte sedimentation rate was frequently elevated.

(5) The morphological features of chronic aggressive hepatitis on laparoscopy and histological examination.

Furthermore, it must be stressed that all of our patients had an organ-specific immunological finding. This consisted of specifically sensitized cells in the liver detected by immuno-fluorescent staining with FITC-labelled specific liver protein. / A liver-specific serum auto-antibody could be identified rarely only. (For references see Dr. Meyer Zum Büschenfelde's paper).

234

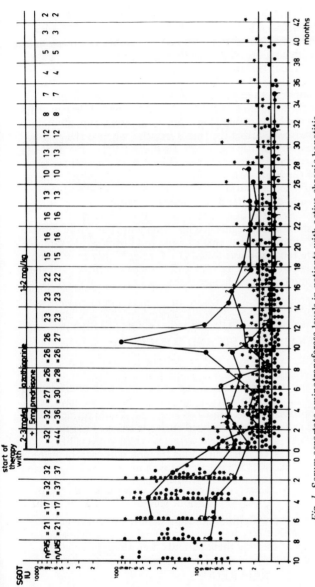

Fig. 1. Serum aspartate aminotransferase levels in patients with active chronic hepatitis before and during treatment with azathioprine and prednisone. The dots indicate patients without fibrotic change and stars those with fibrotic change. Each symbol represents one value for the serum aspartate aminotransferase. Three patients differed in their therapeutic management.

1 1 This case received azathioprine only up to the 10th month. After the addition of prednisone, the aspartate aminotransferase levels returned to normal.

2 2 This case received azathioprine as sole medication. Note that the aminotransferase levels did not return to normal.

⊛⊛ This case with early fibrotic change in the liver discontinued therapy on his own accord after 6 months and developed a highly active relapse, which was reversed promptly after reinstitution of therapy.

RESULTS TO-DATE

As Dr. Popper pointed out yesterday, patients with fibrosis on liver biopsy differ in prognosis from patients without fibrotic change. In our experience also, it seems particularly important when evaluating therapeutic results, to distinguish between cases with and without cirrhosis. In the patients without cirrhosis the serum aminotransferase values rapidly returned to normal within 2 months of starting treatment. In contrast, although the aminotransferase values decreased in the group with cirrhosis, they usually remained slightly above the normal level despite continuous therapy with azathioprine and prednisone (Fig. 1).

The difference in response to therapy becomes still more evident when comparing the course of the albumin and gammaglobulin values of patients with and without cirrhosis. In the latter group (Figs. 2a and 2c) the serum albumin concentrations return to normal during the first 3 months, whereas the gammaglobulin values tend to remain slightly elevated for a much longer time. Patients with active chronic hepatitis and fibrotic changes (Figs. 2b and 2c) behave like patients with cirrhosis of the liver. Despite long term immunosuppressive therapy their serum gammaglobulin concentrations do not return to normal and the albumin concentrations only do so after 5 to 6 months treatment.

The morphological lesions of the disease seem to require a period of 6 months of therapy to show any recognizable improvement (Fig. 3). In some patients without fibrotic change on first laparoscopic and histological examination of the liver, complete remission was found at a further biopsy after 2 and 3 years of continuous treatment (Figs. 4a—4c). Inflammatory infiltrates of the portal tracts were either minimal or no longer visible and piecemeal necrosis was absent.

Specifically sensitized cells could no longer be detected in any patient treated for 18 months, regardless of whether or not cirrhosis was present.

OVERALL BENEFIT AND TOXICITY

All patients treated with azathioprine and prednisone felt well again after a few months and returned to work 6 to 12 months after the start of immunosuppressive therapy, except for the group of patients with uninfluenced cirrhosis of the liver. As far as untoward reactions are concerned, we have never seen gastrointestinal symptoms such as nausea or anorexia. Azathioprine was temporarily reduced in 4 patients with advanced cirrhotic lesions because of the development of megaloblastic anaemia. The anaemia was easily reversible and the patients did well thereafter, on continuous therapy with azathioprine (1 to 2 mg./kg. body weight daily). Care has to be taken in cases with significant intrahepatic cholestasis. These patients were given a preliminary course of prednisone alone at a higher dose until bilirubin levels had fallen below 4 mg. per cent.

As a result of our experience with immunosuppressive treatment in active chronic hepatitis, we believe that it is definitely beneficial in carefully selected cases, and is the best means of treating these patients that we know of at the moment.

REFERENCES

Editorial, (1968) New Engl. J. Med. 278, 277.
Fahrlander, H., Huber, F. and Engelhart, G. (1968) Schweiz. med. Wschr. 98, 363–369.
Mackay, J. R. and Wood, J. J. (1963) Gastroenterology 45, 4–13.
Mackay, J. R. (1968) Quart. J. Med. 37, 379.
Meyer zum Büschenfelde, K. H. Dt. Med. J. 16, 522–527.
Page, A. R., Condie, R. M. and Good, R. A. (1964) Amer. J. Med. 36, 200–213.
Read, A. E., Sherlock, S. and Harrison, C. V. (1963) Gut 4, 378.
Weinreich, J. (1967) Acta hepato-splen. 14, 189–198.

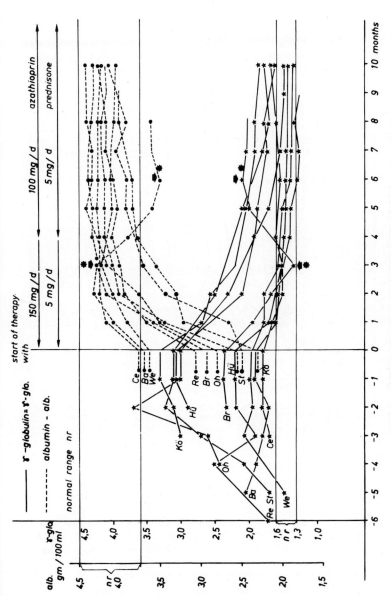

Fig. 2a. Serum albumin and gamma globulin concentrations before and during treatment with azathioprine and prednisone in patients with active chronic hepatitis without fibrosis of the liver. The arrow and* refer to a case who discontinued therapy of his own accord and showed minor improvement only after its reinstitution.

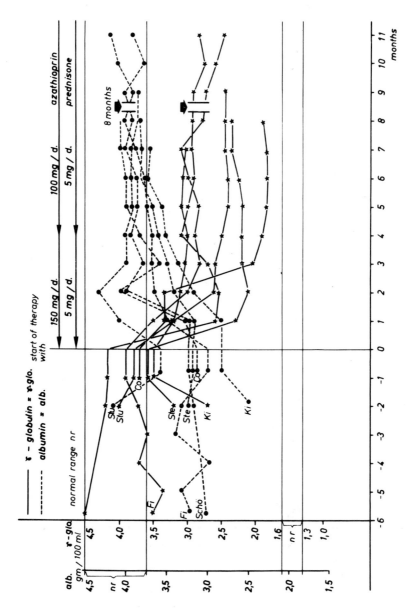

Fig. 2b. Serum albumin and gamma globulin concentrations before and during treatment with azathioprine and prednisone in patients with active chronic hepatitis and fibrotic changes of the liver.

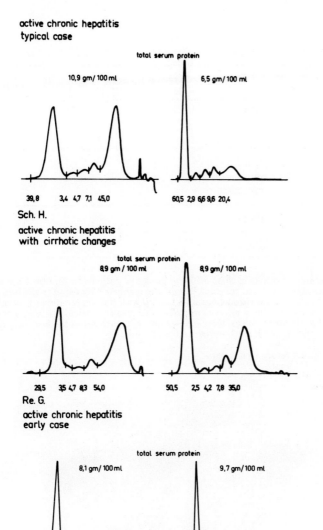

Fig. 2c. Serum electrophoretic patterns in 3 patients with different stages of active chronic hepatitis before and six months after therapy was instituted.

Fig. 3.
Therapeutic Evaluation after a One Year Period of Treatment

Disease	N	Therapy	Transaminasen			φ-globulin			Histology		
			N	I	U	N	I	U	N	I	U
Active chronic hepatitis	25	Azathioprine and prednisone	19	6	—	9	16	—	—	16	—
Cirrhosis of the liver	10	Azathioprine and prednisone	1	—	9	—	1	9	—	—	3
Active chronic hepatitis	10	Prednisone alone	—	8	2	—	2	8	—	—	6

Fig. 3. Summary of results in three different groups of patients treated for 12 months by an uninterrupted and constant therapeutic regimen. Compared to the other groups, the cases of active chronic hepatitis treated with the combination of azathioprine and prednisone show much more favourable results, particularly when considering the histological findings. Only one patient with cirrhosis of the liver benefited from therapy with azathioprine and prednisone.

    N = return to normal
    J = improved
    U = unchanged

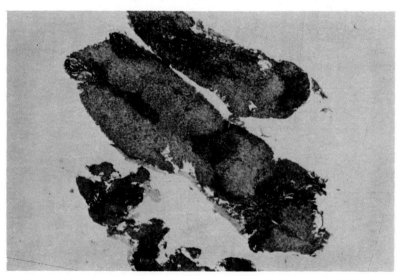

Fig. 4. (a) Initial liver biopsy specimen from a patient with active chronic hepatitis. (Low magnification. Haematoxylin and eosin).

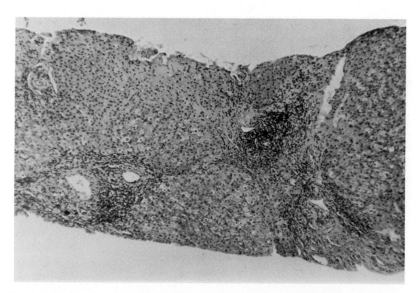

Fig. 4. (b) First re-biopsy specimen of the same patient after a 6-month period of uninterrupted immunosuppressive treatment. (High magnification. Haematoxylin and eosin.)

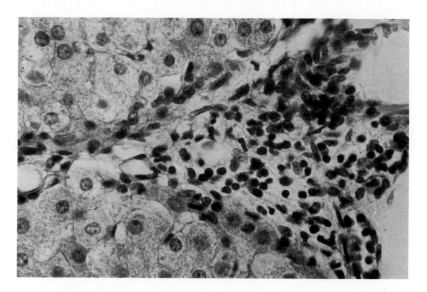

Fig. 4. (c) Second re-biopsy specimen after an 18-month period of uninterrupted immuno-suppressive treatment. (High magnification. Haematoxylin and eosin.)

DISCUSSION
Chairman: Dr. J. Saunders

WILLIAMS

If the patients had deep jaundice you gave them prednisone first. Was this because they became more jaundiced on azathioprine?

KNOLLE

Yes.

WILLIAMS

Did you have any other patients who were not jaundiced when you started azathioprine, but developed jaundice whilst on it? In other words, do you have evidence of a hepatotoxic effect in patients who were not jaundiced?

KNOLLE

This did not occur in our series although it has been reported with 6-mercaptopurine.

TREATMENT OF CHRONIC HEPATITIS WITH AZATHIOPRINE AND PREDNISONE COMBINED

J. De Groote, J. Fevery, and J. Vandenbroucke

80 per cent of our cases with cirrhosis are of the cryptogenic or auto-immune variety. It is important to try to prevent the development of cirrhosis particularly in cases diagnosed at the stage of chronic hepatitis which we consider to be a pre-cirrhotic condition. In a previous study on a group of 34 patients with chronic hepatitis, 4 were found to develop cirrhosis over the course of 3 years. As abnormal immune mechanisms may be instrumental in the pathogenesis of some types of cirrhosis we decided to investigate the therapeutic effect of immunosuppressive agents. The main purpose of the clinical trial to be described now, was to assess the influence of prednisolone and azathioprine on moderately active chronic hepatitis, without overt signs of immunopathology.

SELECTION OF PATIENTS

Laparoscopy and liver biopsy were performed on all patients and, on the basis of these two tests, a macroscopic and microscopic classification was made, the latter according to criteria set out by the pathology group of the European Association for the Study of the Liver (De Groote *et al.,* 1968). In all, 44

Table 1
Diagnosis of Patients
The hepatitis associated antigen (H.A.A.) was determined by complement fixation. One patient with haemophilia had no liver biopsy

	Total No. seen	No. examined	H.A.A. Positive	H.A.A. Negative
Chronic hepatitis				
Aggressive A	28	16	7	9
Aggressive B	3	—	—	—
Haemophiliac ?	1	1	1	—
Cryptogenic cirrhosis				
Class A	7	6	2	4
Class B	3	2	—	2
Primary biliary cirrhosis	2	—	—	—
Total	44	25	10	15

patients were included in the trial (Table 1) and in 93% of cases the disease had been present for more than 1 year (Table 2). Of the 28 patients with moderately active chronic hepatitis, 7 were found to have positive latex tests but none were positive for LE cells or antinuclear factor. Liver function tests in 25 of these 28 patients were observed for at least 2 months prior to the beginning of the trial.

Table 2
Known duration of Liver Disease before Therapy

		6–12 months	1–2 years	2–5 years	5 years	Total
Active chronic hepatitis	A	3	6	13	6	28
	B	–	1	2	–	3
Haemophiliac	?	–	1	–	–	1
Cirrhosis	A	–	–	2	5	7
	B	–	1	1	1	3
Primary biliary cirrhosis		–	1	1	–	2
Total		3	10	19	12	44

RESULTS OF THERAPY

Clinical

In general the patients improved symptomatically very rapidly, usually within the first month and at the moment 39 of these patients are at work. In all those with chronic hepatitis the liver edge became impalpable and was no longer tender. In cirrhotic patients there was often some decrease in liver size which then remained constant.

Biochemical

Liver function tests were measured at monthly intervals throughout the trial. During the first 6 months of treatment there was a statistically significant decrease in serum alanine aminotransferase levels (Fig. 1). This was also true for serum gamma globulin levels, thymol turbidity and zinc sulphate flocculation. A less marked improvement in these tests was noted over the longer period of observation, and this could not be assessed statistically. 33% of the patients now have normal liver function tests, and in a further 23%, only the flocculation tests remain abnormal (Table 3). The time taken for liver function to return to normal ranged from 2–17 months with a mean duration of therapy of 9·2 months. The remission may be sustained and has lasted for more than 1 year in 5 patients and more than 6 months in 2 others (Table 4).

DETAILS OF THERAPEUTIC SCHEDULE

In all cases treatment was started with 15–20 mg. per day of prednisone and in most instances 50 mg. per day of azathioprine. In 3 patients higher initial doses (75–100 mg. per day) were administered. According to the results of various investigations the dose of azathioprine was increased by 25 mg. at approximately 8 week intervals. No patient received more than 100 mg. per day of this drug and only 6 patients with moderately active chronic hepatitis, 1 with the more severe form and 2 with cirrhosis, reached this maximum dose.

Therapy was continued until liver function tests became normal. When this occurred a second liver biopsy was performed. If the histological appearances

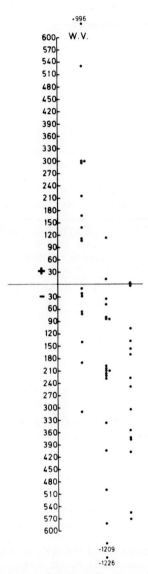

Fig. 1. Illustrating changes in serum alanine aminotransferase. TH, 2m 6m represent the
differences in serum level between that found at the beginning of therapy and that
2 months before (TH), 2 months (2m) and 6 months (6m) afterwards. This difference
was statistically significant (P < 0·01).

Table 3
Present State of Liver Function Tests

		Total No.	Normal	Abnormal flocculation only	Abnormal tests
Chronic hepatitis	A	28	12	4	12
Aggressive	B	3	1	1	1
Haemophiliac	?	1	—	—	1
Cirrhosis	A	7	—	4	3
Class	B	3	1	1	1

Table 4
Duration of Remission and Relation to H.A.A.

		Duration of Remission				
		2 months	2–6 months	6–12 months	12 months	Total
	H.A.A.	+ − ?	1 − ?	+ − ?	+ − ?	14
Active chronic hepatitis	A	1 2 −	1 1 1	1 − 1	− 2 2	12
	B	− − −	− − −	− − −	− − 1	1
Haemophiliac	?	− − −	− − −	− − −	− − −	—
Cirrhosis	A	− − −	− 1 −	− − −	− − −	1
	B	− − −	− − −	− − −	− − −	—

had returned to normal or showed chronic persistent hepatitis, only then was therapy discontinued. At the moment the duration of therapy in the whole group ranges from 2–41 months with a mean duration of 15 months.

Histological

A repeat liver biopsy was performed on 11 patients between 4–18 months after the start of therapy (Table 5). In none were the histological appearances as severe as in the previous biopsy. The laparoscopic appearances also showed there had been no development of the cirrhotic process. In six patients the histological appearances were almost normal and were classified as those of chronic persistent hepatitis. In a cirrhotic with normal liver function tests, there was practically no cellular infiltration remaining.

There is no comparable control group to this treated series. However, in the same hospital we have previously studied a group of 34 patients who had been followed for more than three years. In this group, treated with or without prednisone, 4 patients progressed to cirrhosis and 10 were considered to be in a lasting remission and perhaps to be cured.

Table 5

Changes in Histological Appearances of Liver Biopsy in 11 Patients who had Biopsies During Control and Follow-up Periods

Patient	Histological classification*	Duration months	Follow-up biopsy**	Details of subsequent therapy
D.M.	ACH_a	24	A	Continued
E.V.	ACH_a	18	A	Continued
J.A.	ACH_a	4	P	Stop + resumed
H.A.	ACH_a	12	Nl	Stop
P.H.	ACH_a	12	A	Continued
S.L.	ACH_a	12	P	Stop
C.H.	ACH_a	12	P	Stop
M.E.	ACH_a	16	P	Stop
V.C.	ACH_b	12	P	Stop
C.J.	$Cirrhosis_a$	18	C.A	Continued
Cl.A.	$Cirrhosis_b$	12	C.−	Continued

*ACH_a = Moderately active chronic hepatitis
ACH_b = Very active chronic hepatitis
**P = Chronic persistent hepatitis
A = Chronic aggressive hepatitis (grade a).
C.A. = Cirrhosis with moderate inflammatory activity (grade a).
C.− = Cirrhosis with almost no inflammatory activity (grade −).

DISCONTINUATION OF THERAPY

Therapy was discontinued 18 times in 16 patients (Table 6) and restarted in 5. Two patients with cirrhosis developed serious infections. Therapy was discontinued at once, but both died six months later in liver failure. In one this had developed spontaneously, in the other after a surgical intervention. Five patients suffered significant gastrointestinal intolerance. Only 1 patient developed leucopenia and thrombocytopenia severe enough to discontinue the drug. It should also be noted that one patient with moderately active chronic hepatitis, abnormal liver function tests and with the hepatitis associated antigen in the serum passed through a normal pregnancy and delivered a healthy baby despite continuous therapy with azathioprine and prednisone.

However, in those patients considered to be in remission, liver function tests tended to deteriorate after discontinuation of therapy. In one, a relapse was observed by serial liver biopsies. This patient, a chief nurse in surgery, had initially developed an acute hepatitis in April 1968. By June of that year, liver function tests had reverted to normal but in September she had a relapse. At that time a liver biopsy showed appearances of chronic active hepatitis (Grade a) with an acute exacerbation. Combined treatment with prednisone and azathioprine was started. She felt better very rapidly and resumed full time work whilst on therapy. In January 1969 a follow-up liver biopsy was considered to show mild chronic persistent hepatitis only. The azathioprine was discontinued at the end of May and three weeks later the patient had a clinical and biochemical relapse. Now back on azathioprine the patient is in good health and is working full-time.

Table 6
Number of Patients and Reasons for Discontinuing Azathioprine Together with the Number of Patients Resuming Therapy

| | | | | Ceased | Resumed | |
| | | | | | | |
	Total	Dead	Cirrhosis	Active chronic hepatitis	Cirrhosis	Active chronic hepatitis
Remission	5		—	5	—	1
Gastro-intestinal intolerance	5		4	1	2	1
Infection	2	2	2	—	—	—
Phlebitis	1		—	1	—	1
Influenza epidemic	1		—	1	—	1
Leucopenia	1		1	—	1	—
Miscellaneous	3		2	1	—	1
Suicide	—	1	—	—	—	—

Table 7
Relation of Abnormal Function Tests To H.A.A.

	H.A.A.	Abnormal flocculation only + − ?	Abnormal tests + − ?	Death +
Active chronic hepatitis	A	1 − 3	5 4 3	1*
	B	− − 1	− 1 −	
Haemophiliac	?	− − −	1 − −	
Cirrhosis	A	− − −	2 3 1	1
	B	− 2 −	− − −	1

* This patient committed suicide.

Relation to Hepatitis associated antigen

The relationship between the hepatitis associated (H.A.A.) or Australia antigen and chronic hepatitis is far from clear: it is unlikely in such a small group of patients that a definite answer will be found. In the moderate active chronic hepatitis group 8 of 17 patients were H.A.A. positive and in those that had already developed cirrhosis, 2 out of 8 (Table 1). The presence of H.A.A. in the patients' serum was unrelated to liver function. When all the patients were divided into groups according to the state of liver function tests then we found that, in the group with abnormal tests, the antigen might or might not be present; and that in 3 patients whose liver function tests became normal the antigen remains positive until now (Table 4 and 7).

Conclusions

In patients with chronic active hepatitis with or without cirrhosis, combined azathioprine and prednisone therapy has a favourable influence on general well being and liver function tests. When the latter are compared 2 months before and 6 months after starting theraphy, the difference is statistically significant. Furthermore, a sustained remission is possible. However, a flare-up of the disease may be observed after discontinuation of the therapy especially when therapy is given for less than one year. In the present series there was no progression towards cirrhosis and even in those patients with cirrhosis the rate of deterioration seemed to be less pronounced. Moderately active chronic aggressive hepatitis has an unpredictable and very variable course, and some patients may heal spontaneously. However, others will develop cirrhosis and the combined treatment may influence favourably the course and the general outcome. This study warrants a larger scale trial on a double blind basis with a control series.

REFERENCE

De Groote, J., Desmet, V. J., Gedik, P., Korb, G., Popper, H., Poulsen, H., Scheuer, P. J., Schmid, M., Thaler, H., Vehlinger, E. (1968) Lancet 2, 626.

A CONTROLLED TRIAL OF PREDNISONE AND AZATHIOPRINE IN ACTIVE CHRONIC HEPATITIS

M. G. Geall, R. D. Soloway, A. H. Baggenstoss, L. R. Elveback,
L. J. Schoenfield, B. L. Stubbs and W. H. J. Summerskill

I would like to present some preliminary results of a trial that has been going on at the Mayo Clinic for the last three years under the direction or Drs. Schoenfield and Summerskill.

DESCRIPTION OF TRIAL AND SELECTION OF PATIENTS

The trial consists of a controlled double-blind prospective evaluation of prednisone, azathioprine, a combination of prednisone and azathioprine, and a placebo, in active chronic hepatitis. The criteria for inclusion in the trial included:—

(1) At least 10 weeks duration of liver disease without improvement.

(2) The serum aspartate aminotransferase level had to be persistently greater than 10 times normal or alternatively, persistently greater than 5 times normal if associated with a twice normal serum gamma globulin level.

(3) Histological appearances. Liver biopsy was carried out before treatment in all patients where this was possible and in fact, 90 per cent of patients were biopsied before treatment. These uniformly showed piecemeal necrosis, round cell infiltration and Kupffer cell proliferation; 50 per cent of the patients had cirrhosis at the first biopsy. No patient has subsequently returned to normal.

Post-pubertal patients were selected and informed participation was gained. They were then allocated into 4 subgroups, depending on whether they had had previous treatment with either azathioprine or prednisone, and whether or not the initial biopsy showed cirrhosis. They were then randomized in a double-blind fashion to the treatment groups.

So far we have information on 54 patients followed from three months to three years. There are 14 patients in the placebo group, 16 in the prednisone group (20 mg. per day), 13 in the azathioprine group (100 mg. per day), and 11 in the combination group of prednisone (10 mg. per day), and azathioprine (50 mg. per day).

COMPARABILITY OF CONTROL AND TREATED GROUPS

There is no difference in distribution of patients according to sex, age and duration of the disease between the four treatment groups, as shown in Fig. 1. The comparability of pretreatment study groups with respect to three important biochemical parameters of activity, serum aspartate aminotransferase, bilirubin and gamma globulin levels is shown in Fig. 2. There is no statistically significant difference between the four treatment groups.

There was also no difference in the clinical manifestations of strength, appetite, ascites, bleeding or coma, shown by the four treatment groups. Similarly, the liver biopsies, assessed by Dr. Baggenstoss in a "blind fashion", revealed no differences in the incidence of cirrhosis, piecemeal necrosis, round cell infiltration or Kupffer cell proliferation between the four treatment groups.

COMPARABILITY OF PRETREATMENT STUDY GROUPS

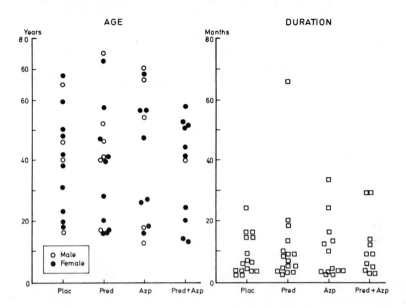

Fig. 1. Comparing the age, sex and duration of disease of the patients in the various treatment groups.

COMPARABILITY OF PRETREATMENT STUDY GROUPS

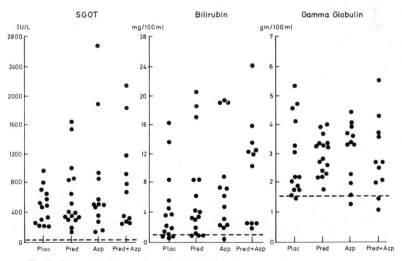

Fig. 2. Comparing the pretreatment liver function tests in the various groups.

CRITERIA FOR IMPROVEMENT

These were predetermined (Table 1). Firstly, considering the serum aspartate aminotransferase levels, there had to be a fall to 33 per cent of the pretreatment value for the improvement to be regarded as "significant". Similarly for the serum bilirubin, if the level dropped to 33 per cent of the pretreatment value, this was regarded as a "significant" improvement. For the gamma globulin concentration, a fall to 67 per cent of the pretreatment value was regarded as "significant". With respect to strength and appetite, these were arbitrarily graded 0–4, 0 being normal. In order to say that a person had improved, they had to improve two grades; therefore they had to have at least a grade of 2 before this could be evaluated. Similar grading and criteria for improvement were taken in the liver biopsy assessment.

Table 1

Criteria for Double-Blind Evaluation of Change

Parameter	Relevant Abnormal Value	Improvement* (% Pretreatment Value)
SGOT <24 IU/ml	>250 IU/ml	33 (e.g.: 600 → 200 IU/ml
Bilirubin <1 mg./100 ml.	>3 mg./100 ml.	33
Gamma globulin <1·6 gm./100 ml.	>2·4 gm./100 ml.	67
		Improvement* in grade
Strength or appetite (graded 0–4)	2 or more	2 grades
Histologic (graded 0–4)	2 or more	2 grades

* Deterioration defined as reciprocal of improvement.

RESPONSE TO TREATMENT

This is shown in Fig. 3. The duration of treatment in patient-months is comparable in the placebo, prednisone and azathioprine group. However, the prednisone/azathioprine combination group was added 14 months ago and although the randomization has been statistically adjusted, our experience with this combination group is much less than with the others.

Firstly, with regard to the clinical improvement, a number in each group improved in strength (Table 2). Similarly, the appetite improved in a number of the patients in each of the 4 groups. However, statistical analysis showed no significant differences in either strength or appetite, and no significant difference in deterioration between the four treatment groups.

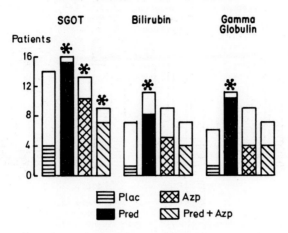

PROPORTION OF PATIENTS SHOWING
BIOCHEMICAL IMPROVEMENT

Fig. 3. Representing the proportion of patients in each group showing biochemical improvement. Columns marked � represent significant differences from the placebo group.

Table 2

Response to Treatment

	Plac.	Pred.	Azp.	Pred. + Azp.
Patients, no.	14	16	13	11
Duration of treatment (patient-months)	214	266	194	49
Clinical improvement				
Strength	5 of 8*	6 of 11	7 of 10	3 of 7
Appetite	2 of 3	7 of 7	5 of 5	1 of 1
Deterioration	No significant difference			

* No. of patients with relevant abnormal values.

Figure 3 illustrates the proportion of patients showing biochemical improvement. It will be seen, with respect to the serum aspartate aminotransferase, that prednisone, azathioprine and the combination of prednisone/azathioprine were superior to placebo in reducing the serum level. In reducing the serum bilirubin level, only prednisone was superior to placebo and similarly prednisone was the only treatment which significantly reduced the serum gamma globulin level. Figure 4 shows that the proportion of patients with

254

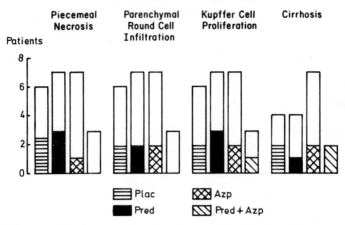

Fig. 4. Representing the proportion of patients showing histological improvement.

Table 3

Overall Response to Treatment

Number of Patients

	Plac.	Pred.	Azp.	Pred. + Azp.
3 Months				
Improvement	0	8	0	4
No change	9	5	11	1
Deterioration	4	1	2	1
Up to 3 years				
Improvement	5	10	5	5
No change	5	4	4	4
Deterioration	4	2	4	1

histological improvement was similar in the four treatment groups. No significant differences in piecemeal necrosis, round cell infiltration, Kupffer cell proliferation and cirrhosis could be found.

The overall response to treatment as judged by the various clinical and biochemical parameters which I have outlined is shown in Table 3. At 3 months, no patient in the placebo group had improved whereas in the prednisone group 8 were better. In the azathioprine group, no patient had improved whereas improvement was noted in 4 with the combination treatment. So that at 3 months, prednisone is clearly superior. However, by 3 years, 5 patients in the placebo group had improved. In the prednisone group 10 had improved but the

Table 4

Severance of Treatment

	Plac.	Pred.	Azp.	Pred. + Azp.
Treatment failure	3	3	5	1
Death	2	1	2	1
Encephalopathy	3	1	2	1
Toxicity	(2)	2	3	
Withdrawal		2	1	

statistically significant advantage that prednisone had at 3 months could no longer be demonstrated at 3 years.

The number of patients in whom treatment was discontinued either because of treatment failure or death, encephalopathy or toxicity is shown in Table 4. There is no significant difference in treatment failure between the 4 groups and no significant difference in the death rate or the complication rate in the groups.

CONCLUSIONS

We need many more patients and more time, but our initial conclusions are clinically that all groups have subjectively improved and there is no significant difference yet. The improvement of the prednisone group at 3 months is lost when the later data is analysed. Biochemically, prednisone in comparison to placebo significantly decreases serum bilirubin, aspartate aminotransferase and gamma globulin levels. Both azathioprine and the combination of prednisone and azathioprine reduce the serum aspartate aminotransferase level. The serial liver biopsies showed that 25 per cent improved but there was no significant difference between the four treatment groups. There was no significant difference in the number of patients who had to be withdrawn because of death or toxicity from the 4 groups of patients.

ADDENDUM

By September, 1970, when 65 patients had enrolled in the study, statistically significant differences had emerged. With regard to survival, prednisone was more effective than azathioprine and placebo ($p < 0.05$). Also, both the prednisone and the prednisone plus azathioprine groups showed significantly better survival and fewer treatment failures ($p < 0.05$) than either the azathioprine alone or the placebo groups. On the other hand, serious toxic effects from prednisone necessitated discontinuation of the medication during the second year of treatment in 3 patients. Azathioprine toxicity presents particular difficulties because of its hepatotoxicity and the difficulty in distinguishing this from hepatic failure due to the disease.

DISCUSSION
Chairman: Dr. S. J. Saunders

BERENBAUM
In the placebo group 2 patients were withdrawn for toxicity. Could you explain that?

GEALL
Any patient who became leucopenic was withdrawn from the trial by the clinicians because, as this was a double blind evaluation, the patient could have been on azathioprine. This is why these two patients were withdrawn. However, as they were in the placebo group the statisticians put them back into the trial. Presumably their leucopenia was due to hypersplenism.

WILLIAMS
We tried to follow your criteria in setting up our own trial and found it very difficult to find such severe biochemical abnormalities in active chronic hepatitis. We often found that the aminotransferase levels fell very quickly after hospitalization, perhaps within a week or even while they were awaiting admission. Would you comment?

GEALL
This is quite true; we could not include many patients with active chronic hepatitis. We were trying to get a homogeneous group of patients to randomize into four groups. Then one could say with some confidence, that any differences demonstrated were probably due to the treatment. Nevertheless, these stringent requirements do make it difficult to obtain a large series.

WILLIAMS
But you may have selected the one end of the spectrum that is not going to respond to prednisone because they are the patients with the most active disease.

GEALL
It may be that people who are inactive respond better to treatment!
(LAUGHTER)

Meyer Zum BÜSCHENFELDE
I must draw attention to the fact that you were using different doses of azathioprine in your groups. The dose of azathioprine alone was 100 mg. daily, whereas in combination with prednisone you gave only 50 mg. per day. It was reported in 1965 that 50 mg. per day had no effect at the beginning of treatment. Furthermore, we have found that reducing the dose too soon leads to a fresh necrotic episode in these patients.

GEALL
What you say is true, but to get a clear cut result you must set your dosage beforehand and not alter it. It may be that 100 mg. of azathioprine with 10 mg. of prednisone is a more effective therapeutic combination. However, with too many groups you will need a still larger series of patients and we are already in difficulty with numbers. It may be significant, however, that in the azathioprine/prednisone group, the serum aspartate aminotransferase has been reduced.

Meyer Zum BÜSCHENFELDE
Perhaps you should remember that Dr. Miescher and also Dr. Good have shown that 50 mg. azathioprine per day is insufficient to treat lupus erythematosus.

TYGSTRUP

When you showed those figures for serum aminotransferase above 10 x normal and gamma globulin above 2 x normal, I thought they were going to provide the definition of active chronic hepatitis. Now you tell us that they select just a small fraction of these patients. What are your definitions then, and why did you choose those patients with the most abnormal values?

GEALL

We have a slight objection to the term "active chronic hepatitis" — the reason being that 50 per cent of the patients have cirrhosis when you first biopsy them; a better term is "chronic active liver disease".

We agree with Dr. Doniach, that we are really looking at an iceberg of chronic liver disease. At the tip of the iceberg the florid cases will be found, presenting with acute hepatitis: then there is a gradation from jaundice with high gamma globulins, high serum aminotransferases, and L.E. cells, to less necrosis down to inactive cirrhosis. If you ask me to define part of the iceberg it will always be arbitrary; we set these criteria simply to get a comparable group of patients in order to study the effect of therapy.

TYGSTRUP

Do you think that the patients with high serum enzymes were the most ill patients? Was that why you took them?

GEALL

Partly, but as you know there are very few ways of defining active chronic hepatitis and this is the problem we have all had: is the definition on biopsy or is it by biochemical tests? We were hoping to define a subgroup who were relatively pure and would therefore all respond similarly.

TYGSTRUP

So it was still by way of definition that you used it?

GEALL

No, not by definition, it was done arbitrarily, to get a pure group to study. The tip of the iceberg.

TYGSTRUP

Why do you think that it is pure? Do you think that the survival of these patients is shorter than those with the low serum enzymes?

GEALL

I don't know.

TYGSTRUP

I don't think so.

EXPERIENCE WITH AZATHIOPRINE IN PRIMARY BILIARY CIRRHOSIS

Alison Ross and Shelia Sherlock

In this paper I shall describe our experience at the Royal Free Hospital of the use of azathioprine in patients with primary biliary cirrhosis over the past 18 months. There is some evidence that there are disorders of immune mechanisms in primary biliary cirrhosis. The successful treatment of active chronic hepatitis with corticosteroids and azathioprine is well established. We therefore thought it reasonable to try some form of immunosuppression in our patients with primary biliary cirrhosis.

Corticosteroid treatment is sometimes effective in reducing the plasma bilirubin and aminotransferase levels in these patients, but we were not happy to give this on a long term basis because of the problems that these patients have with their bones, developing osteomalacia and osteoporosis. The course of primary biliary cirrhosis is exceedingly variable, and we therefore decided to do a controlled trial of azathioprine versus no treatment; a placebo was not given. Patients are allocated to either treatment group randomly, by the use of sealed envelopes. We chose an initial dose of 2 mg./kg. body weight of azathioprine, and this dose has been continued.

SELECTION OF PATIENTS

The patients had to have a history compatible with primary biliary cirrhosis (Table 1). We excluded patients with collagen disease who were found incidentally to have primary biliary-like lesions on liver biopsy. Patients with a history which was more suggestive of active chronic hepatitis were also excluded. The liver histology had to be compatible with the diagnosis, falling into the categories Stage 1 to Stage III of the classification of primary biliary cirrhosis according to Dr. Scheuer. The mitochondrial antibody test also had to be positive, unless the liver histology showed typical granulomatous bile duct destruction, in which case patients without mitochondrial antibodies were included.

Patients in a late stage of the disease were excluded, as these would not be expected to benefit from immunosuppressive therapy. We therefore did not include any patient with evidence of liver failure (hepatic precoma or fluid retention), oesophageal varices, or established cirrhosis on needle biopsy.

DURATION OF TRIAL

At the present time, 30 patients have been admitted to the trial, all during the past 16 months. Three patients on azathioprine had to be withdrawn from the trial within the first month of therapy. One of these had developed a severe anaemia, without leukopenia or thrombocytopenia, and two patients had severe diarrhoea, in one almost certainly precipitated by azathioprine. In one patient in the control group the clinical picture changed into that of active chronic hepatitis, with very high serum transaminase values, and she was also withdrawn from the trial. Excluding these 4 patients, at the present time we have followed 23 patients for longer than 6 months, and 14 of these for longer than 12 months.

Table 1

Selection of Patients for Azathioprine Trial

Present	Absent
1. Compatible history	Liver failure
2. M Antibody + Biopsy Stage I–III	Oesophageal varices
or M Antibody – Biopsy Stage I	(Needle biopsy)

Table 2

Clinical Assessment of Patients Followed for
Longer than Six Months

	Control (11 Patients)	Azathioprine (9 Patients)
Deaths	2	1
Liver failure	2	1
No change	9	8
Pruritus improved	0	6

OVERALL RESULTS

Ultimately, assessment of the value of the drug is going to depend on whether or not survival is prolonged, and for this the trial must continue much longer. However, it is worthwhile trying to assess the effects of azathioprine on liver function, on the immunological status, and on liver histology in the patients treated to-date, to see if there is any arrest of the disease after treatment for one year. Table 2 shows the clinical status of the patients in the trial who have been followed for longer than 6 months. There appears to be very little difference between the two groups; the death in the azathioprine treated patients was from bleeding oesophageal varices – this patient had not developed liver failure.

Pruritus was present in 11 of the control group, requiring treatment with cholestyramine, and it has not been possible to reduce the dose level of cholestyramine in any of these patients. Nine patients in the azathioprine group suffered from pruritus initially; 3 patients have been able to reduce their dose of cholestyramine substantially. These findings may be significant.

Biochemical, Immunological and Histological Assessment

The changes in biochemistry during the trial are shown in Fig. 1. At the start of the trial there was no significant difference between the two groups in any biochemical test. In the treated group, there was a significant fall in serum alkaline phosphatase, aspartate transaminase, and cholesterol, as assessed by a paired t test at 3 and 6 months, but this was no longer significant at 9 months, although at this

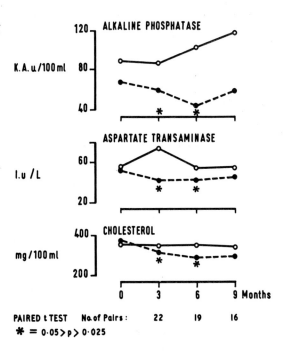

Figure 1.

stage the numbers were rather small. There has been no significant change in the serum bilirubin, albumin, or bile salt levels.

We have also performed serial measurements of the serum immunoglobulin levels in these patients. There was a significant fall in the IgM level at 3 months, but this was not maintained. There was no change in the other immunoglobulins. We estimated the titre of serum mitochondrial antibody by a fluorescent technique both at the start of the trial and at one year, but could find no significant change. Liver biopsy has been repeated at the end of one year in 6 patients on azathioprine and 3 patients on no treatment, and there is no significant change in the histology. One patient on azathioprine has developed cirrhosis, as has one patient in the control group.

CONCLUSIONS

These are of course very preliminary. We are fairly happy that azathioprine is not toxic to our patients at a dose level of 2 mg./kg. In the treated patients there is some evidence of improved biliary excretion as assessed by the liver function tests and there is a possible effect on the immunological factors. So far we have been unable to detect any influence on liver histology.

DISCUSSION
Chairman: Dr. S. J. Saunders

WILLIAMS

I have seen very few patients with primary biliary cirrhosis who have responded to corticosteroids; do you agree? If they do not benefit this is an argument against the idea that auto-immune reactions are important in this condition.

ROSS

To my knowledge, there has been no systematic study made of this. I have seen perhaps 3 patients whose biochemistry appeared to respond to steroids.

EDDLESTON

As you know, azathioprine is metabolized in the liver. Bach from Paris, has shown that the immunosuppressive effect of this drug is very dependent on liver function — it is probably one of the metabolites which is producing the effect. You are trying to treat patients in liver failure with a drug dependent for its action on liver function. You tell us that you have excluded some cases with very severe liver cell failure by your criteria for admission. However, have you grouped the patients on the trial into those with evidence of liver failure and those without and if so, did the latter show more improvement in liver function with azathioiprine?

ROSS

"No" is the answer to that one. How do you define "liver failure"? The bilirubin level is of no help and we have observed a marked fall in alkaline phosphatase in a patient who was severly jaundiced.

Meyer zum BÜSCHENFELDE

We have studied one patient with primary biliary cirrhosis for 18 months. Before the diagnosis had been made she was treated with prednisone elsewhere. We also treated her with prednisone and despite this her liver function deteriorated rapidly. Neither did a combination of azathioprine and prednisone have any beneficial effect, and the patient died within 3 months of starting this combined therapy.

RANEK

We have tried azathioprine in 14 patients — seven with active cirrhosis and seven with biliary cirrhosis. All but one of these had previously been treated unsuccessfully with prednisone. During the therapy, 4 of the cases died from sepsis and one patient died from progressive liver failure, probably not due to azathioprine. Figure 1 shows the serum bilirubin levels; the patients who died had a striking rise in bilirubin as well as high levels at the start of the treatment. The alanine aminotransferase levels fell in all cases, irrespective of the fate of the patients (Fig. 2). I do not think much emphasis should be given to such changes in serum enzyme levels.

ROSS

They can only be compared with a control group.

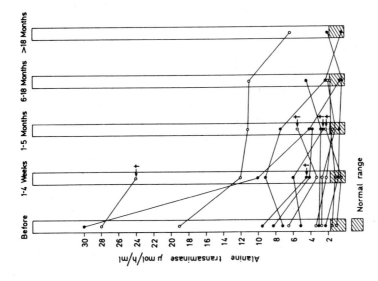

Fig. 2. Serum alanine transaminase levels before and during treatment with azathioprine.

○—○: biliary cirrhosis.
●—●: active cirrhosis.
+: last value before death.

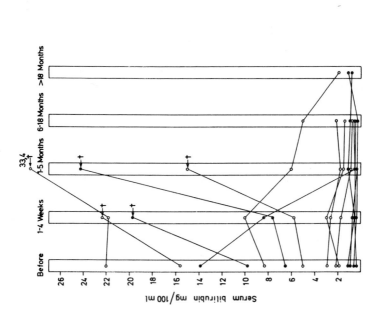

Fig. 1. Serum bilirubin levels before and during treatment with azathioprine.

○—○: biliary cirrhosis.
●—●: active cirrhosis.
l+: Last value before death.

ROUND TABLE DISCUSSION ON RESULTS OF IMMUNO-SUPPRESSIVE THERAPY
Chairman: Dr. S. J. Saunders

CHAIRMAN
It is very clear from these studies that there is a need for very carefully controlled data and for a proper understanding of the natural history of the disease. Our problem seems to be in defining what we are treating.

WILLIAMS
May I ask the panel if they feel we should do as Professor Tygstrup has suggested and study patients with cirrhosis as a whole because in the end all the data is in the computer for analysis? Or should we follow the example of the Mayo Clinic and examine the responses within a small section of that group? This seems to me a fundamental question that must be answered if there is to be any real knowledge gained from these studies. It may well be that the acute group that Dr. Geall has described includes the patients with the greatest tendency to spontaneous remission — we all accept that it may occur in this disease.

De GROOTE
As long as we do not know which group will respond, it is better to do as comprehensive a trial as possible — as has been done in Denmark — and subsequently to analyse all the data in order to detect the subgroups which respond to therapy. We do not yet know the iceberg, and we do not know what part of it to treat. In the past I have selected patients for treatment according to the liver histology regardless of liver function. In the first group that I studied, it seemed that those with low serum enzyme and gamma globulin levels were the ones most likely to develop cirrhosis. There are two main dangers for these patients, first the development of acute insufficiency and secondly the development of cirrhosis. We should bear both possibilities in mind in assessing the results of therapy in chronic hepatitis.

TYGSTRUP
I agree with that and we have tried to include all patients with cirrhosis. However I am worried about the active chronic hepatitis patients who do not have cirrhosis on biopsy, because it is difficult to clearly separate them from chronic persistent hepatitis. Therefore, you do need definition. If you can give us clearcut criteria which can be understood by all our pathologists, so that chronic persistent and active chronic hepatitis may be distinguished, I would prefer to include the latter group. I would not be happy to exclude any cirrhotics, not even the alcoholics, but the important thing is to have a very clear distinction between active chronic and chronic persistent hepatitis.

GEALL
I take a different point of view. Given a homogeneous group of patients selected by well defined criteria, the effect of a treatment which reduces mortality by 20 per cent, could be shown to be statistically significant with approximately 200 patients. With large numbers of patients the data tends to get rather low-grade, one can never be absolutely sure whether it is all being done in a random way. A really effective treatment will show, in a properly conducted trial, with relatively small numbers.

TYGSTRUP

If you have a highly selected and very well defined group, then you will learn how to treat patients in that group only, and you will not learn how to treat the majority of patients that we see. I think the group we study should be the group we want to treat.

GEALL

I entirely agree with that, and therefore you must define the sort of patients that you want. If you want to find out whether a treatment is of value in alcoholic cirrhosis, then you will treat patients with alcoholic cirrhosis. If you want to treat other groups of patients, then you must define them. The definition only assures you of comparable patients and this is its main advantage. But to try and take all patients with cirrhosis introduces too many variables. I would prefer to study smaller groups of patients with preset definitions and preset criteria for improvement. Our difficulty is that we have not enough patients.

TYGSTRUP

Yes, but I do not think you can apply the results to the rest of the patients.

GEALL

No. If we want to find out how to treat alcoholic cirrhosis, then we must do a trial in those patients.

TYGSTRUP

Or on the other cases of active chronic hepatitis with low serum enzyme levels.

SCHAFFNER

I think, Professor Tygstrup that if we are to use the computer, as you suggest, we must utilize and understand the language of the statisticians. One thing they talk about is the signal-to-noise ratio, and your suggestion will certainly accumulate a lot of noise which may drown any signal that is trying to come through. I think that is why it is going to be necessary to sharply define the criteria that we use.

The Research Committee of the American Gastroenterological Association met recently and discussed how to set up a trial in the United States. One thing seems clear from my own observations and from what I have heard to-day: liver function tests in general should be disregarded. They contribute the most noise. The second thing is that at some stage we must decide on the significance of the various histological observations. We must carefully separate cirrhosis which is a vascular, fibrosing disease, from chronic hepatitis which is a mesenchymal disorder involving lymphoid cells. The two may have very different implications and although treatment may influence lymphoid cells, I know of nothing that will remove fibres from the liver. You talk about deaths from encephalopathy and from bleeding varices. Some of these are the result of the cirrhosis and have nothing to do with the hepatitis part. We often are dealing a priori with a two-component illness; that is why your thought of "chronic liver disease" is unacceptable.

The last point has to do with the subjective comfort of the patients. Surely, the ultimate criteria should be the quality and the length of life. Without these, all the rest becomes perfectly meaningless.

WRIGHT

Would this not be the ideal situation for using a system of restricted randomization? Groups in which you are quite certain of the diagnosis may be randomized and the remainder put in a separate group. This has been used very effectively in other situations. Secondly, I have often been unable to biopsy these patients because of a prolonged prothrombin time. What is the effect of the various types of therapy on the prothrombin time? This is surely a good index of liver function.

TYGSTRUP

If we could not obtain a biopsy on a patient, he could not be included in the trial. Of course, this introduces a certain amount of selection because the most ill patients are excluded; therefore the survival time of the control group is longer than has been reported in other series. However, I would not take the prothrombin time as too sure an index of liver function.

CHAIRMAN

Dr. Cook, in your study at the Royal Free the amino transferase levels did not seem to be reduced by prednisone. Were you surprised about that?

COOK

Yes, I was indeed. Actually during the first few weeks there was a significant reduction but this was not borne out by the long term study.

SCHAFFNER

Most of us would accept prothrombin time prolongation in acute liver disease as evidence of severe hepatic dysfunction. This is simply not true in the chronic disease. Whether this is because of complexing of prothrombin factors with the increased globulins, or something else, I do not know. Patients have survived 10 years or more with prothrombin times more than twice the normal value without ill effects.

Secondly, Reynolds and Redeker from Los Angeles found that in the patients with "transaminitis" and minor histological abnormalities, varying doses of prednisone produced no constant effect on the serum enzyme levels.

Meyer zum BÜSCHENFELDE

For patients who do not have cirrhosis evident on liver biopsy, we believe that the occurrence of hypergammaglobulinaemia is an important point in relation to the development of cirrhosis. Before this we do not treat them with immuno-suppressive drugs, however, once hypergammaglobulinaemia is found then therapy with azathioprine and prednisone is instituted.

On the other hand, all patients who already show cirrhosis, receive treatment regardless of the results of biochemical tests.

CHAIRMAN

In Cape Town, a number of our patients die of septicaemia and many get other infections. Are you sure that we are not doing them harm with prednisone and/or azathioprine.

SCHAFFNER

What sort of dose do you use?

CHAIRMAN

We use prednisone to treat their symptoms, to keep them at work if they feel ill, that is all, and therefore the dose is rather variable. We usually start at 20 mg. per day and then reduce it.

SCHAFFNER

One dose daily, or divided? Do you give it every other day?

CHAIRMAN

A divided dose, which we usually give every day. I do not think that really makes a difference to the incidence of sepsis.

SCHAFFNER

Oh, it does!   (LAUGHTER).

WILLIAMS

Do the panel think that there should be a trial of corticosteroid therapy in primary biliary cirrhosis, or should one start with the agent that is in fashion at the moment — azathioprine?

ROSS

I do not think we should try prednisone. I feel it would be unwise to add the osteoporosis of long term steroid therapy to the bone complications of primary biliary cirrhosis.

WILLIAMS

But bone complications are seen in patients with primary biliary cirrhosis not treated with prednisone. Is there any evidence that they are worse on steroid therapy?

ROSS

No.

WILLIAMS

If liver function were better, maybe their bones would improve.

ROSS

Perhaps.

CHAIRMAN

There is also a question built into the programme which has been partially discussed, about the possibility of cooperative trials. Professor Tygstrup described very clearly and accurately the problems of organizing such a trial and the various prejudices which one must successfully overcome. However, to get enough patients for a large study, there is no doubt that a great deal of cooperation is necessary.

TYGSTRUP

Professor Schaffner talked a little about this and mentioned a very important point, namely, the signal-to-noise ratio. Certainly, if many people are involved the evaluation of clinical signs, the laboratory methods and so on may be different, which will introduce noise. Of course, as much as possible must be done to minimize this by standardization before the trial begins. The best way to reduce the signal-to-noise ratio would be to let one man do all the work. Then the noise would at least be unidirectional!

But on the other hand, you can readily calculate how long it would take one man to see a sufficient number of cases with primary biliary cirrhosis to make a controlled study possible. It would be about 200 years, I think So we have to accept a certain signal-to-noise ratio and all we can do is to try to minimize it. I do not think it should prevent us from trying to set up multicentre controlled trials.

The other problem Dr. Schaffner mentioned was whether the fibrosis could be cured. I do not think it is just a problem of curing the patient. He himself said that the problem was to get as good a quality of survival as possible. However, it is very difficult to evaluate the quality of another person's life and we may have to restrict ourselves to assessing the quantity rather than the quality, and to try to prolong survival within reasonable limits. A controlled trial can compare the survival of different groups, although of course other things besides the treatment or the disease may influence survival. However, it is survival we should concentrate on rather than changes in liver function tests, which we cannot evaluate, or changes in the liver biopsy, which we also know very little about.

CHAIRMAN

One essential problem is to make sure that the data being fed into the computer from multiple centres is comparable.

WALKER

May we ask what is going to happen in the States?

SCHAFFNER

The American Association for the Study of Liver Disease will probably set up a controlled trial. We are going to look for parameters to assess the quality of living and these may include such things as days in hospital, days lost from work: these are useful and practical. We have learned from experimental pathology that counting dead ones is a very bad endpoint for the most part! We hope to eliminate some of the signal-to-noise ratio by patient selection. We also have to decide how to do the weighting for that is the other part of computer analysis. How much extra weight do you give a biopsy as compared to a gamma globulin level?

PART V
Some Aspects of the Immunology of Liver
Transplantation

RESULTS WITH RELATION TO TISSUE TYPING AND RECURRENCE OF PRIMARY HEPATOMA

Roger Williams

I am often asked how it was that Professor Calne and I came to be linked in this work. The reasons are twofold, firstly, we had complementary interests in transplantation surgery and in liver disease. Secondly, the availability of donors in any one institution is limited and we have never felt justified in moving a potential donor from one hospital to another for the purposes of organ transplantation; instead, we move the combined team and recipient to the same hospital as the donor. Indeed, in recent months we have moved out to hospitals all round the countryside!

I am going to concentrate entirely on orthotopic transplantation and Table 1

Table 1
The Diagnosis and Number of Patients Treated by Orthotopic Transplantation

Orthotopic Transplantation

	No. patients
Primary Hepatoma	5
Carcinoma of hepatic duct	5
Secondary Deposits	1
Cirrhosis with liver failure	7
Extrahepatic biliary atresia	1
Total	19

shows the diagnosis of the 19 patients operated on to date. Our sole criterion in selecting these patients has been an otherwise hopeless prognosis of a few month's duration only. Indeed each of the conditions has particular problems when it comes to transplantation. Primary hepatomas are highly malignant tumours which metastasise early and I will discuss this aspect later. Carcinoma of the hepatic duct is in many ways an ideal tumour to treat by transplantation because it is slowly growing and metastasises late. However, these tumours are often associated with infection and there have been many problems related to post operative biliary sepsis in this group. Cirrhosis with liver failure will probably constitute the largest group of patients for transplantation in the future, although the removal of a cirrhotic liver from a patient in terminal liver failure is hazardous because of bleeding. In these patients a previous portacaval anastomosis which has lowered portal pressure to normal, is an undoubted advantage.

IMMEDIATE RESULTS

These can be dramatic; liver function tests have returned to normal in a patient whose pre-operative serum bilirubin was 42 mg./100 ml. as a result of

271

a carcinoma of the porta hepatis. A patient with subacute hepatic necrosis
and cirrhosis awoke from hepatic coma within 24 hours of transplantation
(Parkes *et al.*, 1970). In a patient with profound hypoglycaemia due
to massive hepatic secondary deposits, the blood sugar returned to normal from
the time of operation. Hypercalcaemia due to a parathyroid hormone-producing
primary hepatoma disappeared (Knill-Jones *et al.*, 1970) and following transplantation in a patient with primary biliary cirrhosis we observed a fall in titre
of the serum mitochondrial antibody so characteristic of that condition (Fig. 1).

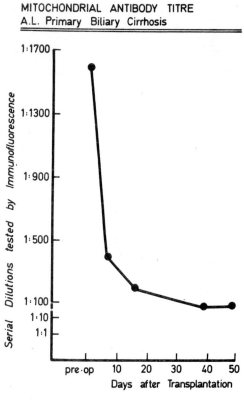

MITOCHONDRIAL ANTIBODY TITRE
A.L. Primary Biliary Cirrhosis

Fig. 1. Changes in serum mitochondrial antibody titre in a patient with primary biliary
cirrhosis following an orthoptic transplantation (by courtesy of Dr. Deborah
Doniach, from Williams, 1970).

Such findings are extremely encouraging but the most important question is
— what are the long term results of liver transplantation and what sort of life
do these patients enjoy?

DETAILS OF TWO LONG TERM SURVIVORS

To give you some idea, I would like to describe briefly the case histories
of two patients whose photographs are shown in Fig. 2. The first is that of
a man aged 57 years, whose liver disease had started with hepatitis in Burma
during World War II. He developed cirrhosis and first showed signs of hepatic
encephalopathy following a portacaval anastomosis. Despite a low protein diet,
neomycin and lactulose, his condition steadily deteriorated and by March 1968,
when transplantation was carried out, he was completely disabled by severe

chronic portal systemic encephalopathy. When the liver was sectioned after removal it was found to contain a multicentric hepatoma.

Following transplantation all signs of encephalopathy disappeared. He was able to go home and in fact he built a greenhouse in the summer! Unfortunately in the 11th month after transplantation he developed a gram-negative septicaemia which proved fatal, the autopsy showing a small biliary fistula to the duodenum with numerous calculi in the biliary system. The only evidence of tumour that

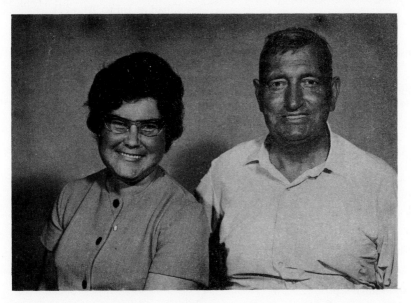

Fig. 2. Clinical photos of the two patients whose case histories are described in test, taken at about 6 months after transplantation.

we were able to find at autopsy was a 2 cm. metastasis in the right adrenal — this was despite a 11 months immunosuppressive therapy post-operatively and a highly malignant hepatoma pre-operatively.

The second patient is now in the 17th month after transplantation. She is a 44-year-old housewife, with children, who developed a primary hepatoma without an underlying cirrhosis. Her liver after removal weighed 4 Kg. In this case the donor liver was from a 4-year-old child, the victim of a road accident. Despite its relatively small size, the functional capacity of the donor liver was always adequate after transplantation. The patient has done extremely well and has gone back to work. Liver function tests and histology are virtually normal and so far there has been no evidence of metastases.

THE OVERALL RESULTS

When the overall results are examined the picture is not so encouraging (Table 2). This is not surprising for the operative mortality of such a major procedure carried out in such sick patients is high. Of the first 17 patients, 11 died without leaving hospital and of those, 7 died during or within the first 6 days from a variety of technical and other complications. The other 4 died at various times up to the 9th week, mainly from infection. The latter, usually secondary to breakdown of the biliary anastomosis, has been the main

Table 2
Overall Results in the 19 Patients Treated to Date

Orthotopic Transplantation — 19 Patients

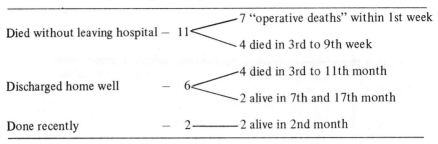

Died without leaving hospital — 11
- 7 "operative deaths" within 1st week
- 4 died in 3rd to 9th week

Discharged home well — 6
- 4 died in 3rd to 11th month
- 2 alive in 7th and 17th month

Done recently — 2 ———— 2 alive in 2nd month

Table 3
Site and Predisposing Factors of the Major Infections which Led to Death of 8 Patients

	No. of cases	Predisposing factors
Fungal meningitis	1	Chronic rejection Heavy immunosuppression
Chest infections	2	Broad spectrum antibiotics Influenza infection
Abdominal sepsis	5	Previous surgery or chemotherapy Biliary fistula

cause of death in our series (Murray-Lyon *et al.,* 1970). The patients with hepatic duct carcinomas were already infected at the time of transplantation, pus being found at the site of previous operations (Table 3).

Of the six patients who were discharged home well, with normal liver function, four died at various times from the 3rd to the 11th month. I have already referred to one of these, the 11 month survivor. Another died as a result of chronic rejection — the only patient with this in our series so far. He developed a cholestatic jaundice, characteristic of chronic rejection, which progressed despite intensive immunosuppressive therapy, and eventually died of a fungal meningitis in the 5th month after transplantation. Two patients are alive and well, the one already described, now in the 17th month and the other in the 6th month after transplantation. To these survivors should be added two patients operated on recently. One, who had secondary hepatic deposits from a primary meningioma treated some years previously, has now been discharged home. The other, operated on for a primary hepatoma, although in good general condition, has developed persistent jaundice and will be described in more detail by Dr. Eddleston and Dr. Mitchell.

OCCURRENCE OF JAUNDICE

Towards the end of the first week, episodes of jaundice due to rejection, have occurred in a number of our patients. In a typical episode there is a rise both in serum bilirubin and aminotransferase levels (Fig. 3). A temporary increase in the dose of prednisone is usually sufficient to control these episodes. Percutaneous liver biopsies at this time have shown changes consistent with rejection. Characteristically, there is centrilobular cholestasis, spotty necrosis of hepatocytes and cellular infiltration of the portal tracts and sinusoids. Large cells of the lymphoid series with pyroninophilic cytoplasm, plasma cells and other mononuclear cells comprise the majority of the infiltrate (Williams *et al.*, 1969).

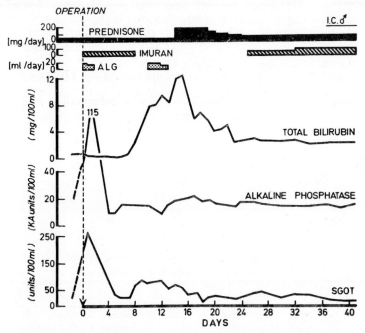

Fig. 3. Liver function tests and immunosuppressive therapy after an orthotopic transplantation showing a characteristic early episode of jaundice attributed to rejection. (From Williams, *et al.*, 1969).

In the patient who died in the 5th month with chronic jaundice due to rejection, the appearances were different. There was marked fibrosis both periportally and around central veins with septum formation but no nodule formation. Dense centrilobular cholestasis was present but the cellular infiltration was minimal. We also observed the characteristic arterial lesion seen with chronic rejection of kidney and heart grafts. Macroscopically the branches of the hepatic artery had thickened walls, and on microscopic examination foamy macrophages containing lipid were seen internal to the inner elastic lamina with cellular fibrous tissue just beneath the intima (Williams *et al.*, 1969).

There are many other causes of jaundice during the first few months after transplantation, including serum hepatitis, azathioprine hepatotoxicity and biliary obstruction. These can sometimes be difficult to distinguish, even with the aid of information from liver biopsy, and it was for this reason that we looked at various *in vitro* immunological techniques for the diagnosis of rejection which Dr. Eddleston will be describing.

RELATION BETWEEN REJECTION AND TISSUE TYPING

Table 4 shows the tissue typing results in 6 patients who lived for more than 2 months after transplantation. The patient with chronic rejection had three major mismatches, but then so did another patient dying at 2½ months from infection related to breakdown of the biliary anastomosis, in whom there was minimal evidence of rejection both during life and at autopsy. In the series as a whole there is no clear correlation between the occurrence and severity of rejection and the results of tissue typing. This may be because the immuno-suppressive therapy has been so effective that almost all the evidence of rejection has been suppressed. There are certainly many other possible factors relating to surgical technique and the presence of infection after the operation which could affect such a correlation. In a series of patients after kidney transplantation in

Table 4

Tissue Typing Results in The 6 Patients Discharged Home and Surviving more than 2 Months (for Typing Methods, see Joysey, 1969)

Case	Course	Rejection	Major mismatches
J.J.	Died, 4½ months	Chronic	HLA1, HLA7, 4b
E.C.	Died, 2½ months	Minimal	HLA1, HLA5, 4b
I.C.	Died, 2½ months	Minimal	4b
G.K.	Died, 11 months	Minimal	HLA7
S.G.	Alive, 7 months	Minimal	HLA12, HLA10
W.S.	Alive, 17 months	Minimal	4a, ? HLA5

Table 5

Data in 5 Patients Relating to Recurrence of Growth after an Orthotopic Transplant for Primary Hepatoma

Case	Course	Recurrence or Metastases
I.C.	1 died, 2½ months	Small metastases in lymph nodes
G.K.	1 died, 11 months	2 cm. metastasis in right adrenal
J.J.	1 died, 4½ months	No growth at autopsy
J.Y.	1 alive, 2 months	No clinical evidence of
W.S.	1 alive, 17 months	recurrence

whom cross matching was done with the same antisera, there was a significant correlation between the results of tissue typing and the subsequent clinical status of the patient. Those with 2 or less mismatches (which was the case in 4 of the 5 patients with minimal evidence of rejection in the present series) fared significantly bettter than those with 3 or more (Batchelor and Joysey, 1969).

It is also difficult to evaluate the exact relation between tissue typing and occurrence of rejection in Starzl's series. Many of his long term survivors have died of metastases and his immunosuppressive regime has changed considerably during the course of the series. It is interesting to note however, that one long term survivor with normal liver function at 254 days had a Terasaki Grade "D" match with 3 major mismatches. Another patient in his series who had a grade "A" match with complete conformity of all 9 antigen groups tested developed irreversible rejection within two weeks which necessitated re-transplantation 68 days after the first operation.

One must also stress that the achievement of a close tissue match with liver transplantation is going to be much more difficult for some time to come than for kidney transplantation. To achieve a close match it is necessary to have a large pool of recipients and, unfortunately, there is as yet no equivalent to renal dialysis which could keep patients with advanced liver failure alive, until a donor with the appropriate tissue match became available.

RECURRENCE OF HEPATOMA AFTER TRANSPLANTATION

Finally, I want to touch on one other aspect of liver transplantation and immunosuppression which has been stressed recently by Starzl — that is the development of recurrence or metastatic spread of a primary hepatoma after transplantation. Starzl has gone so far as to say that patients with primary hepatomas should not be treated by transplantation because of this risk. All 5 patients in his series with malignant hepatic disease who have lived long enough to permit meaningful observations after what was thought to be complete excision of the neoplasm, developed widespread recurrences.

We all know that primary hepatomas are usually very malignant tumours and most patients are dead within 4–6 months of diagnosis. Although it is possible to exclude those with macroscopic secondaries by careful investigation before operaion, it is certainly not possible to exclude the presence of small microscopic metastases. Immunosuppression might well be expected to cause a more rapid proliferation of any remaining neoplastic tissue, but in our series of 5 patients with primary heptoma treated by transplantation we have not observed this (Table 5). One case dying at 2½ months had small metastases in the lymph-nodes and in the patient who died 11 months after operation the only growth found at autopsy was a 2 cm. metastasis. In the patient who died at 4½ months from chronic rejection there was no growth at autopsy despite the very high doses of immunosuppressive drugs he had received. Neither of the 2 patients alive at this present time, including the lady at 17 months, show any evidence of recurrence (Table 5).

Whether our experience differs from Starzl's because we do not use the same immunosuppressive regimen is not known. Starzl relies very much on anti-lymphocyte globulin which he continues for months, whereas we have used it very little and instead have relied on azathioprine and prednisone. Our view at the present time is that patients with primary hepatomas, if they are otherwise suitable should still be considered for transplantation. One will not be surprised if sometimes it proves impossible to remove the growth completely or at other times, that metastases appear during the ensuing months. This applies to all types of surgery for malignant disease but for the individual patient the chance of a cure or worthwhile palliation is suffcent justification.

SUMMARY

We have treated 19 patients by an orthotopic transplant. There are four survivors at the present time, the longest being 17 months — a lady with a primary hepatoma who now has normal liver function and no clinical evidence of metastases. The major cause of death has been abdominal sepsis related to breakdown of the biliary anastomosis. We have seen jaundice due to rejection mainly during the first few weeks after transplantation but one patient developed a relentlessly progressive cholestatic jaundice which was attributed to chronic rejection. The exact relation between tissue-typing and the occurrence of rejection is not clear at the moment and, so far, we have not experienced an explosive spread of hepatoma after transplantation.

ACKNOWLEDGEMENT

I am grateful to Dr. Valerie Joysey for allowing me to show the tissue typing results.

REFERENCES

Batchelor, J. R. and Joysey, V. C. (1969) Lancet 1, 790.
Knill-Jones, *et al.* (1970) New Engl. J. Medicine. 282, 704.
Murray-Lyon, *et al.* (1970) Brit. J. Surgery.
Parkes, J. D., Murray-Lyon, I. M. and Williams, R. (1970) Quart. J. Med. In Press.
Starzl, T. E. (1970) Experience in hepatic transplantation, W. B. Saunders Co., London.
Williams, R. (1970) British Medical Journal 1, 585.
Williams, R., *et al.* (1969) British Medical Journal 3, 12.

DISCUSSION
Chairman: Dr. J. R. Batchelor

TERBLANCHE
At first we thought that most of our transplants would be done for primary hepatoma, because it is very common in the African population. In fact, we have now decided not to do them on the evidence that Starzl has put forward, which I find completely acceptable. I believe that the evidence you have shown us supports his findings. In his hepatoma patients that have died in under 4 months, there has frequently been no autopsy evidence of spread of this disease. It is the patients who have lived longer in whom this occurs and your 17-month survivor is unusual in that there is no evidence of recurrence. When I was in Denver I was shown a young lad of 17 in whom metastases were first noted 15 or 16 months after transplantation. The rapid spread of malignant disease in patients on immunosuppressive therapy can be very impressive. Recently one of the heart transplant patients in Cape Town was operated on for a ruptured aneurysm, and at the time he was found to have a gastric ulcer which looked benign. The ulcer was excised but the histology was reported to be malignant and within 2 months he had died of widespread malignancy within the peritoneal cavity.

Bile duct carcinoma is another story, because this does appear to run a slower course. But there again, one has to be sure that the patients are being offered better treatment by transplantation than by other palliative means, because people have shown that these patients can live for longer than 2 years. Of the 9 patients that we have seen in the last 2½ years with bile duct carcinoma, there are 3 alive at over a year, and one at 2 years; 3 have died but all survived for longer than a year with conservative means. These patients did not have a transplant simply because we could not get donors for them. To have one of them still alive after 2 years, makes us wonder whether she would have been as well after a transplant.

WILLIAMS
I was visiting Starzl a month or so ago and in some of his patients metastases have appeared within a few months of transplantation. What I was trying to emphasize in my presentation concerning primary hepatomas, was that we have not seen the explosive spread after transplantation that Starzl describes. One of our patients still has no sign of recurrence 17 months after operation. Another

who underwent transplantation for a multicentric hepatoma in a cirrhotic liver, had only one small metastasis at autopsy some 11 months later. Now, it seems to me most odd that you have patients such as these on immunosuppression, who have not developed rapid metastases if Starzl's findings are to apply to the whole group of primary hepatomas. I think you have to compare immuno- suppression with immunosuppression: our regime is completely different from his. In Denver, the patients go on week after week having antilymphocyte globulin and it is not really known whether antilymphocyte globulin is different from other immunosuppressive agents in relation to the risks of developing secondary malignant disease.

CHAIRMAN

In view of the work on the pig that Professor Calne has been doing at Cambridge, what made you choose a fairly heavy dose of immunosuppression to treat your patients with, and are you reconsidering this now?

WILLIAMS

We have gone through various phases. At the beginning we used the standard kidney regime, giving similar doses of prednisone — 60 or 100 mg per day — but with smaller doses of azathioprine, because of the problem of hepatotoxicity. Now we are steadily reducing the doses and in fact we have one patient on azathioprine only. But we did go to the other extreme on one occasion in a patient with subacute hepatic necrosis, probably due to viral hepatitis. Because of the latter we did not give azathoprine or prednisone to that patient after his transplant, and almost certainly he died from an acute rejection episode. I am sure these patients do need immunosuppression, but it may be less than for other transplants.

VELASCO

Do you still consider fulminant hepatitis an indication for transplantation?

WILLIAMS

I think I still believe it to be — although Najarian from Minnesota told me that after he had operated on a patient with subacute hepatic necrosis, his own serum bilirubin climbed to more than 20 mg. per cent and several of his team went down with viral hepatitis. So, although transplantation is probably the only method of treatment that can save a patient with fulminant hepatitis where the liver has become completely necrotic, it undoubtedly carries a risk to those involved.

THE LEUCOCYTE MIGRATION TEST IN ASSESSMENT OF REJECTION

A. L. W. F. Eddleston

The problems of the post-operative management of patients after liver transplantation are diverse. The key to success lies in the ability to make an accurate diagnosis of the cause of any disturbance in liver function. This is something which is difficult enough in ordinary patients admitted to the ward with jaundice. When the problem is further complicated by the presence of a graft capable of being rejected and immunosuppressive therapy which not only may modify rejection and immunological defence mechanisms against disease, but also may alter the systemic manifestations of disease, accurate diagnosis is almost impossible.

As Dr. Williams stressed most of our liver transplant patients have died of infections (Murray-Lyon *et al.*, 1970) and the aim must therefore be to keep the level of immunosuppression as low as possible while still protecting the transplanted organ from immunological attack. To do this effectively, rejection must be detected at an early stage. Histological examination of percutaneous liver biopsy specimens is perhaps the most accurate way of making the diagnosis (Williams *et al.*, 1969) but daily biopsies are obviously not practical. Acute rejection is probably mediated by lymphocytes sensitized to the liver graft (Porter, 1969) and a daily test for rejection might be possible if these could be detected in the peripheral blood (Eddleston *et al.*, 1969).

The leucocyte migration test as described by Dr. Søborg (1967) is an *in vitro* measure of cell-mediated immunity and we have used this test to detect alterations in the immune response to liver and histocompatibility antigens in 10 patients after transplantation. Our technique is similar to that described by Dr. Søborg. The liver antigen was obtained by homogenizing pooled foetal livers and the histocompatibility antigens, by freezing and thawing donor leucocytes. The results of the test are expressed in the manner that Dr. Smith described this morning. I would like to illustrate our experience with leucocyte migration after transplantation by describing a few selected examples.

EARLY REJECTION EPISODES

Several of our patients have had rejection episodes of varying severity shortly after the operation. My first example concerns the early post-operative course of a 44-year old woman with a very large primary hepatoma — the survivor at 17 months already referred to by Dr. Williams. Immediately after the operation the serum bilirubin and aminotransferase levels were high but, as liver function was good, these levels fell steadily during the first few days (Fig. 1). However, towards the end of the first week liver function became impaired and the bilirubin and aminotransferase levels rose. Just preceding this deterioration inhibition of leucocyte migration in the presence of foetal liver homogenate was found (Fig. 1). In this case both liver function and the migration index appeared to respond to an increased dose of prednisone and returned slowly to normal over the succeeding days. This is the typical timing of an early rejection episode with the histological changes on liver biopsy that Dr. Williams has just described.

The next slide illustrates the findings in a lady who had been operated on for a carcinoma of the hepatic duct. In this patient the changes in migration index occurred earlier and were much more marked (Fig. 2). Her early liver function

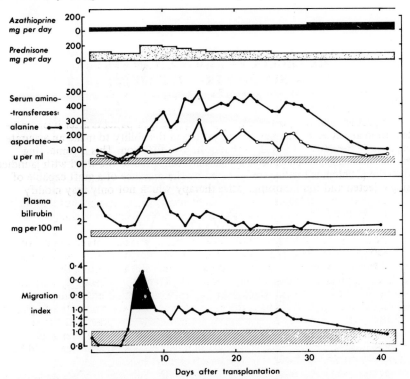

Fig. 1. Serial data in a patient showing a characteristic early rejection episode. Inhibition of leucocyte migration using foetal liver homogenate as antigen precedes the development of jaundice. (From Eddleston *et al.*, 1970).

was never satisfactory for although the serum bilirubin level fell initially, it then progressively rose. Furthermore, the serum aminotransferase level remained very high from the time of operation. Inhibition of leucocyte migration was first found on the fourth day and there followed a 12 day period in which inhibition was consistently found to both histo-compatibility and foetal liver antigens. Neither increasing the dose of prednisone nor administering anti-lymphocyte globulin had any affect on liver function and did not significantly alter migration index. Not until a second course of antilymphocyte globulin was started on the 13th day was there a fall in aminotransferase levels and return to normal of migration index. The serum bilirubin level fell more slowly later. This patient had apparently overcome this severe episode and was ambulant when she unfortunately developed an overwhelming staphylococcal septicaemia and died on the 23rd day. The liver histology at autopsy was consistent with resolving rejection.

From such results as these, it appeared that the observed changes in leucocyte migration were reflecting rejection. However, it could be equally well argued that leucocyte migration was affected as a result of liver damage. A prerequisite of an effective test for rejection, is that it must not be affected by similar deterioration in liver function due to other causes.

A patient without change in migration index

Figure 3 concerns a man also with a carcinoma of the hepatic duct who had undergone several operations on the biliary tree and had residual chronic infection

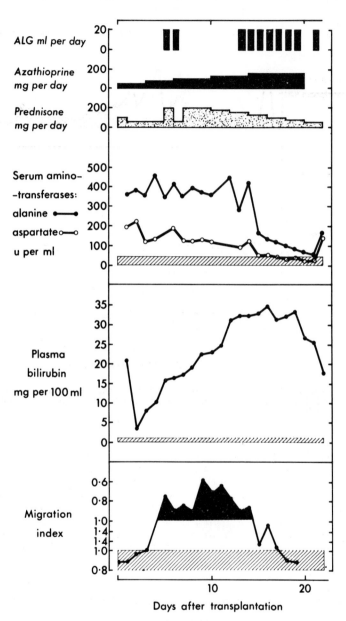

Fig. 2. Serial data in a patient showing a severe early episode of rejection accompanied by inhibition of leucocyte migration. (From Eddleston *et al.*, 1970).

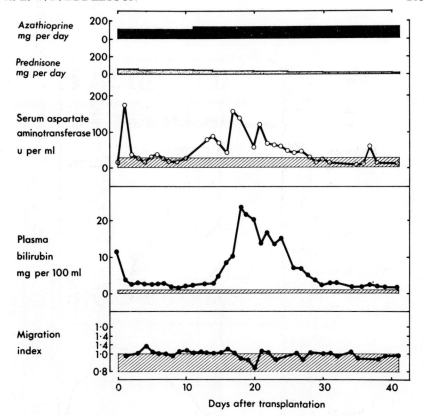

Fig. 3. Serial data in a patient with probable extrahepatic biliary obstruction showing no change in leucocyte migration despite the development of jaundice. (From Eddleston *et al.*, 1970).

prior to liver transplantation. In view of the risk of infection more azathioprine than had previously been given was adminstered from the time of operation in the hope that the prednisone dose could be rapidly reduced. The initial liver function was quite satisfactory in this man, but on the 11th day he developed a biliary fistula. Subsequently the serum bilirubin level rose accompanied by a modest elevation in the aminotransferase level. At laparotomy a large intra-abdominal collection of bile was found. This was drained and with intense antibiotic therapy the liver function returned to normal. A liver biopsy taken at the height of the jaundice, showed no evidence of rejection and the likely explanation for this episode was extrahepatic biliary obstruction. For the purposes of this discussion, the most striking feature was that throughout this period there was no significant change in the migration index to either antigen.

LATER CHANGES

After the early weeks alteration in the migration index has been found which has not been mirrored by deterioration of liver function. Figure 4 shows the first 250 days after operation in the patient whose early rejection episode was described earlier. To-date she is alive and well some 17 months after receiving her

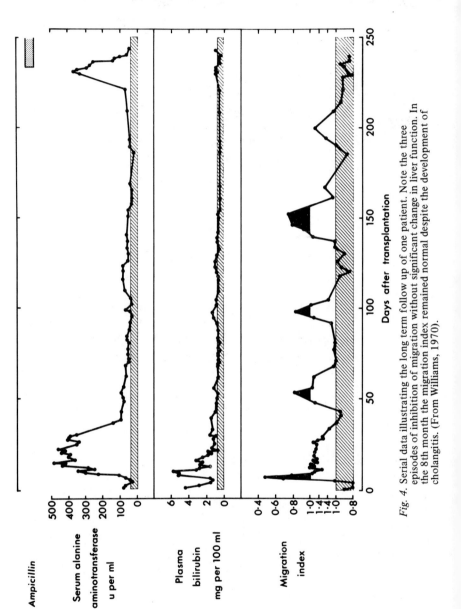

Fig. 4. Serial data illustrating the long term follow up of one patient. Note the three episodes of inhibition of migration without significant change in liver function. In the 8th month the migration index remained normal despite the development of cholangitis. (From Williams, 1970).

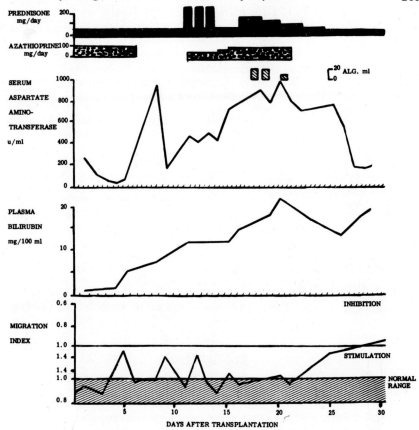

Fig. 5. Serial data in one patient with evidence of severe hepatocellular damage of unknown aetiology.

transplant. Three short episodes of inhibition of migration have occurred during which there was little or no change in the serum bilirubin or aminotransferase level.

If the leucocyte migration test truly detects sensitized effector lymphocytes in the peripheral blood, ipso facto some peripheral protective mechanism must have developed preventing the cells from damaging the graft. A similar mechanism has been postulated by others to explain the phenomenon of organ adaptation in certain experimental animal transplants. Murray *et al.*, (1964) have described the survival of an established graft during the active rejection of a second, more recent organ graft, taken from the same original donor. Our findings, if substantiated by further observations in other patients, provide an interesting corollary to these experiments.

In the 8th month after transplantation this same patient was readmitted to hospital with fever and right hypochondrial pain. A clinical diagnosis of cholangitis was made, which was probably correct as she responded rapidly, clinically and biochemically, to antibiotic therapy. Throughout this episode the leucocyte migration test remained normal despite the high serum amino-transferase levels (Fig. 4).

CONFLICTING FINDINGS IN ONE PATIENT

The results of the leucocyte migration are not always quite so clear cut and it would be a mistake if I were to give you the impression that this has revolutionized our management of transplant patients. To illustrate how complicated the situation after transplantation can be, I would like to describe a recent case in which the cause of the disturbance in liver function and histology is still unknown. The patient is a young man aged 28, with a primary hepatoma of the liver operated on recently, as Dr. Williams has mentioned. All was well until the fourth post operative day when the liver function began to deteriorate (Fig. 5). Severe hepatocellular damage developed, the aminotransferase levels rising to more than 1,000 units per ml.

At this time there was no inhibition of leucocyte migration despite the fact that a biopsy taken on the 11th day showed some evidence of rejection. There was a mild mononuclear cell infiltrate in the portal tracts with considerable hepatocellular necrosis. However, an increased dose of prednisone and azathioprine and the addition of antilymphocyte globulin did not produce any improvement in liver function tests. A few days later a second liver biopsy showed less cellular infiltrate but more hepatocellular necrosis. The suggestion that azathioprine hepatotoxicity was responsible seemed to be confirmed as there was a fall in the aminotransferase levels and a transient decrease in the bilirubin after the drug was withdrawn. Unfortunately the serum enzymes have since risen again and the bilirubin level is increasing, and this time inhibition of migration has occurred. Confused results of this nature are difficult to analyse.

CONCLUSIONS

Finally, I should like, to summarize the findings in our patients after transplantation. One of these patients has shown no inhibition and no evidence of rejection. 5 patients have shown one or more early rejection episodes with preceding inhibition of leucocyte migration. In one patient with histological evidence of chronic rejection, to whom Dr. Williams has referred, inhibition of migration was found. Another patient with probable extrahepatic biliary obstruction had no evidence of rejection either histological or from leucocyte migration. Finally, neither of the two remaining patients have shown significant inhibition of leucocyte migration, but in each case the liver biopsy histology has been equivocal with some features suggesting rejection. It may be significant that in both these cases when azathioprine was stopped liver function improved, in one case only temporarily but in the other liver function returned to normal.

From our results, it appears that the leucocyte migration test can indicate the development of acute rejection. Negative results during an episode of jaundice do not, of course, help in discriminating between the other possible causes but probably do exclude the diagnosis of rejection. Further work is obviously needed to determine the meaning of the later episodes in which inhibition of leucocyte migration occurred.

REFERENCES

Eddleston, A. L. W. F., Smith, M. G. M., Mitchell, C. G. and Williams, R. (1970) Transplantation, In Press.
Eddleston, A. L. W. F., Williams, R. and Calne, R. Y. (1969) Nature 222, 674.
Murray, J. E., Ross Sheil, A. G., Moseley, R., *et al.* (1964) Ann. Surgery, 160, 449.

A. L. W. F. EDDLESTON   287

Murray-Lyon, I. M., (1970) Brit. J. Surg. 57, 280.
Porter, K. A. (1969). In Experience in Hepatic Transplantation By Starzl, T. E., W. B.
    Saunders and Co., Philadelphia.
Søborg, M. and Bendixen, G. (1967) Acta Med. Scand. 181, 247.
Williams, R. (1970) B.M.J. 1, 585.
Williams, R. and Calne, R. Y., et al. (1969) B.M.J. 3, 12.

DISCUSSION
Chairman: Dr. J. R. Batchelor

CHAIRMAN

I did not quite understand whether you used two antigens for your leucocyte migrations. You mentioned that 5 patients with signs of rejection had shown inhibition of leucocyte migration: to which antigen did they show this inhibition or was it to both antigens?

EDDLESTON

In 2 of these 5 patients inhibition of migration was found both with foetal liver homogenate and donor leucocyte extract. In the other patients we were not able to obtain donor leucocytes and so in these cases the inhibition was to foetal liver only.

CHAIRMAN

There was inhibition using foetal liver antigens?

EDDLESTON

Yes. In the cases where we have used both antigens the results were very similar. This does raise a difficult point about the interpretation of the changes to foetal homogenate. They could be due to the presence of histocompatibility antigens, as the homogenate is prepared from 16–18 week foetuses by which time these antigens are present. This may explain the similarity to the changes found with donor leucocyte extract. However, it is just possible that there are differences in organ-specific antigens between individuals.

CHAIRMAN

It would be interesting to compare the results of using a leucocyte extract from normal people known from tissue typing to cross react with the donor, with a leucocyte extract from people who do not cross react. One would expect to find a difference.

EDDLESTON

Falk has recently written up just this experiment. He found that when the antigen to which the recipient had become sensitized, was present in the normal individual's cells, then an extract from those cells could inhibit leucocyte migration.

MacLAURIN

Does the addition of azathioprine in a very low dose to the tissue culture medium influence macrophage migration? I gather that the presence of prednisone in low concentrations does not impair migration.

EDDLESTON

We have not tried this. Because the cells are washed so many times, it is very unlikely that anything present in the patient's serum would remain unless it was very firmly attached to the surface membrane of the cells. Also, we have had patients in whom the dosage of azathioprine has been increased, without the migration index returning to normal.

MacLAURIN

I wanted to know whether azathioprine impairs lymphocyte behaviour to such a degree that they do not produce migration inhibition factor?

EDDLESTON

I do not know.

DYKES

As it is so important to characterize the system satisfactorily, have you made any other comparison? We saw a beautiful correlation from Dr. Søborg this morning, with the skin tests — I don't suppose you have tried skin-testing a patient?

EDDLESTON

This is an attractive idea but we felt that by introducing histocompatibility antigens into the skin a rejection episode might be provoked.

DYKES

You might perhaps choose another *in vitro* test for the correlation.

EDDLESTON

Initially I was doing lymphocyte transformation tests concurrently with leucocyte migration, using the same antigens. The difficulty with transformation was that it took 5 days to get the results, and this was considerably behind the clinical picture. For a test to have any clinical use a more immediate answer must be available. However, in one patient I did find lymphocyte transformation by foetal liver homogenate at the time that the migration index became abnormal.

PODDA

An adaptation of the lymphocyte transformation test which gives results in 8 hours has recently been reported after renal transplantation.

EDDLESTON

Using which antigens?

PODDA

This is spontaneous transformation without antigens.

EDDLESTON

And is it specific for rejection? Would not infection also produce a response?

PODDA

That is correct, but the amount of transformation, measured by uptake of tritiated thymidine, during rejection crises was much greater than during infective episodes.

ASSAY OF SERUM IMMUNOSUPPRESSIVE ACTIVITY AFTER LIVER TRANSPLANTATION

Christine Mitchell

One of the principal drugs used in the immunosuppression of patients receiving a transplant has been azathioprine, but its use is complicated by the possibility of its toxicity. The drug is metabolized *in vivo* (Fig. 1), to give mainly 6-mercaptopurine, and a small amount of 1-methyl-4-nitrothioimidazole (Hitchings and Elion, 1969): 6-mercaptopurine has been found to be hepatotoxic

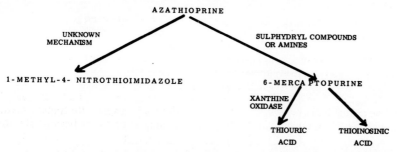

Fig. 1. Some compounds initially formed in the metabolism of azathioprine.

but evidence on the toxicity of azathioprine is less conclusive. The conversion to 6-mercaptopurine is brought about by amines and sulphydryl compounds which are widely distributed in the body. The 6-mercaptopurine is then converted to compounds such as thio-inosinic acid and thiouric acid, the formation of thiouric acid being dependent on xanthine oxidase which in man is found mainly in the liver. It is not known how many or which of the metabolites are responsible for immunosuppression, but there is some evidence that the toxic metabolites of azathioprine are different from those which possess immunosuppressive activity, for pretreatment with allopurinol (a xanthine oxidase inhibitor), in mice increases the immunosuppressive potency of azathioprine more than its toxicity (Elion et al., 1963).

Since the liver appears to be involved in the production of some of these metabolites, it is likely that liver function will influence the degree of immunosuppression obtained after azathioprine administration. In support of this, Bach and Dardenne (1969) found no, or very little, immunosuppressive activity in the serum of patients with severe liver failure given azathioprine. These facts indicated that it was important to determine immunosuppressive levels in the serum of patients after liver transplantation, especially during periods of impaired liver function.

THE TEST SYSTEM

This was based on the ability of certain mouse spleen cells to form rosettes when they are mixed with sheep red cells *in vitro,* and the capacity of serum from immunosuppressed subjects to inhibit this rosette formation. The technique is shown in Fig. 2. Serial dilutions (1/2 to 1/256) of the subject's serum were set up (after absorption with sheep red cells to remove the

289

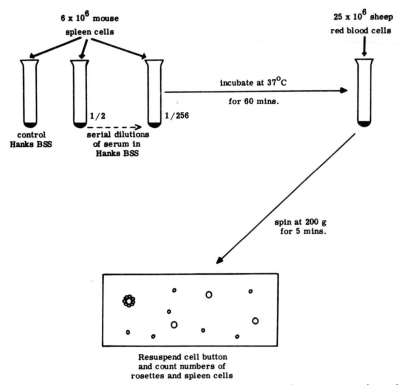

Fig. 2. In vitro rosette inhibition technique for measuring serum immunosuppressive activity.

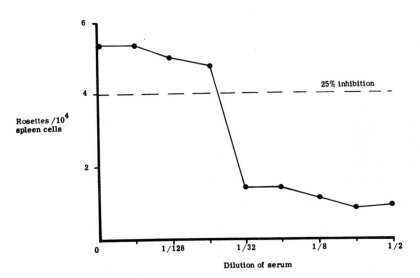

Fig. 3. Typical result of a rosette test, using serum from a patient 1 hour after an oral dose of 125 mg. azathioprine.

anti-SRBC antibodies which are frequently found in human sera) and 6×10^6
spleen cells in Hanks balanced salt solution. After incubation at $37°C$ for 60
minutes 25×10^6 sheep red blood cells were added to each tube, and these were
then centrifuged at 200 g. to facilitate rosette formation. The cell button was
re-suspended by tapping the tube and the numbers of rosettes and spleen cells
were counted in a haemocytometer. A rosette was defined as a lymphocyte to
which 10 or more sheep red cells were adhering. A typical result is shown in
Fig. 3. The number of rosettes/10,000 spleen cells is calculated for the control
and each dilution of serum, and the maximum dilution of serum at which more
than 25 per cent of rosette formation is prevented is taken as the titre of
immunosuppressive activity, in the case illustrated 1/32.

Inhibitory effect of control sera

If serial dilutions of serum from normal subjects are incubated with spleen
cells it is found that serum dilutions of 1/2 or 1/4 will inhibit rosette formation.
If serum is taken one hour after an oral dose of azathioprine in a normal subject
it is found that much greater dilutions (1/64 or 1/128) will cause inhibition. The
cause of the slightly inhibitory effect of control sera is not known, but two
possible explanations are natural antibody directed against mouse lymphocytes,
or cross-reacting antigens between human serum and sheep red blood cells. Like
the normal subjects, the majority of the transplant patients have also had
control titres of 1/2 or 1/4 but one had a higher titre of 1/8 to 1/16. Bach and
Dardenne (1969) have found that patients with hepatic dysfunction have higher
control titres, and patients with primary biliary cirrhosis or active chronic
hepatitis whom we have studied, have had very high control titres. These
patients have antibodies against sheep red blood cells and mouse red blood cells,
and it seems possible that they may also have antibodies against mouse spleen
cells and these could prevent rosette formation.

SERUM LEVELS AFTER TRANSPLANTATION

Bach *et al.*, (1969a) have used the rosette inhibition technique for assaying
the activity of various immunosuppressive drugs and antilymphocyte sera
in vitro, and it is relevant to our test that prednisone does not cause inhibition
of rosette formation. It has also been shown that there is good correlation
between the ability of antilymphocyte sera to inhibit rosette formation and to
prolong skin graft survival time in mice, and this suggests that rosette inhibition
capacity is closely related to immunosuppressive activity (Bach *et al.,* 1969b).
We have now measured serum immunosuppressive levels in 6 patients after liver
transplantation. Serum samples were routinely taken one hour after azathioprine
had been given, since peak immunosuppressive activity has been found to occur
at this time. Figure 4 shows the activity over a complete 24 hour period, in a
patient who had received an oral dose of 125 mg. of azathioprine. She was in the
9th month after transplantation and had normal liver function. There was a high
immunosuppressive titre of 1/128 at 1 hour and by 24 hours all immunosuppressive activity had disappeared.

Table 1 shows the serum bilirubin levels and immunosuppressive titres of 3
patients. W. S. whose liver function was normal, had a high titre of 1/128: G. K.
was in the 7th month after transplantation, and had had a recent cholangitis.
He was mildly jaundiced with a serum bilirubin of 3·5 mg./100 ml. and had a
titre of 1/64. The serum immunosuppressive titre of a child (G. P.) with a
heterotopic transplant was 1/4, 1 hour after a body/weight dose of azathioprine
equivalent to that of the adults. At the time, this child had poor liver function
with a plasma bilirubin of 12·3 mg./100 ml., and a few days later, when the graft
was removed, histological examination showed extensive hepatocellular necrosis.

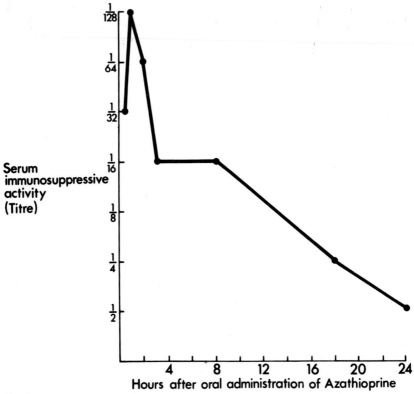

Fig. 4. Measurements of serum immunosuppressive activity over a 24-hour period after oral administration of 125 mg. azathioprine. (From Mitchell *et al.,* 1970.)

Table 1

	Serum Bilirubin	Azathioprine	Serum Immunosuppressive Activity 1 Hour Later
	(mg./100 ml.)	(mg.)	(titre)
W. S.	0·8	125	1/128
G. K.	3·5	125	1/64
B. P.	12·3	25	1/4
Control Serum			1/2-1/4

Table 1. Serum bilirubin levels and immunosuppressive titres of 3 patients with liver transplants, receiving azathioprine. (From Williams, 1970).

Serial readings in three patients

In 3 other patients serum immunosuppressive activity was measured daily, starting on the day after transplantation. In one patient (Case OL16) liver function was excellent at first (Fig. 5). The plasma bilirubin fell to 2·5 mg./100 ml. by the second day, and for the first fortnight remained at about

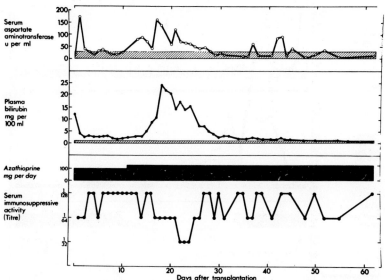

Fig. 5. Case OL16: serial data after orthotopic transplantation. (From Mitchell *et al.,* 1970.)

this level. During this period he had high immunosuppressive titres of 1/128 or 1/64. He then developed a biliary fistula and the plasma bilirubin level rose. There was a fall in the serum immunosuppressive activity, the lowest titres occurring 4–6 days after the highest plasma-bilirubin level. Laparotomy revealed a large intra-abdominal collection of bile and several small infarcts in the left lobe of the liver. A biopsy showed no histological evidence of rejection, and he was therefore given intensive antibiotic therapy. After peritoneal drainage and lavage his liver function steadily improved, and the serum immunosuppressive titres also returned to normal levels. Since then, liver function has been virtually normal, and the high immunosuppressive titres have been maintained.

In the second patient (Case OL17) initial liver function was poor (Fig. 6). There was a very brief drop in plasma bilirubin, but the level then rose to 30 mg. per 100 ml. by the 11th day. Throughout this time the immunosuppressive titre did not rise above 1/32 after an initial titre of 1/64. A laparotomy indicated that the cholestasis was intrahepatic in origin as there was no dilatation of the intrahepatic bile ducts. The possibility of rejection was raised by a biopsy which showed some mononuclear cell infiltrate in the portal tracts, but the periportal hepatocytes appeared to be normal. Another possibility was azathioprine hepatotoxicity and when this drug was discontinued the plasma bilirubin level immediately fell. By the 32nd day the level was 5 mg./100 ml. and azathioprine was restarted. The dose was gradually increased from 25 to 100 mg. and the corresponding rise in serum immunosuppressive activity from 1/4 to 1/16 showed a dose/response relationship. From the 43rd day when the plasma bilirubin level fell within the normal range, higher near-normal titres of 1/32 and 1/64 were recorded.

The third patient (Case OL19) had a higher control immunosuppressive titre (1/8 to 1/16) than the previous patients (1/2 to 1/4). On the 2nd day the titre after azathioprine was 1/256, when the plasma bilirubin was near the normal range (Fig. 7). From the 4th day the plasma bilirubin level began to increase, and

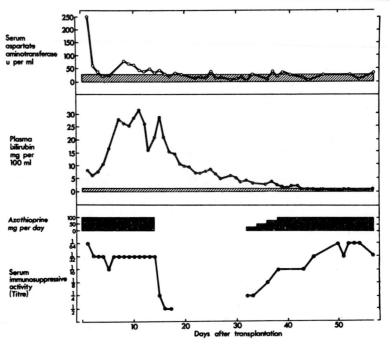

Fig. 6. Case OL17: serial data after orthotopic transplantation. (From Mitchell *et al.*, 1970.)

there was a sharp rise in the serum enzyme levels. Slightly lower immunosuppressive titres of 1/128 and 1/164 were obtained during this time. The
platelet count then dropped and azathioprine was stopped after the 6th day, and
as expected the titre dropped to the control level of 1/8. Azathioprine was
restarted on day 11, and as with the previous patient there was a rise in the
immunosuppressive titre which appeared to correspond with the increasing dose.
Liver function became increasingly bad from the 15th day, the high enzyme
levels suggesting hepatocellular damage. Serum immunosuppressive activity
decreased at this time and control titres of 1/8 and 1/16 were obtained although
azathioprine was still being given. Once again, it was felt that azathioprine could
be responsible for the deteriorating liver function and so the drug was
discontinued after day 20.

SERUM ASSAY RELATED TO TYPE OF DISTURBED LIVER FUNCTION

   The results with these 6 patients demonstrate the dependence of serum
immunosuppressive activity on adequate liver function. As shown in Table 2, the
titre obtained when liver function was normal was as high (1/128) as that
obtained by Bach in normal subjects given azathioprine. When serum
immunosuppression was measured in patients during periods of cholestasis the
titres were reduced, but only to 1/32 or 1/16, these levels being considerably
higher than the control value of 1/2. However, in the case shown in Fig. 6, where
there was hepatocellular damage, a titre of 1/8 was obtained after azathioprine
and this was as low as the control value for this patient. Also, in the child with
severe hepatocellular damage, the serum immunosuppressive activity remained
at the control level of 1/4 after azathioprine. These results are of interest since
cholestasis, whether intrahepatic or extrahepatic would not be expected to
impair the metabolism of azathioprine as much as hepatocellular damage.

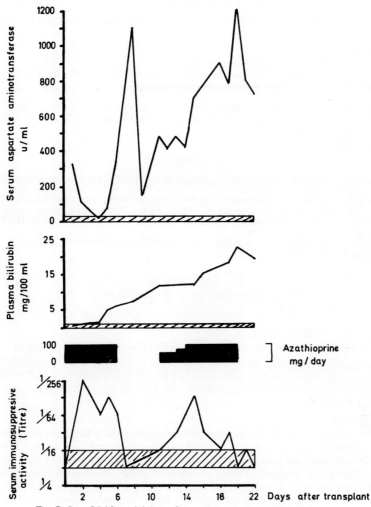

Fig. 7. Case OL19: serial data after orthotopic transplantation.

Table 2

	Type of Jaundice	Control Titre	Titre after Azathioprine
W. S.	None	1/2	1/128
G. K.	Cholestatic	1/2	1/32
S. G.	Cholestatic	1/2	1/32
T. K.	Cholestatic	1/2	1/16
J. Y.	Hepatocellular	1/8	1/8
B. P.	Hepatocellular	1/4	1/4

Table 2. Relationship between the type of jaundice and the level of serum immunosuppressive activity after azathioprine.

CONCLUSIONS
When liver function is normal or only slightly impaired azathioprine should therefore provide effective immunosuppression after liver transplantation, but when liver function is more severely impaired azathioprine appears to be ineffective. If the hepatocellular damage is due to rejection, the serum immunosuppressive activity due to azathioprine is likely to decrease just at the time when increased immunosuppression is needed.

Some of the data given in this communication is taken from: Mitchell, C. G., Eddleston, A. L. W. F., Smith, M. G. M. and Williams, R. (1970) Lancet, 1196.

REFERENCES

Bach, J. F. and Dardenne, M. (1969) Paper read at the Nephrology Congress held in Stockholm in June (In Press).
Bach, J. F., Dardenne, M., Dormount, J. and Antoine, B. (1969) Transplant Proc. 1, 403.
Bach, J. F., Dardenne, M. and Fournier, C. (1969) Nature, London, 222, 998.
Elion, G. B., Gallahan, S., Nathan, H., Bicar, S., Rundles, R. W. and Hitchings, G. H. (1963) Biochem. Pharmac. 12, 85.
Hitchings, G. H. and Elion, G. B. (1969) Accounts of Chemical Research, 2, 202.
Williams, R. (1970) B.M.J. 1, 585.

DISCUSSION
Chairman: Dr. J. R. Batchelor

Meyer Zum BÜSCHENFELDE
Could this be the explanation for the ineffectiveness of azathioprine in primary biliary cirrhosis? We have seen a rise in bilirubin and alkaline phosphatase levels during treatment with azathioprine when liver function is very poor. We now control severe hyperbilirubinaemia with prednisone before introducing azathioprine.

WILLIAMS
It would seem simple to decide whether azathioprine is hepatotoxic or not, but at present there is considerable controversy concerning its toxicity. This is a particularly difficult problem after liver transplantation because the liver is almost certainly damaged to some extent during the operation. We should really study the effects of azathioprine toxicity in relation to various degrees of ischaemic liver damage. With the small number of transplant operations being done, a trial is virtually impossible. This is why it is so important that the metabolism of azathioprine should be studied in patients with active chronic hepatitis and primary biliary cirrhosis.

CHAIRMAN
Is there any information from experimental animal transplantations?

WILLIAMS
Professor Calne showed that azathioprine could be hepatotoxic in the dog with a renal transplant, in just the same way as 6-mercaptopurine. There is good evidence in man that 6-mercaptopurine can produce jaundice, but there is no human study in which azathioprine has been proved to be hepatotoxic. Occasionally renal transplant patients treated with azathioprine may develop jaundice, which disappears when the drug is stopped; but in some of these cases the jaundice has not returned when the azathioprine was restarted. However, that does not mean too much, as the same phenomenon may be observed with chlorpromazine.

WINCH

Azathioprine would not seem to be an ideal immunosuppressive drug on the grounds of its possible hepatotoxicity. Starzl considers that a combination of azathioprine and prednisone predisposes to the development of sepsis after liver transplantation. Bearing this in mind, would Dr. Williams comment on the group of patients with sepsis that he has spoken of this afternoon?

WILLIAMS

That is an awkward question coming from somebody in my own unit! Unfortunately, the two series are not strictly comparable. He has operated mainly on patients with extrahepatic biliary atresia who have not had sepsis before transplantation; we have included in our series patients with carcinoma of the bile duct who have been grossly infected beforehand. So you cannot relate the incidence of sepsis which we found with the incidence in his series. Moreover, his post-operative regime is different from ours.

TERBLANCHE

Using unimmunosuppressed animals, both we, and the group from Denver, have shown a higher incidence of sepsis in those with liver allografts than in those with autografts. There may be a more fundamental reason for the high incidence of sepsis after human liver transplantation than just the immunosuppressive therapy.

WILLIAMS

But any patient with liver disease is probably susceptible to infection. Certainly the cirrhotic is. After all, the liver graft is damaged to some extent.

IMMUNOLOGICAL ASPECTS OF ORGAN GRAFTING
IN THE PIG
R. Y. Calne

I had intended to confine this paper to immunological studies in relation to liver transplantation in the pig. However, as our more recent studies have also concerned renal transplantation, I have decided to broaden the subject matter to include this aspect.

The pig is fully immunologically competent at birth; in fact, during the last third of uterine life competence is developing. Unlike the rat it has a rather short period of immunological maturation and from then onwards the pig will reject skin grafts like any other species. Our interest in organ transplantation in the pig really originated from experiments carried out by Richard Binns at Babraham. He was attempting to produce classical immunological tolerance by injecting pig foetuses in the first half of intrauterine life with lymphoid cells. Subsequently, animals that survived this procedure were to a variable degree tolerant of skin grafts from the cell donor. We then investigated these animals to see whether kidney grafts would also be accepted. In one of his animals that was partially tolerant to a skin graft which was rejected only after 56 days, a kidney graft was accepted apparently permanently.

At this time we had also been doing some preliminary work on liver grafting in the dog. However, it was reported from Bristol, that the pig was an excellent model in which to study liver transplantation as it withstood surgery well, and some of their animals had survived for long periods without rejecting their livers. We were soon able to confirm these findings.

PROLONGED SURVIVAL OF LIVER ALLOGRAFTS IN THE PIG

Pigs usually reject skin allografts within 5–10 days. Heart and pancreas allografts are also rejected in about the same time although we have not done enough to be dogmatic about this. Kidney grafts, of which we have done many, are consistently rejected in the same way as in other species. On the other hand, rejection of liver allografts has been mild or minimal up to two and a half years. We have not seen the parenchymatous destruction of classical first set rejection in an orthotopic porcine liver graft, despite the fact that three different breeds of pigs have been used in various combinations. Another important immunological point is that prior to liver transplantation, killed donor lymphocytes stimulate a proliferative response in recipient lymphocytes when set up in mixed lymphocyte cultures, except in approximately 25 per cent of litter-mates. This is what one would expect if the pig has a strong histocompatibility locus similar to that found in the mouse, the rat and man.

Apart from the peculiarity with the liver, there is nothing strange in the immunological behaviour of pigs. In every species of animal so far studied, some organs seem to be accepted less easily than others: the skin is the most difficult to maintain, marrow may also be difficult, then the heart and then the kidney. In every species the liver has been the organ most easily accepted. However, the pig is remarkable for the ease with which liver grafts are accepted as compared with other organs.

The surgical technique we use in orthotopic liver transplantation may differ in certain minor respects from that used by others. The inferior vena cava is anastomosed above and below the liver. Donor portal vein is linked to recipient portal vein, and the donor hepatic artery is joined by a Carrel patch to the aorta. The recipient and donor common bile ducts are connected directly so as to prevent cholangitis, which can make the histology very difficult to intepret. Some of the pigs find the operation a stressful procedure! — and develop ulcers, and so a vagotomy and drainage procedure is carried out at the same time.

In most of the experiments donor blood has been transfused to the recipient at the time of operation. However, it cannot be this that was affecting the immunological responses as we have one pig surviving more than a year after transplantation which received no blood transfusion during the operation. Nearly all the livers get a sprinkling of lymphocytes in the portal triads and a little increase in fibrous tissue, but the parenchyma remains intact. As time goes by, the cell infiltration tends to disappear. None of these animals has had any immunosuppressive drugs.

That the transplanted liver is functioning adequately, I can only show you in gross terms. The pigs are usually 3 months old at operation and afterwards they are able to grow as usual. By 9 months we have observed as much as a total of eightfold increase in weight of pig and in weight of liver. A liver allograft is also compatible with a happy family life! One of our pigs had a liver allograft 18 months before giving birth to nine happy little piglets — until they realized they were for transplantation experiments!

Some people have suggested that we use closely matched pigs. This is not true; we have transplanted from a Large White to a Saddleback Wessex pig, which are very different in appearance and behaviour. The third breed of pig we have used in the Landrace.

PROTECTIVE EFFECT OF A LIVER GRAFT

Not only is the liver allograft *not* rejected in the pig unlike other tissues, it also has a remarkable protective effect on other tissues transplanted from the same donor. Allografts of skin, heart and kidney from the same donor are protected from rejection. The protection for skin allografts is least effective and the protection of kidney allografts is the most profound of the organs that we have studied. In every case, donor tissue has been protected better than other grafts from different animals. Since there has been this specific donor-protection in every experiment that we have done, I feel that transplantation antigens must be involved. It is almost a question of semantics: if the protective effect is donor-specific then it is difficult to imagine anything other than transplantation antigens relating to both donor and the recipient, that could be responsible.

The protection of kidney allografts, though better than the other tissues that we have investigated, is nevertheless variable. In the worst rejection that we had seen of a kidney graft in the presence of a liver graft from the same donor, there was cellular infiltration, damage to tubules and fibrosis around the glomeruli. This occurred at 70 days and was of the same severity as the rejection that was seen at 5 days in a litter-mate not receiving a liver graft. In another case, the protection of the kidney appeared to have been complete as there was no evidence of rejection at 6 months. Another animal is still alive at two and a half years following bilateral nephrectomy and hepatectomy, and then a liver and kidney transplant from the same donor.

The next series of experiments were designed to discover how long it was necessary, if at all, for the donor liver to remain in the recipient in order for protection of other donor grafts to be achieved. Accessory livers were placed in pigs together with a kidney graft or a skin graft, and after a given period of time the accessory liver was removed. If the accessory liver was left in for only two hours there was no protection and kidney or skin graft rejection went

on relentlessly. If it was left in for 24 hours or longer, then protection seemed
to be, in a small number of experiments, almost as good as if the liver had
been left in indefinitely. This was rather a surprising finding and seemed to us
important in trying to understand the mechanism involved.

The accessory livers were transplanted in the right side of the abdomen with
end-to-side portal vein, vena cava and aorta with coeliac artery, and gall
bladder to gall bladder. It was interesting that these livers showed more
histological evidence of rejection, which at times was quite severe, than was
observed in orthotopic livers. Nevertheless even in this situation the donor liver
could protect donor kidney, skin or heart grafts. The better the initial function
of the liver and the less ischaemic damage it suffered, the greater the protective
effect appeared to be for the liver itself and for other tissues.

Our experiments had reached about this stage when Van Rood et al., (1970)
reported a finding relevant to our work — that small amounts of HLA antigen, a
human transplantation antigen, was present in a soluble form in the albumin
fraction of normal human serum. We have confirmed this finding and using,
multispecific pig-typing sera, preliminary results suggest that the pig equivalent
of HLA (PLA) may be present in pig serum and in a much higher concentration
that HLA in man. This could be very pertinent to the ideas that we have in mind
concerning the pig liver allografts. About a year ago, we suggested that the pig
liver might release into the blood transplantation antigens in a soluble form,
which might then induce partial immunological tolerance. It is known—and
perhaps the most clearcut experiments are those from the Walter and Eliza Hall
Institute — that flagellin, which is a large molecule obtained from the typhoid
bacillus, will produce immunity if it is injected into mice. If the molecule is
broken up into smaller particles then, instead of producing immunity, it produces
specific tolerance. There are a variety of other experiments on similar lines.

STUDIES WITH ANTIGEN EXTRACTS

The next series of experiments, carried out in collaboration with Dr. Alan
Davies, were to investigate possible immunosuppressive properties of donor
soluble cell membrane extracts, which presumably contain PLA antigen, and
of donor blood or serum on recipient pigs.

The experiments were quite simple: three month old pigs underwent
bilateral nephrectomy followed by an orthotopic renal allograft; donor cell
membrane extract or a litre of donor blood or 500 cc. serum was injected
intravenously at the time of grafting. The amount of cell membrane extract
given varied from 50–5,000 mg. of protein, a tremendous variation, but no
relationship was found between the dose given and effects observed. However,
the relationship between total protein content and actual specific transplantation antigen content is unknown. The controls consisted of two series of pigs:
firstly, 17 bilaterally nephrectomized pigs given renal allografts without any
other form of treatment; and secondly, 14 animals in whch the grafted kidney
was removed after 1–2 weeks. Of those 31 controls, all but one had rejection
at the time that the kidney was examined. 9 of the 17 bilaterally nephrectomized control pigs received grafts from litter-mates, whereas in the other
experimental groups none of the donor/recipient combinations were litter-mates.
The longest control survival was 33 days, and all those that survived beyond
15 days received their graft from a litter-mate. The only control animal that
did not show evidence of rejection had received a graft from a litter-mate and
died from hydronephrosis at 12 days.

17 bilaterally nephrectomized animals received a renal graft and cell
membrane extract from donor pigs, none of which were litter-mates of the

recipients. In this group the difference in survival from that in the control group was marked. At 40 days nearly 50 per cent of the animals were still surviving. To-date 4 are alive between 105–258 days. Of the 6 animals given blood instead of cell membrane extract 3 are alive between 78–85 days. Two of the donors of the 3 surviving animals were unrelated to their respective recipients and one was of a different breed. Of the 6 animals given serum, one who also had an unrelated donor, is alive at 91 days. If the 12 animals receiving either blood or serum are considered as a group, the survival is not quite as good as that in the group receiving the cell membrane extract, as only 30 per cent survived beyond 40 days. Nonetheless this was much longer than the mean control survival. Thus, evidence of an immunosuppressive effect of all three agents investigated has been demonstrated beyond doubt, as far as we are concerned. All these findings are compatible with the initial hypothesis, although they by no means prove it.

APPLICATION OF FINDINGS TO OTHER SPECIES

Altough the pig shows this phenomenon most readily, similar mechanisms may be operative in the Rhesus Monkey. Of 4 Rhesus monkeys receiving orthotopic liver allografts without any immunosuppression, three rejected their livers between 10–15 days. The fourth lived for 7 months and finally died of infective cholangitis. Tissue typing had shown definite incompatibilities between recipient and donor in this case. The Rhesus monkey usually promptly rejects other tissues, such as skin, heart or kidney. So perhaps the phenomenon although not so easy to demonstrate in this particular species, may also exist in primates.

What then is the relevance of all this? Is it just good news for pigs that need grafts? Or has it a more general application? What is special about the pig? The pig has a different lymphocyte circulation from other species; it has a much higher lymphocyte count in the peripheral blood and a much lower lymphocyte count in the thoracic duct. The actual organization of the lymphoid follicles is rather different from other species – the cortex and medulla look as though they are reversed. Because of this arrangement it is possible – and this is a speculation – that if a pig is confronted with transplantation antigen in a soluble form, the antigen may gain access to the important parts of the lymphoreticular system in a more comprehensive way than in other species. In the latter a similar confrontation with antigen might not affect all the lymphocytes and some will then become immune, although others may become tolerant.

The other question that is bound to be asked is, why should there be such variation in the reported incidence of rejection after pig liver transplantation? Although some people get results very similar to ours, others observe a fairly consistent rejection pattern. I do not know the answer, but I will not accept the suggestion that our findings are due to chance histocompatibility in our animals. This is principally because of the widely disparate breeds of animals that we have used, the results of mixed lymphocyte cultures and the reaction of these animals to other grafts. It could be that some animals secrete into their circulation more transplantation antigen than others and this might be due to simple environmental factors including the composition of the diet. Currently, we are testing our hypothesis by means of the production of tissue-typing sera to define whether PLA antigen is in fact produced by the liver, and whether this is the substance actually responsible for the observed immunosuppressive effects.

The substance of this talk is derived from the following publications:—

Calne, R. Y., Davis, D. R., Hadjiyannakis, E., Sells, R. A., White, D., Herbertson, B. M., Millard, P. R., Joysey, V. C., Davies, D. A. L., Binns, R. M. and Festenstein, H. (1970) Nature (Lond.) 227, 903.
Calne, R. Y., White, H. J. O., Binns, R. M., Herbertson, B. M., Millard, P. R., Pena, J., Salaman, J. R., Samuel, J. R., and Davis, D. R. (1969) Transpl. Procs. 1, 321.
Calne, R. Y., White, H. J. O., Yoffa, D. E., Maginn, R. R., Binns, R. M., Samuel, J. R., and Molina, V. P. (1967) Brit. Med. J. 2, 478.

and the reference to Professor Van Rood is as follows:—

Van Rood, J. J., Van Leeuwen, A., Van Santen, M. C. T. (1970) Nature (Lond.) 226, 366.

DISCUSSION
Chairman: Dr. J. R. Batchelor

TERBLANCHE

It is interesting that there is such variability in the amount of rejection reported from different centres. In Bristol we have found very much the same picture as you have just shown us. In Cape Town, also using Large White and Landrace pigs, a mild cellular rejection almost invariably occurs at about 2 weeks. However, even though immunosuppressive therapy is not given the cellular infiltrate disappears as can be shown by biopsies taken at 2-day intervals. Figure 1 shows a needle biopsy taken at about 2 weeks in one of our

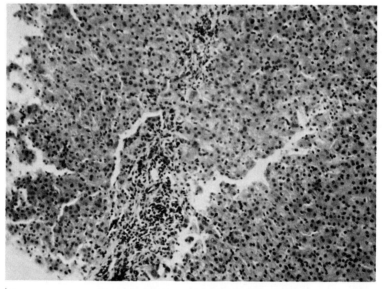

Fig. 1. The histology of a liver biopsy taken two weeks after liver transplantation showing a mild portal infiltration by mononuclear cells. (H & E x 88).

animals; at a higher power, one can see the infiltration particularly in the periportal areas. This animal died a few weeks later of complications unrelated to rejection, and histological examination of liver sections taken at autopsy showed only an increase in connective tissue in the portal tracts without any cellular infiltration (Fig. 2). However, in 5 – 15 per cent of the pigs we see classical biochemical evidence of rejection (Fig. 3). This particular pig died on the 6th day, and the liver histology (Fig. 4) was very reminiscent of

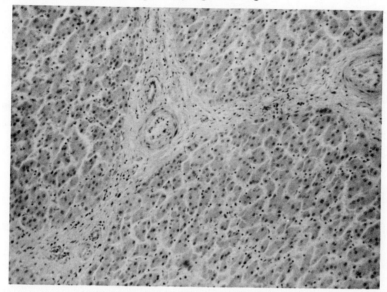

Fig. 2. Autopsy liver histology in the same animal showing connective tissue in the portal tracts without significant cellular infiltration. (H & E x 88).

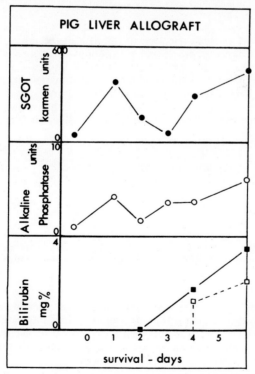

Fig. 3. Illustrating the biochemical changes accompanying acute rejection in the pig dying on the 6th post-operative day.

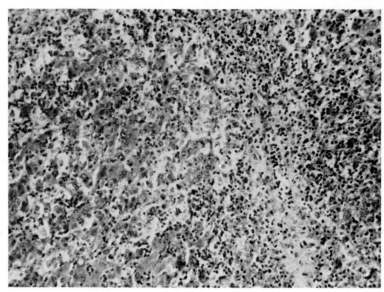

Fig. 4. Autopsy liver histology showing florid rejection with widespread hepatocyte necrosis and accompanying round cell infiltration in the pig dying on the 6th post-operative day. (H & E x 88).

the picture seen in classical rejection of the liver in the unimmunosuppressed dog. The explanation for these peculiar variations is unknown. I agree with Professor Calne that it may well be related to the unusual anatomical con-figuation of the pig's lymphatic system so beautifully described many years ago by Binns and Hall, and subsequently confirmed by Hunt from Bristol. However, it is interesting that more than one group has shown in the *rat* a longer survival for liver allografts than for other allografts. Perhaps the liver is itself responsible.

CALNE
    Are you still using pigs of the same original stock?

TERBLANCHE
    The pigs we use come from a wide range of places as we get them commercially.

CALNE
    One thing, apart from the climate, that is probably different is the food that you give them. It is unlikely to be exactly the same kind, and it may be that the protein content has some relevance.

TERBLANCHE
    We do see quite a lot of sepsis in the animals that survive and some of them develop rough coats and resemble runted animals. It is interesting to speculate whether they get infected first and then refuse to eat or whether there might be a true graft versus host reaction occurring. This does not seem to happen in your pigs, so again there are differences through the world.

Meyer zum BÜSCHENFELDE
    Could you tell us more about your membrane protein? Is it a lipoprotein?

CALNE

It is probably a glycoprotein, and it has a molecular weight that lies between 50–150,000.

MacLAURIN

Professor Calne's suggestion that the soluble antigen might produce a state of tolerance rather than of immunity is of interest to me. It has been demonstrated that in mixed lymphocyte culture it is more difficult to produce high levels of transformation when using disrupted rather than intact lymphocytes on one side of the reaction. The suggestion is that the antigen must be presented in the correct way, and if it is in the soluble form tolerance might be produced. Have you set up mixed lymphocyte cultures in your pigs, and can you tell us whether the serum added to the cultures makes any difference?

CALNE

I cannot answer the second question, as we have not done it. However, Festenstein at the London Hospital has done some mixed lymphocyte culture work on our pigs. Unfortunately it has all been done away from Cambridge and the lymphocytes have not always travelled unharmed. But two patterns have emerged, which Festenstein has described. The reaction of recipient cells to killed donor cells is generally positive before liver transplantation. After liver transplantation, there is a nonspecific depression of the lymphocyte reaction even to phytohaemagglutinin. The reason for this is unknown, but it could possibly be due to the anaesthetic used which is halothane. Then the response to phytohaemagglutinin returns, and two things may happen without the liver being rejected. The first is that specific nonreactivity to donor cells persists for a long time, which is what one would expect if classical tolerance had been produced. Secondly, in other animals the response against donor lymphocytes as well as against indifferent lymphocytes returns, without the liver being rejected. We do not understand this second type of response. Perhaps enhancement is also playing a part, although enhancing antibodies have not been found to date. I can think of no reason why enhancement and tolerance should not co-exist, and the experiments of Stuart in rats with renal allografts confirm this. He found that donor lymphocytes alone produced some prolongation of graft survival; specific enhancing antibody also produced some increase but the combination of the two produced a profound increase in survival time. This fits in quite well with our ideas but I would be very interested to hear what Professor Batchelor has to say.

BATCHELOR

As you know, I believe that enhancement plays a part in some pigs with prolonged graft survival. In the rat kidney transplants that we have been doing at East Grinstead, we find that if you start by giving the recipient rat a dose of antigraft antibody, then the target kidney is not rejected although the animal is quite clearly immunized. Antibody which is definintely of host origin is detectable in the circulation. Later on you can also demonstrate a secondary response in these grafted animals by giving donor type spleen cells. From the few experiments on rats bearing long-surviving enhanced kidneys that we have done, it looks as though the reactivity against donor type antigens has been reduced. If you do the Elkins type of experiment, and put spleen cells from the grafted rats under the kidney capsule of the appropriate donor-type rat, then you do not get anything like as much of a reaction as using cells from an animal without a graft. So I think you may get some degree of tolerance, *pari passu* with enhancement.

INDEX

Agglutination in mechanism of migration
  inhibition, 130
Agglutination test, venereal diseases research
  laboratory antigen, 73
Albano, O., 204
American Association for the Study of Liver
  Disease, 267
American Gastroenterological Association,
  Research Committee of, 264
American Rheumatism Association, 194
Anabolic reaction, 50
  of hepatocytes, 19
  of lymphocytes, 18–19
Antibodies, antiglomerular, 67
  antinuclear, incidence of, 57
  humoral, reaction in mitochondrial
    fractions 103–13; discussion,
    113–16
  mitochondrial, clinical diagnosis, 61
  in drug reactions, 68
  without overt liver disease, 59–65
  occurrence of, 117–21
  pattern in chronic liver disease, 57–59
  reacting with homologous liver protein,
    175
  reacting with intracellular antigens, 114
  related to mitochondria, 69–79; discus-
    sion, 79–81
  role of, 117–21
  smooth muscle, 119
Antigen/antibody complexes in relation to
  fibrosis, 210
Antigen dilution immunoelectrophoresis, 106
Antigens, transplantation, extracts of,
  300–01
Antigens, foetal liver, migration inhibition
  using, 287
  isolation of liver specific, 170
Antinuclear factors, 120
Arthus reaction, 213
Ascites and prednisone treatment, 219
Asherson, G. L., 83
Ashkenazi cells, 50
Atresia, biliary, 66
Auer hepatitis, 211
Australia antigen, and chronic hepatitis, 248
  and smooth muscle antibody, in active
    chronic hepatitis, 33
  and smooth muscle antibody, in acute
    viral hepatitis, 32–33
  electron microscopic observations,
    47–49
  factors determining frequency in active
    chronic hepatitis, 32–34

Australia antigen (*contd.*)
  in auto-immune liver disease 28–37;
    discussion; 37–38
  in Chile, 39–44; discussion, 44–46
  antibody to, 42–44
  family studies, 39–40
  incidence in active chronic hepatitis, 29
  incidence in acute and chronic liver
    disease, 40–41
  incidence in acute viral hepatitis, 28–29
  long tubular forms of, 30
  negative active chronic hepatitis,
    aetiology of, 35–36
  positive and negative differences in
    active chronic hepatitis, 34–35
  positive staining technique for, 47–49
  presence in surgical liver biopsy, 30–32
  relation of particle size to prognosis, 50
  transmission from mother to child,
    30–32
Auto-immune disease, primary, features of, 1
Auto-immune periductular fibrosis, induction and transfer of, 155–66;
  discussion, 166–68
Auto-immunity, and multiple organ involvement, 51
  cellular versus antibody, 165
  hepatic diseases, criteria for, 1–8
  human and animal experiments, 114–15
  multi-system involvement in, 194–202;
    discussion, 202–03
  role of delayed hypersensitivity responses,
    143–44
Azathioprine, 234
  general dosage, 256
  in primary biliary cirrhosis, 258–71;
    discussion, 262
  biochemical, immunological and
    histological assessment of,
    259–70
  duration of trial, 258
  overall results, 259–60
  metabolism of, 262, 289
  therapeutic trial of prednisone against,
    143
  toxicity of, 296
Azathioprine and prednisone, combined
  treatment with, 243–49
  controlled trial, 250–55; discussion,
    256–57
  controlled trial criteria for improvement,
    252
  controlled trial response to treatment,
    252–255

307